Deep Brain Stimulation

Techniques and Practices

William S. Anderson, MA, MD, PhD
Associate Professor of Neurosurgery and Biomedical Engineering
Department of Neurosurgery
Johns Hopkins School of Medicine
Baltimore, Maryland

The Society for Innovative Neuroscience in Neurosurgery
An educational nonprofit organization founded by a group of
functional neurosurgeons dedicated to promoting technological
advances and research in the field

98 illustrations

Thieme
New York • Stuttgart • Delhi • Rio de Janeiro

Acquisitions Editor: Timothy Y. Hiscock
Managing Editor: Prakash Naorem
Director, Editorial Services: Mary Jo Casey
Production Editor: Rohit Dev Bhardwaj
International Production Director: Andreas Schabert
Editorial Director: Sue Hodgson
International Marketing Director: Fiona Henderson
International Sales Director: Louisa Turrell
Senior Vice President and Chief Operating Officer: Sarah Vanderbilt
President: Brian D. Scanlan

Library of Congress Cataloging-in-Publication Data

Names: Anderson, William S. (William Stanley), 1968- editor. |
Society for Innovative Neuroscience in Neurosurgery.
Title: Deep brain stimulation : techniques and practices / [edited by]
   William S. Anderson ; the Society for Innovative Neuroscience in
   Neurosurgery.
Other titles: Deep brain stimulation (Anderson)
Description: New York : Thieme, [2019] | Includes bibliographical
referneces and index. |
Identifiers: LCCN 2019005781 (print) | LCCN 2019006937 (ebook) |
   ISBN 9781626237988 () | ISBN 9781626237971 (hardcover)
Subjects: | MESH: Deep Brain Stimulation
Classification: LCC RC386.6.D52 (ebook) | LCC RC386.6.D52 (print) |
   NLM WL 368 | DDC 616.8/0475–dc23
LC record available at https://lccn.loc.gov/2019005781

© 2019 Thieme Medical Publishers, Inc.

Thieme Publishers New York
333 Seventh Avenue, New York, NY 10001 USA
+1 800 782 3488, customerservice@thieme.com

Thieme Publishers Stuttgart
Rüdigerstrasse 14, 70469 Stuttgart, Germany
+49 [0]711 8931 421, customerservice@thieme.de

Thieme Publishers Delhi
A-12, Second Floor, Sector-2, Noida-201301
Uttar Pradesh, India
+91 120 45 566 00, customerservice@thieme.in

Thieme Publishers Rio de Janeiro
Thieme Publicações Ltda.
Edifício Rodolpho de Paoli, 25º andar
Av. Nilo Peçanha, 50 – Sala 2508
Rio de Janeiro 20020-906 Brasil
+55 21 3172-2297

Cover design: Thieme Publishing Group
Cover image: Ahmed Jorge
Typesetting by Thomson Digital, India

Printed in the United States of America by   5 4 3 2 1
King Printing Co., Inc.

ISBN 978-1-62623-797-1

Also available as an e-book:
eISBN 978-1-62623-798-8

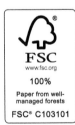

Contents

Contents

Preface

This book represents the attempt of a small, passionate group of functional neurosurgeons to describe the rapidly changing practice of deep brain stimulation (DBS) as it pertains to movement disorders and other emerging conditions. The Society for Innovative Neuroscience in Neurosurgery (SINN) was founded in 2014 in Baltimore by members of this group in an effort to improve communication and collaboration within the field of functional neurosurgery. This group has grown over time, and has now adopted an educational role along with a research and clinical practice emphasis.

Within the context of this rapidly growing and technologically dependent field, we present chapter topics covering the basic application of DBS techniques for movement disorders. Over the last 5 years, our field has been transformed by the introduction of intraoperative imaging-guided lead placement techniques (utilizing intraoperative computed tomography or magnetic resonance [MR] imaging) for lead placement in patients under general anesthesia; a discussion of these techniques is included in this book in addition to discussions of standard frame-based techniques. Moreover, the resurgence of lesioning techniques has taken a prominent role in the treatment of essential tremor in adults and dystonia in children, and we include further discussion of MR-guided focused ultrasound treatment. Importantly, several chapters are included describing the emerging role of DBS for a variety of psychiatric and neurological conditions. Finally, we conclude with practical discussions of intraoperative research implementation, the use of DBS in pediatrics, and some pearls regarding the establishment of a DBS practice for the new surgeon.

It is our hope that this text is useful for neurosurgical residents, functional neurosurgery fellows, and the new DBS practitioners.

The Society for Innovative Neuroscience in Neurosurgery
Founding Members:
William S. Anderson, MA, MD, PhD
Wael F. Asaad, MD, PhD
Jason Gerrard, MD, PhD
Timothy H. Lucas, MD, PhD
R. Mark Richardson MD, PhD, FAANS
Sameer A. Sheth, MD, PhD
Travis S. Tierney, MD, PHD

Contributors

Joseph Adachi, BS
Medical Student
Department of Neurosurgery
Stony Brook University Hospital
Stony Brook, New York

Ahmad Alhourani, MD
Neurosurgery Resident
Department of Neurological Surgery
University of Louisville
Louisville, Kentucky

William S. Anderson, MA, MD, PhD
Associate Professor of Neurosurgery and Biomedical
    Engineering
Department of Neurosurgery
Johns Hopkins School of Medicine
Baltimore, Maryland

Wael F. Asaad, MD, PhD
Associate Professor
Department of Neurosurgery and Neuroscience
Director of Functional and Epilepsy Neurosurgery
Brown University Alpert Medical School and
    Rhode Island Hospital
Providence, Rhode Island

Bradley Ashcroft, BS
Medical Student
Department of Neurosurgery
Stony Brook University Hospital
Stony Brook, New York

Garrett P. Banks, MD
Neurosurgical Resident
Department of Neurosurgery
Columbia University
New York, New York

Vivek P. Buch, MD
Resident
Department of Neurosurgery
Perelman School of Medicine
University of Pennsylvania
Philadelphia, Pennsylvania

Ankur Butala, MD
Assistant Professor
Department of Neurology
Johns Hopkins University School of Medicine
Baltimore, Maryland

H. Isaac Chen, MD
Assistant Professor
Department of Neurosurgery
Perelman School of Medicine
University of Pennsylvania
Philadelphia, Pennsylvania

Jennifer Cheng, MD, MS
Assistant Professor
Department of Neurosurgery
The University of Kansas Medical Center
Kansas City, Kansas

Fatu S. Conteh, BS
Research Assistant
Department of Neurosurgery
Johns Hopkins University School of Medicine
Baltimore, Maryland

Dwaine Cooke MBBS, DM
Consultant Neurosurgeon
Department of Neurosurgery
University of the West Indies–Mona
Kingston, Jamaica, West Indies

W. Jeffrey Elias, MD
Professor of Neurosurgery
Department of Neurological Surgery
University of Virginia School of Medicine
Charlottesville, Virginia

Jason Gerrard, MD, PhD
Assistant Professor of Neurosurgery and Neuroscience
Director, Stereotactic and Functional Neurosurgery
Department of Neurosurgery
Yale School of Medicine
New Haven, Connecticut

June Y. Guillet, MD, PhD
Assistant Professor
Department of Neurosurgery
University of Texas Medical Branch
Galveston, Texas

Abhijeet Gummadavelli, MD
Neurosurgery Resident
Department of Neurosurgery
Yale University School of Medicine
New Haven, Connecticut

Christina Jackson, MD
Resident in Neurosurgery
Department of Neurosurgery
Johns Hopkins University School of Medicine
Baltimore, Maryland

Jordan F. Karp, MD
Associate Professor of Psychiatry, Anesthesiology, and
    Clinical and Translational Science
Department of Psychiatry
University of Pittsburgh School of Medicine
Pittsburgh, Pennsylvania

Ian H. Kratter, MD, PhD
Psychiatry Resident
Western Psychiatric Hospital
University of Pittsburgh Medical Center
Pittsburgh, Pennsylvania

Alexander Ksendzovsky, MD
Resident Physician
Surgical Neurology Branch
National Institute of Neurologic Disorders and Stroke
National Institutes of Health
Bethesda, Maryland;
Department of Neurosurgery
University of Virginia Health System
Charlottesville, Virginia

Peter M. Lauro, BA
MD/PhD Student
Department of Neuroscience
Warren Alpert Medical School
Brown University Carney Institute for Brain Science
Providence, Rhode Island

Shane Lee, PhD
Post-doctoral Fellow
Department of Neuroscience
Warren Alpert Medical School
Brown University Carney Institute for Brain Science
Providence, Rhode Island

Fred A. Lenz, MD, PhD
Professor of Neurosurgery
Department of Neurosurgery
Johns Hopkins University School of Medicine
Baltimore, Maryland

Nir Lipsman, MD, PhD, FRCSC
Neurosurgeon, Sunnybrook Health Sciences Centre
Scientist, Sunnybrook Research Institute
Assistant Professor, Department of Surgery
Associate Member, Institute of Medical Science
University of Toronto
Toronto, Ontario, Canada

Timothy H. Lucas, MD, PhD
Assistant Professor
Co-Director, Penn Center for Neuro-Engineering and
    Therapeutics
Director, Translational Neuromodulation Laboratory
Department of Neurosurgery
Perelman School of Medicine
University of Pennsylvania
Philadelphia, Pennsylvania

Charles B. Mikell, MD
Clinical Assistant Professor
Department of Neurosurgery
Stony Brook University Hospital
Stony Brook, New York

Jonathan P. Miller, MD, FAANS, FACS
George R. and Constance P. Lincoln Professor and
    Vice Chairman
Director, Functional and Restorative Neurosurgery Center
Department of Neurological Surgery
University Hospitals Cleveland Medical Center
Case Western Reserve University School of Medicine
Cleveland, Ohio

Kelly Mills, MD, MHS
Assistant Professor
Department of Neurology
Johns Hopkins University School of Medicine
Baltimore, Maryland

Shayan Moosa, MD
Neurosurgery Resident
Department of Neurological Surgery
University of Virginia School of Medicine
Charlottesville, Virginia

Pranav Nanda, MD
Neurosurgical Resident
Department of Neurosurgery
Massachusetts General Hospital
Boston, Massachusetts

Joseph S. Neimat, MD, MS
Professor and Chairman
Department of Neurological Surgery
University of Louisville
Louisville, Kentucky

Ruchit V. Patel, BS
Undergraduate Student
Department of Neuroscience
Johns Hopkins University
Baltimore, Maryland

Taylor E. Purvis, BA
Medical Student
Johns Hopkins University School of Medicine
Baltimore, Maryland

R. Mark Richardson, MD, PhD, FAANS
Director of Epilepsy and Movement Disorders Surgery
Department of Neurological Surgery
University of Pittsburgh School of Medicine
Pittsburgh, Pennsylvania

Sarah Ridge, BA
Medical Student
University of Cincinnati College of Medicine
Cincinnati, Ohio

Shenandoah Robinson, MD
Professor of Neurosurgery, Neurology and Pediatrics
Division of Pediatric Neurosurgery
Johns Hopkins University School of Medicine
Baltimore, Maryland

Margot Samson, BS
Medical Student
University of Central Florida College of Medicine
Orlando, Florida

Meghal Shah, MD
Medical Student
Department of Neuroscience
Warren Alpert Medical School
Brown University Carney Institute for Brain Science
Providence, Rhode Island

Smit Shah, BA
Medical Student
Rutgers, Robert Wood Johnson Medical School
Piscataway, New Jersey

Sameer A. Sheth MD, PhD
Associate Professor and Vice-Chair of Clinical Research
Director, Psychiatric Neurosurgery
Department of Neurosurgery
McNair Scholar
Baylor College of Medicine
Houston, Texas

Michael D. Staudt, MD, MSc
Neurosurgery Resident
Department of Clinical Neurological Sciences
London Health Sciences Centre
London, Ontario, Canada

Jennifer A. Sweet, MD
Stereotactic and Functional Neurosurgeon
University Hospitals Cleveland Medical Center;
Assistant Professor
Department of Neurosurgery
Case Western Reserve University School of Medicine
University Hospitals
Cleveland, Ohio

Travis S. Tierney, MD, PHD
Senior Lecturer
Department of Brain Sciences, Imperial College London
Department of Neurosurgery, Nicklaus Children's Hospital
Miami, Florida

Teresa Wojtasiewicz, MD
Neurosurgery Resident
Department of Neurosurgery
Johns Hopkins University School of Medicine
Baltimore, Maryland

Andrew I. Yang, MD
Resident
Department of Neurosurgery
Perelman School of Medicine
University of Pennsylvania
Philadelphia, Pennsylvania

Brett E. Youngerman, MD, MS
Chief Resident
Department of Neurosurgery
Columbia University Medical Center
New York, New York

Kareem A. Zaghloul, MD, PhD
Surgical Neurology Branch
National Institute of Neurologic Disorders and Stroke
National Institutes of Health
Functional and Restorative Neurosurgery Unit
Bethesda, Maryland

1 Introduction to Deep Brain Stimulation: History, Techniques, and Ethical Considerations

Teresa Wojtasiewicz, Nir Lipsman, Jason Gerrard, Travis S. Tierney

Abstract

Deep brain stimulation (DBS) is a procedure that developed as a result of decades of work in stereotactic guidance, neurophysiology, and neuroanatomy. Now, DBS is a validated, Food and Drug Administration (FDA)-approved treatment for a number of neurological and psychiatric disorders including Parkinson's disease, essential tremor, dystonia, obsessive compulsive disorder, and epilepsy. Further applications remain an area of ongoing investigation. Lesioning is once again regaining interest, particularly with development of minimally invasive techniques such as laser interstitial thermal therapy and transcranial focused ultrasound. There are several methods for lead placement and procedural techniques will continue to evolve with time. A multidisciplinary team is critical for optimal patient evaluation, target selection, and postoperative follow-up. Medical ethics is a key part of the multidisciplinary management, particularly in case of children, patients with psychiatric disorders, and patients who are severely debilitated from their movement disorders.

Keywords: deep brain stimulation, functional neurosurgery, ethics

1.1 Introduction

Over the past three decades, deep brain stimulation (DBS) has become a widely used treatment for a variety of conditions since Benabid and colleagues first popularized the technique for the treatment of tremor.[1] Even before this, early neuromodulation studies targeted the hypothalamus and somatosensory thalamus, for treatment of pain disorders.[2,3,4] High-frequency stimulation in the thalamus led to discovery that stimulation of the thalamus could reduce tremor.[5,6,7] Further studies showed that modulation or ablation by lesioning had the potential to treat patients with movement disorders.[8,9,10,11] DBS is now a validated, Food and Drug Administration (FDA)-approved treatment for neurological disorders including Parkinson's disease, essential tremor, dystonia, obsessive compulsive disorder, and epilepsy. Additional applications in other conditions remain an area of active investigation. Stereotactic lesioning is regaining additional interest, particularly with development of minimally invasive techniques such as the Gamma Knife and MRI-guided focused ultrasound.[12,13] DBS systems can now be implanted using several different methods, with a range of options of stereotactic frames, image-guided targeting, and intraoperative microelectrode recordings (MERs) and testing. There are now multiple hardware and software options available for use in DBS, including different leads and implanted generators. A multidisciplinary team is critical to decide who is an optimal surgical candidate and what treatment strategy will be most suited for individual patient. Multidisciplinary collaboration maximizes the chance of successful DBS through appropriate preoperative evaluation of potential surgical candidates and continued postoperative care after DBS hardware placement. Medical ethics is an important part of the multidisciplinary management, particularly in case of children, patients with psychiatric disorders, and patients who are severely debilitated from their movement disorders.

1.2 History of Deep Brain Stimulation

Electricity has been a captivating possibility in treatment of human disorders for centuries, beginning with the earliest descriptions of treatment of pain with torpedo fish in Greek and Egyptian medicine, and investigations of contractions in frog muscle by Galvani.[14,15,16] For thousands of years, many civilizations believed that targeting the brain could treat spiritual and mental ailments. Examples range from the earliest attempts at trepanation to 15th century artistic renditions of extracting "mental stones" from unstable people.[17] Interestingly, attempts at lesions of the brain predated an understanding of functional organization of the brain but electric stimulation was key to this knowledge. Anecdotal studies of pathology, such as the frontal lobe disconnection and behavior changes seen in the case of Phineas Gage, suggested that complex behaviors could be attributed to specific areas of the brain.[17,18] Physicians such as Jean Bouillaud, Simon Aubertin, and Paul Broca observed, from cases of patients with aphasia, that speech could be localized to specific regions of the brain.[19,20] These developments inspired researchers Gustav Fritsch and Eduard Hitzig, who proved localization theory by stimulating the exposed cortical surface in dogs and localizing motor and nonmotor functions of the brain.[21] David Ferrier conducted further experiments in monkeys by localizing hearing, visual attention, and secondary motor areas.[20,22] The first use of neurostimulation in a human patient is attributed to Roberts Bartholow who stimulated the parietal lobes in an awake patient with an erosive basal cell cancer in 1874, producing contralateral movements and, subsequently, seizures.[23] Shortly after that, Sir Victor Horsley, a pioneer in many aspects of neurosurgery, published a case of electric stimulation of an occipital encephalocele in 1884 and he and other neurosurgeons began using cortical stimulation for functional mapping.[16,24,25] Horsley would also subsequently perform the first movement disorder surgery in 1908, successfully treating a patient with hemiathetosis by resecting the precentral gyrus, which cured the movement disorder but caused hemiplegia.[26]

For the next few decades after Horsley's resection of the precentral gyrus, attempts at treating movement disorders were aimed at interrupting the pyramidal motor tracts, but with a high degree of morbidity and mortality.[15,16] Abnormalities in deep brain structures, including atrophy of basal ganglia, were identified in anatomic studies of patients with movement disorders, but the basal ganglia was thought to be a dangerous target and the physiology of basal ganglia circuits was not yet well understood.[27] Dr. Meyers reported several approaches to the basal ganglia, including sectioning the ansa lenticularis, but these approaches were accompanied by a 12% mortality which he felt was unacceptable.[28] Despite the complications accompanying an open surgical approach, Meyers' contributions definitively demonstrated that basal ganglia lesions could effectively treat tremor *without* causing paralysis or coma. These notions challenged the prevailing dogma of Dandy who believed that encroachment into the basal ganglia always resulted in coma, and previous ideas that only lesions to the pyramidal tract could alleviate tremor. Meyers' important observations set the stage for future stereotactic surgical methods in targeting extrapyramidal subcortical structures for the treatment of refractory movement disorders. Still working with an open approach to the descending tracts, Irving Cooper in 1952 inadvertently encountered and was forced to ligate the anterior choroidal artery while attempting a pedunculotomy.[29] Serendipitously, the resultant choroidal infarct relieved tremor without causing hemiparesis.[29] He was able to reproduce his results with anterior choroidal artery ligation, ascribing the benefit of this procedure to interruption of efferent pathways from the globus pallidus.[30] Despite the well-known introduction of frame-based stereotaxy by Spiegel and Wycis in 1947, Cooper continued to create lesions in the basal ganglia and thalamus with an essentially free-hand method.[31,32] Cooper's approaches were intermittently successful and may have had a lower risk of complications than other prior open approaches. Though his work did little to advance technical refinements in the field of movement disorders surgery, his findings finally reduced further attacks on the descending cortical spinal tracts as a treatment for tremor.

Lesioning for psychiatric conditions also blossomed in the early to mid 20th century. Developments in neuroanatomy showed function could be localized to certain areas and anecdotal evidence of patients with frontal lobe damage and behavior changes led to a perception that psychopathology could be localized to the frontal lobes.[17] A few early attempts at frontal lobe resection, such as Gottlieb Burckhardt's report of six patients published in 1891 and Lodovicus Puusepp's report of three patients he operated on in 1910, had high rates of mortality and low rates of success in alleviation of symptoms and did not inspire enthusiasm for psychosurgery.[17,33,34] The era of psychosurgery would begin in earnest when, at the Second International Neurologic Congress in London in 1935, John Fulton and Carlyle Jacobsen presented results of chimpanzee experiments showing that frontal lobe resection reduced "frustration behavior" associated with not receiving an anticipated reward.[35] The audience for this meeting included Walter Freeman and Antonio Egas Moniz, who were keen to clinically translate these results. Moniz, in collaboration with Almeida Lima, successfully performed the first frontal lobotomies to treat patients with psychosis, first with alcohol injections and subsequently with a new instrument—the leukotome.[36] Soon after, Walter Freeman and James Watts would replicate Moniz' lobotomy technique, finding that it was successful in treating psychosis and other disorders including depression.[37,38] Freeman and Watts refined Moniz' technique and produced a calibrated instrument—the precision leukotome—and reported initial positive results; though 14% of patients had a poor outcome and there were high rates of uncontrolled bleeding, seizures, and the apathetic "frontal lobe syndrome."[38] Freeman, enthusiastic about these results, modified a transorbital technique developed by Amarro Fiamberti, which he could perform without assistance from a neurosurgeon or anesthesiologist in patients rendered unconscious from an electroshock treatment.[39] These techniques were admonished by the academic medical establishment, including his former collaborator Watts, but Freeman ignored this criticism and began performing his transorbital leukotomies with portable machines around the United States in various settings, including offices, asylums, and motels.[40] His procedural complications, seemingly indiscriminate patient selection, lack of sterility, and inability to recognize his own limitations began to attract significant negative attention from the medical community and general population.[17,41] Ultimately, the development of chlorpromazine and other antipsychotics brought an end to transorbital leukotomies.[17] Though the legacy of frontal lobotomy would permanently mar psychosurgery, many of Freeman's contemporaries recognized that more precise frontal lobe resection could alleviate psychiatric symptoms, including John Fulton who remarked, "Why not use a shotgun?" in describing the crude Freeman lobotomy and William Scoville who developed a method of cortical undercutting.[42,43] Stereotaxy would allow a much higher level of precision in treating targets for psychiatric surgery.

The development of stereotactic frames allowed more precise and safe neurosurgical procedures that had the potential to treat neurological diseases. Sir Victor Horsley collaborated with Robert Clarke to develop the first stereotactic frame (▶ Fig. 1.1a). This frame was used in animal experiments to successfully insert a probe.[44,45] This initial frame was based on a three-dimensional (3D) Cartesian coordinate system and included a needle holder to insert into a specified structure, which would allow entry to a specified target with minimal injury to surrounding tissue.[44,45] However, the Horsley-Clarke frame relied on external cerebral landmarks, which was not reliable and it was not used in human subjects.[44,45] Spiegel and Wycis addressed this problem by creating a similar frame at Thomas Jefferson Hospital in Philadelphia (▶ Fig. 1.1b). Together with stereoencephalographic methods, they used their frame to perform true stereotactic approaches to thalamotomy, pallidotomy, ablation of the Gasserian ganglion, and ablation of the spinothalamic tract.[46] After viewing the Spiegel-Wycis frame, Lars Leksell created a novel frame with an arc center target and published his results in 1951 (▶ Fig. 1.1c).[44,47] The Leksell frame had ring and arc angle that could be used to easily create trajectories to a target from virtually any point on the skull.[44,47] Leksell, like the Wycis and Spiegel group, used his stereotactic methods to perform anterior capsulotomies and treated patients with obsessive compulsive disorder.[48] The advent of stereotaxy allowed neurosurgeons to safely target deep regions of the brain for stimulation and other treatment modalities, including capsulotomies, cingulotomies, subcaudate tractotomies, and limbic leukotomies.[49] In the 1960s and 1970s, as lobotomy was beginning to fall out of favor, several other groups attempted to perform stereotactic lesioning procedures to treat psychiatric illness. The anterior capsule, first targeted by Talairach and colleagues and later refined by Leksell and others, could be ablated with an approximate efficacy of 50 to 70% in treating obsessive compulsive disorder.[50,51] Anterior cingulotomy could also be

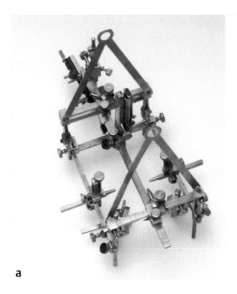

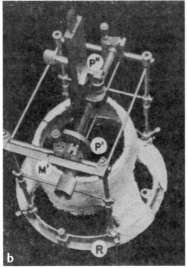

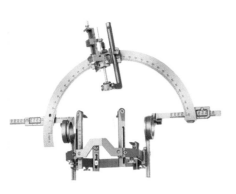

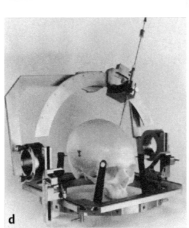

Fig. 1.1 Stereotactic frames. (a) Horsley-Clarke frame (from the Science Museum, London). (b) Spiegel-Wycis frame (from Spiegel et al.[46]). (c) Leksell® Coordinate Frame and Leksell® Multipurpose Stereotactic Arc (Elekta, Inc). (d) Cosman-Roberts-Wells frame (from Couldwell and Apuzzo[55]).

used to interrupt limbic projections with reasonable efficacy in a variety of conditions including obsessive compulsive disorder, anxiety, depression, and bipolar disorder.[49] Studies suggest a reasonable, i.e., 33 to 60% efficacy and a low risk of complications in patients with medically refractory disease with anterior capsulotomy.[49] Subcaudate tractotomy, first introduced by Geoffrey Knight in 1964, targeted anterior white matter tracts connecting the orbitofrontal and limbic regions. The procedure was used for obsessive compulsive disorder, anxiety, depression, and bipolar disorder with 40 to 60% efficacy, comparable to cingulotomy, with a similarly low rate of complications[52,53] A combination of anterior cingulotomy and subcaudate tractotomy lesions called the limbic leucotomy was also used for obsessive compulsive disorder and depression with reasonable efficacy and a low incidence of side effects.[54] The ablation procedures made possible with stereotactic surgery would lay a foundation to perform DBS for treatment of psychiatric illness. Both movement disorder surgery and psychosurgery led to the development of DBS.

Though the birth of modern DBS is typically attributed to Benabid's 1987 paper on thalamic stimulation, neurosurgeons had been using acute stimulation long before that.[1,15] DBS gained acceptance in the 1950s, after the rise of stereotaxy. In the 1940s and early 1950s, many surgeons, including Spiegel

and Wycis, would stimulate stereotactic trajectories before ablation as a method of ensuring safety.[15] Soon, electrode stimulation began to be used for psychiatric indications, starting with Dr. Pool's studies of hypothalamic stimulation and continuing to Robert Heath's cerebellar stimulation for psychosis.[2,56,57] Although enthusiasm for movement disorder and psychiatric surgery diminished in the 1970s after the introduction of levodopa[58] and chlorpromazine, respectively, investigation into ablation and neurostimulation for these neurological disorders continued at select centers. DBS was also investigated for use in other conditions, such as chronic pain disorders.[2,3,4] Attempts at stimulation for pain in the somatosensory thalamus then led to the discovery that thalamic stimulation could reduce tremor.[5,6,7] In 1987, Dr. Benebid and his group showed that thalamic DBS could alleviate medication-refractory tremor symptoms in Parkinson's disease patients. Subsequent investigation proved the safety and efficacy of thalamic DBS for tremor and led to FDA approval of thalamic DBS in 1997 for essential tremor.[8,9,10] Randomized-controlled and large prospective trials confirmed the efficacy of thalamic DBS in essential tremor.[59,60,61] Over the next several years, other DBS targets would be established for movement disorders, including the globus pallidus interna (GPi)[11,62] and subthalamic nucleus (STN).[9,63] The FDA approved both GPi and STN DBS in Parkinson's disease in 2002.

Subsequently randomized-controlled trials verified that DBS in the GPi and STN were effective in Parkinson's disease.[64,65,66,67]

1.3 Ablative Procedures

Ablative procedures started to fall out of favor when DBS was introduced, but lesioning has remained an option for certain patients. Lars Leksell's initial use of the Leksell frame included radiosurgical pallidotomies and thalamotomies,[68,69] and stereotactic radiosurgery continues to be used for these purposes.[70,71,72] Lesioning has regained some interest in psychiatric treatment, despite its negative association with earlier psychiatric ablative procedures.[73] Stereotactic radiosurgery can be used for focused ablation of structures including the anterior cingulate, substantia innominate, and the anterior limb of the internal capsule, and it may alleviate symptoms of obsessive compulsive disorder, anxiety, and depression.[74] Laser interstitial therapy (LITT), in which a laser fiber is passed through a burr hole and an ablation trajectory can be defined, has also been used anecdotally for pallidotomy.[75] Finally, MRI-guided focused ultrasound for unilateral thalamotomy has been shown to be effective in treatment of essential tremor[12] and tremor-dominant Parkinson's disease[13] with low complication rates.[76] Though there is no current procedure that can supplant DBS, these new applications and methods of DBS will continue to be an active area of investigation.

1.4 Operative Techniques

DBS can be successfully performed in many different ways, with several options for targeting and hardware placement. Between centers, there is significant heterogeneity in how the procedure is performed, with differences in many elements of surgery including preoperative target and trajectory planning, frame usage, incision and burr hole planning, intraoperative clinical and stimulation testing, and postoperative imaging for confirmation.[77] The majority of surgeons perform DBS as a staged procedure with electrode placement and extension cabling/pulse generator implantation as separate procedures.[77] The rationale for staging may be related to the duration of the procedure, the need for different anesthesia techniques and patient positioning, and a concern for increased risk of infection. At the present time, both staged and single-operation DBS are appropriate techniques.[77,78] As the companies that offer DBS devices compete with each other, more hardware choices are available and will continue to develop. Directional leads with segmented contacts can be programmed to "steer" current to avoid delivering current to unwanted structures, such as the internal capsule, while maintaining current delivery to therapeutic targets.[79,80] Rechargeable implanted pulse generators are now available which last longer before needing replacement and may be a good option for patients who are willing to recharge their devices.[81,82]

1.4.1 Frame-based versus Frameless Approaches

Accurate targeting is critical to successful DBS. DBS can be performed with frame-based approaches and there are several frames available including the Leksell (▶ Fig. 1.1c) and Cosman-Roberts-Wells (CRW) frames (▶ Fig. 1.1d). It has been shown that DBS can also be safely and accurately performed with frameless technology, and there are several options available including NexFrame and StarFix. The procedures and technology for frameless DBS will be discussed at length in other sections in this text. Experimental studies with skull models suggested frameless technology could exceed the accuracy of frame-based approaches (with a mean of 1.25 mm of localization error for frameless techniques, compared to 1.8 mm for CRW and 1.7 mm error for Leksell frames).[83,84,85] However, some studies of frameless technology in patients have shown that frameless technology may not be as accurate as frame-based approaches, though the outcomes for patients appear comparable.[86,87] Nowadays, surgical robot assistance may offer another accurate technique in stereotactic cranial procedures and may be useful for electrode placement in DBS.[88,89]

1.4.2 Microelectrode Recording and Intraoperative Monitoring

Another topic of debate is whether DBS performed with MER and intraoperative testing ("awake") or DBS performed solely with anatomic/image-guided targeting ("asleep") is more accurate and effective. There is some controversy regarding whether MER is an indispensable tool for accurate lead placement or current image-guided techniques are sufficiently accurate.[90,91,92] Studies have shown that MER frequently provides data that leads to a revision in the final lead location, suggesting that the information gathered by MER is vital to accurate lead placement.[93,94,95] There is no consensus of whether the revisions in lead location suggested by MER lead to improved outcomes and studies of DBS without MER indicate good results.[96,97] In addition, the proponents of direct image guidance techniques suggest that the corrections made with intraoperative recordings are done at the time of image-based target selection, which often varies somewhat from the indirect coordinates. A recent meta-nalysis showed that MER and awake surgery is associated with more lead passes and a higher rate of complications, but a lower rate of stimulation-induced side effects.[98] The overall motor outcomes appear comparable with both "awake" and "asleep" procedures, though there is some suggestion that patients may improve more quickly after "awake" procedures.[98] Patients seem to have a preference for DBS performed under general anesthesia.[99] Some patients are either unwilling or unable to tolerate being awake and participating in testing during a long procedure so further improvement in accuracy of asleep procedures, such as robotic guidance, will be of great benefit.[100]

1.4.3 Description of Surgical Procedure

As described above, there are various methods of performing DBS, with new technology providing additional options that may make surgery more comfortable, convenient, safer, and more accurate. We will describe the surgical procedure for frame-based DBS, using MER and intraoperative stimulation. For other excellent reviews of surgical techniques, please see (Kramer et al)[101] and (Machado et al).[102] Other sections in this textbook will detail alternatives, including frameless stereotaxy and magnetic resonance imaging/computed tomography (MRI/CT) localization without intraoperative recording or stimulation.

Preoperative planning

Patients are scheduled for a preoperative MRI, with thin-cut axial T1- and T2-weighted images as well as 3D volumetric T1 post-gadolinium-contrast images. Shortly before the surgical procedure, a CT scan with 1.5-mm axial slices at zero gantry angle is obtained. On the day of the procedure, a commercial computerized stereotactic planning station (e.g., FrameLink, Medtronic, Minneapolis, MD or iPlan Stereotaxy, Brainlab Inc., Westchester, IL) can be used to coregister the CT and MRI and plan the trajectory to the target. Fusion of MRI and CT helps in improving the spatial accuracy of targeting.[103] The anterior commissure (AC) and posterior commissure (PC) are identified and compared with atlas-based coordinates to estimate DBS target locations.[104,105] Once target, entry point, and trajectory have been planned, the stereotactic planning station can be used to obtain X, Y, Z, and arc and ring angle coordinates.

Frame placement

On the morning of the procedure, the stereotactic frame is assembled. For the Leksell frame used at our institution, the set-up is as follows: the face plate is fixed in the anterior aspect of the frame with the curve directed superiorly. Two long, angled posts are fixed in the two anterior corners of the frame with the base fixed at the 6-cm mark. Two short posts are fixed into the posterior corners of the frame with the base fixed at the 2-cm mark (▸ Fig. 1.2 and ▸ Fig. 1.3). Adjustments may be made to these measurements as needed so that the frame is in line with the patient's zygoma and parallel to the canthomeatal line. Once the frame has been assembled, the patient is prepared for frame placement. Anxiolytic medications may be given prior to positioning and frame placement, if required. The patient should be positioned upright (at 90 degrees) in a wheelchair or stretcher. The frame is positioned over the patient's head and marks with a skin marker are made at the preliminary target points where the screws will be placed. The sites are

prepared with iodine or chlorhexidine and local anesthetic is administered. At our institution, we use approximately 15 to 30 cc of a 1:1 mixture of quick-acting and long-acting local anesthesia (i.e., lidocaine and bupivacaine) that is injected subcutaneously. After local anesthetic is administered, the frame is aligned (▸ Fig. 1.4), again with a goal of positioning parallel to the canthomeatal line which should ideally also be parallel to the AC-PC line. The frame should also be positioned so that its center corresponds to the patient's midline. Once the frame position appears satisfactory, appropriate length screws are chosen and then the screws are positioned and inserted, using

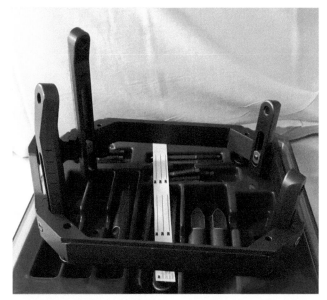

Fig. 1.3 Frame set up, lateral view.

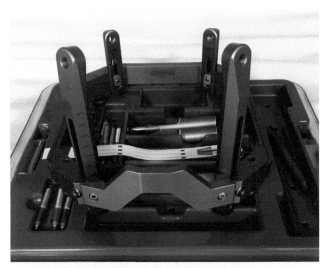

Fig. 1.2 Frame placement, frame set up, anterior view.

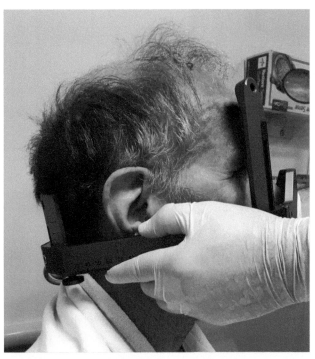

Fig. 1.4 Frame positioned on patient.

the screwdriver, in the frame kit. Contralateral anterior and posterior screws are applied together (e.g., right anterior and left posterior applied simultaneously, (▶ Fig. 1.5)) until there is appropriate bone purchase, with appropriate resistance from the screwdriver. Additional local anesthetic is applied if patients report continued discomfort when screws are applied. Care should be taken to monitor for vasovagal responses which may occur after local anesthetic administration or after screw placement. After the frame has been positioned (▶ Fig. 1.6, anterior view and ▶ Fig. 1.7, lateral view), the fiducial localizer box is placed over it and a high-resolution CT scan is obtained. Alternately, the patient can be brought to the operating room and this CT scan can be obtained using intraoperative O-arm, if available.

Preparation for localization

The CT scan with the patient in the frame is merged with the preoperative imaging and coordinates for a target and trajectory are refined. After CT scan, the patient is brought to the operating room and the frame is fixed to the table using the Mayfield adapter. Padding is applied as needed to ensure the patient is comfortable. The scalp is shaved, prepped, and draped with preliminary marking of incisions. At our institution, we mark two parallel incisions approximately 3 to 3.5 cm lateral to midline along the coronal suture. The stereotactic arc is prepared with holes created in a large, clear drape to attach the arc to the Leksell frame. The frame is attached to the base ring of the frame. The frame is moved to the appropriate coordinates for the target and trajectory, beginning on the patient's most affected or most dominant side for initial lead placement. The incision on each side is made to facilitate a burr hole at the calculated entry point. After the burr hole is created, the area around the burr hole can be further drilled so that the plastic fixation rings are recessed and flush with the surrounding skull. The dura is incised and underlying pia gently coagulated to facilitate insertion of an introducer cannula for each microelectrode. Each high-impedance platinum-iridium microelectrode is threaded into a parallel trajectory and connected to the microdrive mounted on the stage. At this point, MER can be started (▶ Fig. 1.8).

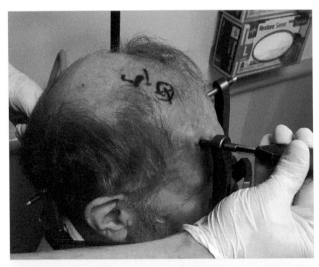

Fig. 1.5 Appropriate technique for pin placement.

Physiologic localization—microelectrode recording

After verification of the electrode impedance, the microelectrode is slowly advanced, while a clinician physiologist monitors the MER. The deep grey matter structures exhibit characteristic neuronal firing patterns which are utilized to track the pathway. Neuronal responses such as the kinesthetic

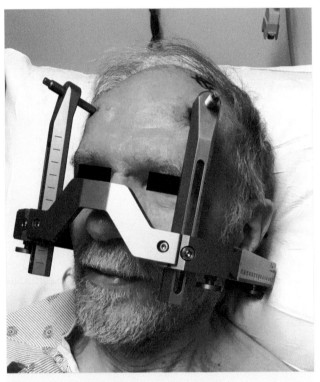

Fig. 1.6 Frame placed on patient, anterior view.

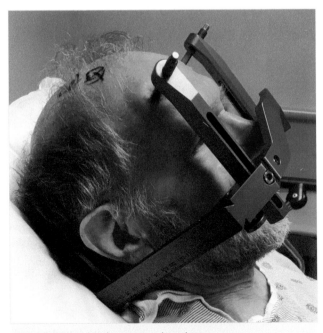

Fig. 1.7 Frame placed on patient, lateral view.

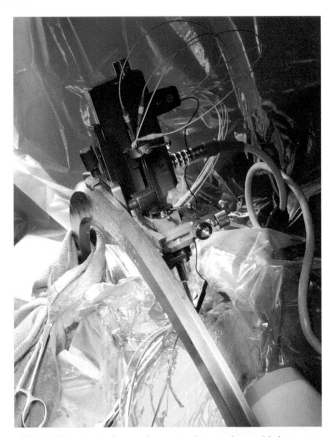

Fig. 1.8 Microelectrode recording, microdrive, and assembled stage.

response to movement, sensory response to stimulation, or tremor oscillations are used to confirm that the electrode is proceeding along the appropriate trajectory.[106] The microelectrode is advanced through the target nuclei or 3 to 5 mm below the target. Following MERs subcortical mapping is done with micro- or macrostimulation. Microstimulation is performed while an examiner assesses the patient, monitoring for therapeutic benefit and, more importantly, stimulation-induced side effects that can be useful to identify the relative positions of the optic tract, internal capsule, sensory thalamic nuclei, and medial lemniscus in reference to the trajectories. Data from different trajectories can be compared and the initial planned location for lead placement may be refined based on this information.

Electrode placement

The microelectrodes are removed and the lead is placed in the final trajectory determined by MER. Intraoperative fluoroscopy is used to verify lead location. Stimulation of the lead can be performed at various settings to ascertain symptom relief and any side effects from adjacent structures. Once the lead position is verified, the lead is secured. Once both leads have been placed, temporary lead covers are placed and the leads are tunneled along the scalp toward the planned pulse generator site.

Implantation of pulse generator

The implantable pulse generator (IPG) can be placed immediately after the DBS leads are placed or in a delayed fashion in the following weeks. The patient is placed under general anesthesia with the head turned away from the side of the distal electrode connector(s) and planned IPG placement. An incision is made over the tunneled leads and the distal electrode connectors are gently pulled out of the incision and a site is prepared for the connection fixture to the lead extension cabling. The infraclavicular incision is made and a pocket is prepared above the pectoralis fascia to house the pulse generator. A trough can be drilled in the skull to make the connection fixture less prominent and reduce the tension on the overlying skin. The lead extension cabling is tunneled in the subcutaneous space between the two incisions and connected to the electrode on the cranial end and the pulse generator in the chest. The pulse generator is placed into the infraclavicular pocket with wire slack loops placed behind the pulse generator. The connection fixture and pulse generator are secured with sutures to prevent migration and the incisions are closed.

1.5 Multidisciplinary Committees

DBS has been shown to be an effective and safe therapy and is increasingly utilized in the treatment of movement disorders and other neurological diseases. An interdisciplinary preoperative assessment and discussion has become critical. Most patients are referred for DBS by their neurologist, who will begin assessing a patient for surgery with a comprehensive neurology assessment to ensure a patient is appropriately diagnosed and appropriately medically optimized. A potential candidate for DBS is referred to a neurosurgeon for evaluation and for the discussion of the procedure, operative risks, and expected benefit. Assessment of medical comorbidities and safety of surgery is important and may require collaboration with other medical specialists. Cognitive, memory, and psychological assessment with a neuropsychologist and, if appropriate, psychiatrist, is essential to identify any comorbid cognitive impairment, and any psychiatric or behavioral issues (such as compulsive gambling or severe anxiety) that would reduce a patient's ability to benefit from DBS. Some analysis of multidisciplinary tiered assessment indicates that approximately 27% of patients with Parkinson's disease referred for DBS are deemed not fit candidates based on this preoperative assessment, with cognitive impairment being the most common exclusion factor.[107] Though metanalysis and randomized trials seem to indicate that suicidality is generally unchanged or improved after DBS,[108,109] patients at imminent risk of suicidal behaviors should be stabilized prior to consideration of DBS implantation. In psychiatric patients, preoperative assessment includes appropriate utilization of all prior resources for treatment, including appropriate psychiatric care and careful consideration of psychosocial factors that can be strained in the perioperative period.[110]

1.6 Ethics

The use of DBS, particularly in emerging indications, raises several important ethical questions.[111] These include issues of consent in early phase clinical trials, involving especially the application of novel technology to potentially vulnerable, treatment-refractory populations.[112] As interest in treating psychiatric disorders with DBS has grown, we remember the ethical violations by previous generations and aim for stringent ethical guidelines for future procedures. There were significant advances in medical ethics not long after the era of Walter Freeman. In 1966, Henry Beecher, an anesthesiologist, noted widespread failure of clinical researchers to obtain appropriate consent and to protect their subjects from harm from experimental procedures.[113,114] This, alongside the scandal of the Tuskegee Syphilis Study, generated widespread organizational efforts to protect patients.[115] The National Research Act in 1974 and the National Commission for the Protection of Human Subjects generated the Belmont Report of 1979 which outlined the three principles of ethics that continue to guide clinical ethics today: respect for persons, beneficence, and justice. Since the Belmont Report, there have been many proposed frameworks for protecting patients who might undergo psychiatric surgical procedures.[116,117,118] These guidelines consistently emphasize that patients must able to fully consent to their procedures, the safety and expected efficacy of a treatment should be carefully studied before a treatment is implemented, and that researchers must collaborate to ensure patients are appropriately cared for before, during, and after a procedure.[116,117,118] The use of multidisciplinary committees can provide ethics oversight for patients considered for DBS surgery and therapy, especially when utilized for neuropsychiatric conditions. Further, the optimal design of DBS trials remains unclear, as the ethics of sham surgery or blinded brain stimulation in psychiatric or other conditions is an area of active investigation. Designing trials that optimally balance potential benefit with not only surgical risks, but the risk of blinded stimulation is critical to determining the place of DBS in emerging indications. Patient registries have been suggested to capture the global DBS experience, especially in rare or investigational studies, where large single-center trials may not be possible.[119] Managing relationships between investigators and industry sponsors, selecting optimal patients for pivotal trials of DBS in emerging indications, and the implications of DBS trials for resource allocation, especially in developing countries, are key ethical and practical questions requiring careful, rigorous study in the years ahead.

1.7 Conclusion

The history of DBS neuromodulation has evolved from the early recognition of the utility of electrical stimulation and consideration of ablative lesions to treat various movement and psychiatric disorders. Currently approved indications for DBS include essential tremor, primary dystonia, Parkinson's disease, obsessive compulsive disorder, and partial seizures with ongoing clinical trials in a number of other conditions including major depression, chronic pain, and Tourette's syndrome. The techniques for implantation of leads has also evolved over time from classic physiologically guided placement to purely anatomically guided approaches. Incremental changes in DBS technology also continue with improvements in lead and IPG design as competing companies join the market. The future of DBS therapy is certainly one of expanding indications where multidisciplinary collaboration and careful attention to ethical principles will ensure optimal outcomes for the individual patient.

References

[1] Benabid AL, Pollak P, Louveau A, Henry S, de Rougemont J. Combined (thalamotomy and stimulation) stereotactic surgery of the VIM thalamic nucleus for bilateral Parkinson disease. Appl Neurophysiol. 1987; 50(1–6):344–346

[2] Pool JL, Clark WK, Hudson P, Lombardo M. Hypothalamic-hypophysial dysfunction in man. Laboratory and clinical assessment. In: Guillemin R, Guillemin R, Carton CA, eds. Hypothalamic-hypophysial interrelationships. Springfield: Thomas; 1956:114–124

[3] Mazars G, Mérienne L, Ciolocca C. [Intermittent analgesic thalamic stimulation. Preliminary note]. Rev Neurol (Paris). 1973; 128(4):273–279

[4] Hosobuchi Y, Adams JE, Rutkin B. Chronic thalamic and internal capsule stimulation for the control of central pain. Surg Neurol. 1975; 4(1):91–92

[5] Jasper HH, Bertrand G. Thalamic units involved in somatic sensation and voluntary and involuntary movements in man. In: Purpura DP, Yahr MD, eds. The Thalamus. New York: Columbia University Press; 1966:365–390

[6] Merienne L, Mazars G. [Treatment of various dyskinesias by intermittent thalamic stimulation]. Neurochirurgie. 1982; 28(3):201–206

[7] Tasker RR, Organ LW, Hawrylyshyn P. The thalamus and midbrain in man: a physiologic atlas using electrical stimulation. Springfield, IL: Thomas; 1982

[8] Benabid AL, Pollak P, Gervason C, et al. Long-term suppression of tremor by chronic stimulation of the ventral intermediate thalamic nucleus. Lancet. 1991; 337(8738):403–406

[9] Benabid AL, Pollak P, Gross C, et al. Acute and long-term effects of subthalamic nucleus stimulation in Parkinson's disease. Stereotact Funct Neurosurg. 1994; 62(1–4):76–84

[10] Siegfried J, Lippitz B. Chronic electrical stimulation of the VL-VPL complex and of the pallidum in the treatment of movement disorders: personal experience since 1982. Stereotact Funct Neurosurg. 1994; 62(1–4):71–75

[11] Siegfried J, Lippitz B. Bilateral chronic electrostimulation of ventroposterolateral pallidum: a new therapeutic approach for alleviating all parkinsonian symptoms. Neurosurgery. 1994; 35(6):1126–1129, discussion 1129–1130

[12] Elias WJ, Lipsman N, Ondo WG, et al. A randomized trial of focused ultrasound thalamotomy for essential tremor. N Engl J Med. 2016; 375(8):730–739

[13] Bond AE, Shah BB, Huss DS, et al. Safety and efficacy of focused ultrasound thalamotomy for patients with medication-refractory, tremor-dominant Parkinson disease: a randomized clinical trial. JAMA Neurol. 2017; 74(12):1412–1418

[14] Bresadola M. Animal electricity at the end of the eighteenth century: the many facets of a great scientific controversy. J Hist Neurosci. 2008; 17(1):8–32

[15] Gildenberg PL. Evolution of neuromodulation. Stereotact Funct Neurosurg. 2005; 83(2–3):71–79

[16] Schwalb JM, Hamani C. The history and future of deep brain stimulation. Neurotherapeutics. 2008; 5(1):3–13

[17] Robison RA, Taghva A, Liu CY, Apuzzo ML. Surgery of the mind, mood, and conscious state: an idea in evolution. World Neurosurg. 2013; 80(3–4):S2–S26

[18] Harlow JM. Recovery from the passage of an iron bar through the head. Boston Med Surg J. 1848; 39:389–393

[19] Broca PB. Perte de la parole, ramollissement chronique et destruction partielle du lobe antérieur gauche du cerveau. Bull Soc Anthropol. 1861; 2:235–238

[20] Finger S. Chapter 10 The birth of localization theory. In: Aminoff MJ, Boller F, Swaab DF, eds. Handbook of clinical neurology. Elsevier; 2009:117–128

[21] Kerr PB, Caputy AJ, Horwitz NH. A history of cerebral localization. Neurosurg Focus. 2005; 18(4):e1

[22] Ferrier D. The localisation of function in the brain. Proc R Soc Lond. 1874; 22:229–232

[23] Morgan JP. The first reported case of electrical stimulation of the human brain. J Hist Med Allied Sci. 1982; 37(1):51–64

[24] Vilensky JA, Gilman S. Horsley was the first to use electrical stimulation of the human cerebral cortex intraoperatively. Surg Neurol. 2002; 58(6):425–426

[25] Horsley V. Case of occipital encephalocele in which a correct diagnosis was obtained by means of the induced current. Brain. 1884; 7:228–243

[26] Horsley V. The linacre lecture on the function of the so called motor area of the brain: delivered to the Master and Fellows of St. John's College, Cambridge, May 6th, 1909. BMJ. 1909; 2(2533):121–132

[27] Lanska DJ. Chapter 33: the history of movement disorders. Handb Clin Neurol. 2010; 95:501–546

[28] Meyers R. The modification of alternating tremors, rigidity and festination by surgery of the basal ganglia. In: Putnam TJ, ed. The Diseases of the Basal Ganglia. New York: Hafner Publishing; 1966:602–665

[29] Cooper IS. Ligation of the anterior choroidal artery for involuntary movements; parkinsonism. Psychiatr Q. 1953; 27(2):317–319

[30] Cooper IS. Anterior choroidal artery ligation for involuntary movements. Science. 1953; 118(3059):193

[31] Cooper IS, Bravo G. Chemopallidectomy and chemothalamectomy. J Neurosurg. 1958; 15(3):244–250

[32] Cooper IS, Bravo GJ, Riklan M, Davidson NW, Gorek EA. Chemopallidectomy and chemothalamectomy for parkinsonism. Geriatrics. 1958; 13(3):127–147

[33] Burckhardt G. Ueber Rindenexcisionen, als Beitrag zur operativen Therapie der Psychosen. Allg Zeschr f Psychiatr. 1891; 47:463–548

[34] Puusepp L. Alcune considerazioni sugli interventi chirurgici nelle malattie mentali. Giorn Accad Med Torino. 1937; 100:3–16

[35] Fulton JF, Jacobsen CF. The functions of the frontal lobes: a comparative study in monkeys, chimpanzees, and man. Abstracts of the Second International Neurological Congress; 1935:70–71

[36] Moniz E. Essai d'un traitement chirurgical de certaines psychoses. Bull Acad Med. 1936; 115:385–392

[37] Freeman W, Watts J. Psychosurgery. In: Thomas C, ed. the Treatment of Mental Disorders and Intractable Pain. 2nd ed. Springfield; 1950

[38] Freeman W. Psychosurgery; retrospects and prospects based on 12 years' experience. Am J Psychiatry. 1949; 105(8):581–584

[39] Freeman W. Transorbital leucotomy. Lancet. 1948; 2(6523):371–373

[40] Caruso JP, Sheehan JP. Psychosurgery, ethics, and media: a history of Walter Freeman and the lobotomy. Neurosurg Focus. 2017; 43(3):E6

[41] Hoffman JL. Clinical observations concerning schizophrenic patients treated by prefrontal leukotomy. N Engl J Med. 1949; 241(6):233–236

[42] Fulton JF. Frontal lobotomy and affective behaviour: a neurophysiological analysis. New York: W. W. Norton; 1951

[43] Scoville WB. Selective cortical undercutting as a means of modifying and studying frontal lobe function in man; preliminary report of 43 operative cases. J Neurosurg. 1949; 6(1):65–73

[44] Rahman M, Murad GJ, Mocco J. Early history of the stereotactic apparatus in neurosurgery. Neurosurg Focus. 2009; 27(3):E12

[45] Horsley V, Clarke RH. The structure and functions of the cerebellum examined by a new method. Brain. 1908; 31:45–124

[46] Spiegel EA, Wycis HT, Marks M, Lee AJ. Stereotaxic apparatus for operations on the human brain. Science. 1947; 106(2754):349–350

[47] Leksell L. The stereotaxic method and radiosurgery of the brain. Acta Chir Scand. 1951; 102(4):316–319

[48] Leksell L, Backlund EO. [Radiosurgical capsulotomy—a closed surgical method for psychiatric surgery]. Lakartidningen. 1978; 75(7):546–547

[49] Ballantine HT, Jr, Cassidy WL, Flanagan NB, Marino R, Jr. Stereotaxic anterior cingulotomy for neuropsychiatric illness and intractable pain. J Neurosurg. 1967; 26(5):488–495

[50] Herner T. Treatment of mental disorders with frontal stereotaxic thermolesions: a follow-up study of 116 cases. Acta Psychiatr Scand. 1961; 36(Suppl 158):1–140

[51] Leiphart JW, Valone FH, III. Stereotactic lesions for the treatment of psychiatric disorders. J Neurosurg. 2010; 113(6):1204–1211

[52] Göktepe EO, Young LB, Bridges PK. A further review of the results of stereotactic subcaudate tractotomy. Br J Psychiatry. 1975; 126:270–280

[53] Knight G. Stereotactic tractotomy in the surgical treatment of mental illness. J Neurology, Neurosurgery Psychiatry. 1965; 28:304–310

[54] Sweet WH. Treatment of medically intractable mental disease by limited frontal leucotomy—justifiable? N Engl J Med. 1973; 289(21):1117–1125

[55] Couldwell WT, Apuzzo ML. Initial experience related to the use of the Cosman-Roberts-Wells stereotactic instrument. Technical note. J Neurosurg. 1990; 72(1):145–148

[56] Delgado JM, Hamlin H, Chapman WP. Technique of intracranial electrode implacement for recording and stimulation and its possible therapeutic value in psychotic patients. Confin Neurol. 1952; 12(5–6):315–319

[57] Heath RG. Depth recording and stimulation studies in patients. In: Winter A, ed. The Surgical Control of Behavior. 1971:21–37

[58] Cotzias GC, Papavasiliou PS, Gellene R. Modification of parkinsonism—chronic treatment with L-dopa. N Engl J Med. 1969; 280(7):337–345

[59] Koller WC, Lyons KE, Wilkinson SB, Troster AI, Pahwa R. Long-term safety and efficacy of unilateral deep brain stimulation of the thalamus in essential tremor. Mov Disord. 2001; 16(3):464–468

[60] Sydow O, Thobois S, Alesch F, Speelman JD. Multicentre European study of thalamic stimulation in essential tremor: a six year follow-up. J Neurol Neurosurg Psychiatry. 2003; 74(10):1387–1391

[61] Schuurman PR, Bosch DA, Bossuyt PM, et al. A comparison of continuous thalamic stimulation and thalamotomy for suppression of severe tremor. N Engl J Med. 2000; 342(7):461–468

[62] Ghika J, Villemure JG, Fankhauser H, Favre J, Assal G, Ghika-Schmid F. Efficiency and safety of bilateral contemporaneous pallidal stimulation (deep brain stimulation) in levodopa-responsive patients with Parkinson's disease with severe motor fluctuations: a 2-year follow-up review. J Neurosurg. 1998; 89(5):713–718

[63] Hamani C, Richter E, Schwalb JM, Lozano AM. Bilateral subthalamic nucleus stimulation for Parkinson's disease: a systematic review of the clinical literature. Neurosurgery. 2008; 62 Suppl 2:863–874

[64] Deuschl G, Schade-Brittinger C, Krack P, et al. German Parkinson Study Group, Neurostimulation Section. A randomized trial of deep-brain stimulation for Parkinson's disease. N Engl J Med. 2006; 355(9):896–908

[65] Follett KA, Weaver FM, Stern M, et al. CSP 468 Study Group. Pallidal versus subthalamic deep-brain stimulation for Parkinson's disease. N Engl J Med. 2010; 362(22):2077–2091

[66] Weaver FM, Follett K, Stern M, et al. CSP 468 Study Group. Bilateral deep brain stimulation vs best medical therapy for patients with advanced Parkinson disease: a randomized controlled trial. JAMA. 2009; 301(1):63–73

[67] Williams A, Gill S, Varma T, et al. PD SURG Collaborative Group. Deep brain stimulation plus best medical therapy versus best medical therapy alone for advanced Parkinson's disease (PD SURG trial): a randomised, open-label trial. Lancet Neurol. 2010; 9(6):581–591

[68] Laitinen LV. Leksell's unpublished pallidotomies of 1958–1962. Stereotact Funct Neurosurg. 2000; 74(1):1–10

[69] Steiner L, Forster D, Leksell L, Meyerson BA, Boëthius J. Gammathalamotomy in intractable pain. Acta Neurochir (Wien). 1980; 52(3–4):173–184

[70] Frighetto L, Bizzi J, Annes RD, Silva RdosS, Oppitz P. Stereotactic radiosurgery for movement disorders. Surg Neurol Int. 2012; 3 Suppl 1:S10–S16

[71] Kondziolka D, Flickinger JC, Lunsford LD. Stereotactic radiosurgery for epilepsy and functional disorders. Neurosurg Clin N Am. 2013; 24(4):623–632

[72] Niranjan A, Raju SS, Kooshkabadi A, Monaco E, III, Flickinger JC, Lunsford LD. Stereotactic radiosurgery for essential tremor: retrospective analysis of a 19-year experience. Mov Disord. 2017; 32(5):769–777

[73] Cleary DR, Ozpinar A, Raslan AM, Ko AL. Deep brain stimulation for psychiatric disorders: where we are now. Neurosurg Focus. 2015; 38(6):E2

[74] Patel SR, Aronson JP, Sheth SA, Eskandar EN. Lesion procedures in psychiatric neurosurgery. World Neurosurg. 2013; 80(3–4):31.e9–31.e16

[75] Gross RE, Stern MA. Magnetic resonance-guided stereotactic laser pallidotomy for dystonia. Mov Disord. 2018

[76] Fishman PS, Elias WJ, Ghanouni P, et al. Neurological adverse event profile of magnetic resonance imaging-guided focused ultrasound thalamotomy for essential tremor. Mov Disord. 2018; 33(5):843–847

[77] Abosch A, Timmermann L, Bartley S, et al. An international survey of deep brain stimulation procedural steps. Stereotact Funct Neurosurg. 2013; 91(1):1–11

[78] Rezai AR, Kopell BH, Gross RE, et al. Deep brain stimulation for Parkinson's disease: surgical issues. Mov Disord. 2006; 21 Suppl 14:S197–S218

[79] Alonso F, Latorre MA, Göransson N, Zsigmond P, Wårdell K. Investigation into deep brain stimulation lead designs: a patient-specific simulation study. Brain Sci. 2016; 6(3):6

[80] Steigerwald F, Müller L, Johannes S, Matthies C, Volkmann J. Directional deep brain stimulation of the subthalamic nucleus: a pilot study using a novel neurostimulation device. Mov Disord. 2016; 31(8):1240–1243

[81] Rizzi M, Messina G, Penner F, D'Ammando A, Muratorio F, Franzini A. Internal pulse generators in deep brain stimulation: rechargeable or not? World Neurosurg. 2015; 84(4):1020–1029

[82] Niemann M, Schneider GH, Kuhn A, Vajkoczy P, Faust K. Longevity of implantable pulse generators in bilateral deep brain stimulation for movement disorders. Neuromodulation. 2018; 21(6):597–603

[83] Henderson JM, Holloway KL, Gaede SE, Rosenow JM. The application accuracy of a skull-mounted trajectory guide system for image-guided functional neurosurgery. Comput Aided Surg. 2004; 9(4):155–160

[84] Cheng CY, Hsing MT, Chen YH, et al. Deep brain stimulation for Parkinson's disease using frameless technology. Br J Neurosurg. 2014; 28(3):383–386

[85] Maciunas RJ, Galloway RL, Jr, Latimer J, et al. An independent application accuracy evaluation of stereotactic frame systems. Stereotact Funct Neurosurg. 1992; 58(1–4):103–107

[86] Bjartmarz H, Rehncrona S. Comparison of accuracy and precision between frame-based and frameless stereotactic navigation for deep brain stimulation electrode implantation. Stereotact Funct Neurosurg. 2007; 85(5):235–242

[87] Bot M, van den Munckhof P, Bakay R, Sierens D, Stebbins G, Verhagen Metman L. Analysis of stereotactic accuracy in patients undergoing deep brain stimulation using nexframe and the leksell frame. Stereotact Funct Neurosurg. 2015; 93(5):316–325

[88] Mazzone P, Arena P, Cantelli L, et al. Experimental new automatic tools for robotic stereotactic neurosurgery: towards "no hands" procedure of leads implantation into a brain target. J Neural Transm. 2016; 123(7):737–750

[89] Vadera S, Chan A, Lo T, et al. Frameless stereotactic robot-assisted subthalamic nucleus deep brain stimulation: case report. World Neurosurg. 2017; 97:762.e11–762.e14

[90] Hariz MI. Safety and risk of microelectrode recording in surgery for movement disorders. Stereotact Funct Neurosurg. 2002; 78(3–4):146–157

[91] Kocabicak E, Alptekin O, Ackermans L, et al. Is there still need for microelectrode recording now the subthalamic nucleus can be well visualized with high field and ultrahigh MR imaging? Front Integr Nuerosci. 2015; 9:46

[92] Chen T, Mirzadeh Z, Ponce FA. "Asleep" deep brain stimulation surgery: a critical review of the literature. World Neurosurg. 2017; 105:191–198

[93] Zonenshayn M, Rezai AR, Mogilner AY, Beric A, Sterio D, Kelly PJ. Comparison of anatomic and neurophysiological methods for subthalamic nucleus targeting. Neurosurgery. 2000; 47(2):282–292, discussion 292–294

[94] Guridi J, Rodriguez-Oroz MC, Lozano AM, et al. Targeting the basal ganglia for deep brain stimulation in Parkinson's disease. Neurology. 2000; 55(12) Suppl 6:S21–S28

[95] Starr PA, Christine CW, Theodosopoulos PV, et al. Implantation of deep brain stimulators into the subthalamic nucleus: technical approach and magnetic resonance imaging-verified lead locations. J Neurosurg. 2002; 97(2):370–387

[96] Kochanski RB, Sani S. Awake versus asleep deep brain stimulation surgery: technical considerations and critical review of the literature. Brain Sci. 2018; 8(1):8

[97] Chen T, Mirzadeh Z, Chapple KM, et al. Clinical outcomes following awake and asleep deep brain stimulation for Parkinson disease. J Neurosurg. 2018: 1–12

[98] Ho AL, Ali R, Connolly ID, et al. Awake versus asleep deep brain stimulation for Parkinson's disease: a critical comparison and meta-analysis. J Neurol Neurosurg Psychiatry. 2018; 89(7):687–691

[99] LaHue SC, Ostrem JL, Galifianakis NB, et al. Parkinson's disease patient preference and experience with various methods of DBS lead placement. Parkinsonism Relat Disord. 2017; 41:25–30

[100] Lefranc M, Zouitina Y, Tir M, et al. Asleep robot-assisted surgery for the implantation of subthalamic electrodes provides the same clinical improvement and therapeutic window as awake surgery. World Neurosurg. 2017; 106:602–608

[101] Kramer DR, Halpern CH, Buonacore DL, et al. Best surgical practices: a stepwise approach to the University of Pennsylvania deep brain stimulation protocol. Neurosurg Focus. 2010; 29(2):E3

[102] Machado A, Rezai AR, Kopell BH, Gross RE, Sharan AD, Benabid AL. Deep brain stimulation for Parkinson's disease: surgical technique and perioperative management. Mov Disord. 2006; 21 Suppl 14:S247–S258

[103] Alexander E, III, Kooy HM, van Herk M, et al. Magnetic resonance image-directed stereotactic neurosurgery: use of image fusion with computerized tomography to enhance spatial accuracy. J Neurosurg. 1995; 83(2):271–276

[104] Schaltenbrand G, Walker AE. Stereotaxy of the human brain. New York: Thieme-Stratton; 1982

[105] Talairach J, Tournoux P. Co-planar stereotaxic atlas for the human brain: 3-D proportional system: an approach to cerebral imaging. New York: Thieme; 1988

[106] Anderson WS, Winberry J, Liu CC, Shi C, Lenz FA. Applying Microelectrode Recordings in Neurosurgery. Contemp Neurosurg. 2010; 32(3):1–7

[107] Abboud H, Mehanna R, Machado AG, et al. Comprehensive, multidisciplinary deep brain stimulation screening for Parkinson patients: no room for "short cuts". Mov Disord Clin Pract. 2014; 1(4):336–341

[108] Weintraub D, Duda JE, Carlson K, et al. CSP 468 Study Group. Suicide ideation and behaviours after STN and GPi DBS surgery for Parkinson's disease: results from a randomised, controlled trial. J Neurol Neurosurg Psychiatry. 2013; 84(10):1113–1118

[109] Combs HL, Folley BS, Berry DT, et al. Cognition and depression following deep brain stimulation of the subthalamic nucleus and globus pallidus pars internus in Parkinson's disease: a meta-analysis. Neuropsychol Rev. 2015; 25(4):439–454

[110] Schrock LE, Mink JW, Woods DW, et al. Tourette Syndrome Association International Deep Brain Stimulation (DBS) Database and Registry Study Group. Tourette syndrome deep brain stimulation: a review and updated recommendations. Mov Disord. 2015; 30(4):448–471

[111] Lozano AM, Lipsman N. Probing and regulating dysfunctional circuits using deep brain stimulation. Neuron. 2013; 77(3):406–424

[112] Lipsman N, Giacobbe P, Bernstein M, Lozano AM. Informed consent for clinical trials of deep brain stimulation in psychiatric disease: challenges and implications for trial design. J Med Ethics. 2012; 38(2):107–111

[113] Beecher HK. Consent in clinical experimentation: myth and reality. JAMA. 1966; 195(1):34–35

[114] Beecher HK. Ethics and clinical research. N Engl J Med. 1966; 274(24):1354–1360

[115] Jones DS, Grady C, Lederer SE. "Ethics and Clinical Research"—The 50th Anniversary of Beecher's Bombshell. N Engl J Med. 2016; 374(24):2393–2398

[116] Gostin LO. Ethical considerations of psychosurgery: the unhappy legacy of the pre-frontal lobotomy. J Med Ethics. 1980; 6(3):149–154

[117] Nuttin B, Wu H, Mayberg H, et al. Consensus on guidelines for stereotactic neurosurgery for psychiatric disorders. J Neurol Neurosurg Psychiatry. 2014; 85(9):1003–1008

[118] Park RJ, Singh I, Pike AC, Tan JO. Deep brain stimulation in anorexia nervosa: hope for the hopeless or exploitation of the vulnerable? The Oxford Neuroethics Gold Standard Framework. Front Psychiatry. 2017; 8:44

[119] Synofzik M, Fins JJ, Schlaepfer TE. A neuromodulation experience registry for deep brain stimulation studies in psychiatric research: rationale and recommendations for implementation. Brain Stimul. 2012; 5(4):653–655

2 Customized Platform-Based Stereotactic DBS Lead Placement Technique (FHC STarFix, Medtronic Nexframe, and Robotic System Placement)

Ahmad Alhourani, Margot Samson, Joseph S. Neimat

Abstract

Traditional rigid frame-based systems have been the gold standard in stereotactic surgery for decades. Several customized platform-based stereotactic systems have recently been developed to overcome some of the limitations of traditional frames. These new systems offer comparable accuracy and precision along with added patient comfort. In this chapter, theoretical basis behind each system and its workflow for deep brain stimulation (DBS) lead placement has been described. The advantages and disadvantages between these systems and traditional frames have also been compared.

Keywords: frameless, deep brain stimulation, Nexframe, robotic, STarFix, stereotaxis

2.1 Background

The advent of stereotaxis in neurosurgery marked a huge leap by offering minimally invasive corridors to access the brain. Pioneering work by Zernov[1] in 1889 and Clarke and Horsley[2] in 1906 paved the way for the first routinely applied stereotactic system by Spiegel and Wycis[3] in 1947. Improved frame designs, such as the Leksell frame that integrated Cartesian targeting and polar trajectory selection[4] and the enhanced imaging of computed tomography (CT) and magnetic resonance imaging (MRI), made accurately reaching subcortical structures feasible. Stereotactic neurosurgery traditionally relied on a coordinate system contained within the frame itself and a method to relate those coordinates with those of the patient and their imaging. This relationship is calculated by acquiring patient imaging while in the frame. Although these traditional frame-based approaches remain accurate and reliable, they have several drawbacks. The main drawback is the need for the patient to be rigidly fixed in the frame throughout the procedure to maintain this relationship. This can be cumbersome for awake movement disorder patients as the weight of the frame itself requires frame and patient to be bolted to the operative table. For this reason, several stereotactic systems have been developed to allow greater patient comfort with equivalent accuracy and precision. In this chapter, we describe the three most commonly used systems, the theoretical basis for their design, and their practical workflow. We also describe the clinical results from reported experience with each system. In addition, we highlight the advantages and disadvantages to compare across systems.

2.2 Frame versus Imaging-based Coordinate Systems

The principle innovation that has enabled novel frame technologies was the advancement of imaging modalities for three-dimensional (3D) acquisition that incorporates an inherent coordinate space. Almost all CT and MRI scans currently acquired incorporate a precise parametric coordinate system such that each point on the scan has a distinct X, Y, Z designation. With this innovation, frames no longer had to provide an independent Cartesian coordinate system that was so critical when using X-ray ventriculography or 2D CT slice acquisitions (▸ Fig. 2.1a). New frame systems have been developed that essentially co-opt the 3D CT space as their own inherent coordinate system (▸ Fig. 2.1b). All platforms and trajectories within this system are simple mathematical transforms relating points of attachment and registration to targets and trajectories in the same 3D space. This is the same innovation that have made the commonly used frameless stereotactic guidance systems feasible. All the systems described below share and benefit from this simple innovation. The application of this strategy has taken different forms, each with their own unique advantages.

2.2.1 Surgical Targeting Fixture (STarFix) Platform

The STarFix system (FHC Inc., Bowdoin, ME) is an alternative method of stereotaxy that relies on custom microtargeting platforms (MTP) (▸ Fig. 2.2). Rather than giving the trajectory coordinates as input into the standard frame, an MTP is generated which incorporates one or more trajectories into a lightweight fixture that is directly attached to the skull. This process became feasible in the clinical setting with the emergence of

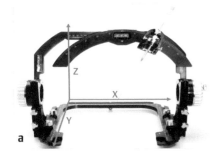

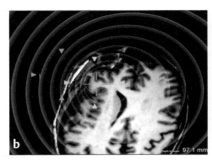

Fig. 2.1 Frame versus imaging-based coordinate systems. Traditional frames rely on an inherent coordinate Cartesian coordinate system contained within the frame (**a**). On the other hand, new frameless systems use the coordinate system inherent in the 3D image volumes (**b**).

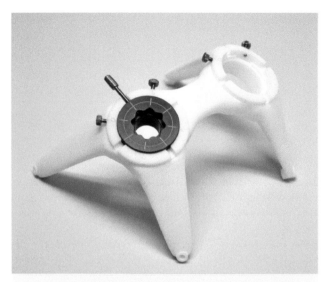

Fig. 2.2 Surgical Targeting Fixture platform. A bilateral STarFix frame (FHC Inc., Bowdoin, ME) is shown with the associated guide tube.

rapid prototyping technology to allow the manufacture and delivery of an MTP in a relatively short time, as little as 3 days. The complete system includes planning software and bone fiducial markers. The bone fiducial markers initially used for registration become anchors for the MTP to couple to during surgery, while the planning software generates the instruction file for manufacturing of an MTP.

The STarFix system retains the basic principles of traditional stereotactic frames, in that (1) the fiducial points are incorporated into the platform itself, and (2) there is a rigid relationship between registration points and the trajectory fixture. It relies on three key data points: bone fiducial anchor locations (made more accurate by recording bone fiducial anchor orientation), the target location, and the trajectory to target. Based on these data points, a transform is generated to translate the imaging space to the patient's physical space. In addition, the orientation of the trajectory with respect to the anterior commissure-posterior commissure line and midline are taken into account to allow for trajectory translation.

In contrast to traditional frames, the general workflow of the STarFix system is broken into two discrete steps over a period of 1 to 2 weeks. In Stage I (termed Step 0 at some centers), the bone fiducial markers are implanted in a separate surgical procedure. This can be performed under local or general anesthesia. At least 3 are required for unilateral cases and 4 are typically used for bilateral frames. (Implantation of 6 or more anchors may be used for specialized applications such as stereotactic electroencephalography, SEEG.) They serve as a rigid reference point for image registration and rigid attachment for the MTP later on. By necessity, the fiducials must remain fixed in the same location between procedures. The bony anchors went through several transformations from externalized MRI-detectable posts and caps to the current internalized bone posts that are buried completely under the scalp. The anchors are placed into the outer table of the skull through simple stab incisions and closed with a single suture or staples. CT scan is obtained immediately following the procedure while the patient is still under general anesthesia or immediately after the procedure. The CT is then registered to any additional imaging that has been acquired. A high-resolution MRI is typically used and can be obtained under the same general anesthesia (if used) for outstanding motion-free images. This enables the acquisition of higher quality imaging free from motion artifact. Patients are usually discharged home with instructions to keep the anchor sites clean.

Surgical planning follows similar steps as for traditional frames where the CT and MR images are coregistered, identifying the target locations and selecting the optimal entry points. However, instead of generating coordinates, the planning software creates a customized MTP design. The design file is sent to the manufacturer and the MTP is delivered to the hospital within a few days. Several compatible planning software are available to generate the design files such as Voxim, WayPoint planner, and StimPilot.

Stage II is usually performed about a week after stage I. Most commonly, this stage is done under local anesthesia, with intravenous sedation. The bone marker incisions are opened and the MTP is rigidly connected to the bone anchors using couplers with submillimetric tolerance. This obviates the need to lock the patient's head to the operating table. A guide is used to mark the entry point on the scalp and skull through the ring opening of the MTP. The steps afterwards from burr hole creation, microelectrode mapping, electrode implantation and macrostimulation are done in a standard fashion.

The STarFix system offers some distinct advantages and disadvantages. First, both trajectories can be mounted and mapped simultaneously through separate microdrives. This can potentially save significant time as both sides are explored and recorded at once. Second, although the frame is nondeformable around the planned trajectory, the trajectory can be adjusted using various offset adapters for the drive assembly allowing for a maximum offset of 11 mm from the central target in all directions which is typically sufficient for any deep brain stimulation (DBS)-type procedure. No final confirmation fluoroscopic imaging is used due to the lack of stable reference imaging with the patient's head not being locked to the operating table. Moreover, the STarFix system is compatible with most microdrives and cannula systems, although the frame height from the skull is different from the Leksell frame and that difference needs to be accounted for when the microelectrodes and cannulas are mounted to calculate the correct distance to target.

The STarFix system was approved by the Food and Drug Administration (FDA) in 2001 and the largest reported experience comes from Vanderbilt where it has been adopted since 2002. The largest case series of 265 patients covered cases performed from 2002 to 2008 using several iterations of the system including its current mature form.[5] The system showed high accuracy with a targeting error of 1.99 ± 0.9 mm across 75 patients. The targeting error was further reduced to 1.24 ± 0.4 mm when accounting for brain shift. The case series demonstrated the safety of the system with less than 0.2% complication rate across the entire cohort. Specifically, 0.1% of patients had dislodgment of the bony fiducial. However, this occurred in earlier versions of the system that had externalized posts and caps in patients with severe dyskinesia. This complication is not seen in the current internalized version of the bony fiducials. There was one case of bone marker infection (0.004%) that was simply treated by removal of the fiducials and a short course of antibiotics. Also, the custom MTP for one patient (0.004%) could not couple to the bone anchors. That was traced back to anchor localization error during planning rather than a manufacturing error.

The clear benefit of the STarFix system is the superior patient comfort it affords by allowing patients to move freely especially in case of patients with severe tremors or dyskinesias. This can help a lot of patients overcome the anxiety of being in a rigid frame for extended periods of time. There is no limitation on head size to fit inside the frame. Finally, it allows for simultaneous bilateral cells microelectrode mapping which increases the speed and efficiency of the operation and may open many opportunities for scientific research.

A recent innovation on the STarFix platform is the advent of the Microtable. This fixture employs the same basic strategy of bone marker insertion and subsequent fixture application. The fixture is a Lexan plate that has holes of various depths drilled into it to hold legs of different length (▶ Fig. 2.3). The resulting geometry can reproduce any single stereotactic trajectory with accuracy equivalent to the STarFix platform. The advantage of the Microtable is that the fixture can be created in just a few minutes and therefore be available for same day surgeries. To date it has been utilized in more than 20 surgeries and publications on safety and accuracy are anticipated in the coming year. (M Fitzpatrick, personal communication).

2.2.2 Nexframe

The Nexframe (Medtronic Inc, Minneapolis, MN), while in the same category as the STarFix system, is the only true frameless system available currently (in the sense that there is no rigid attachment between the reference points and the trajectory)

(▶ Fig. 2.4). It also uses bone fiducial markers for image registration, but they are used as markers for optical tracking to manually register and align the trajectory during surgery[6] and are not incorporated in the fixture itself. It utilizes principles similar to infrared-guided biopsy probes. However, it relies on rigid registration markers and more tightly controlled guide tower allowing for the precision that is required for DBS lead implantation. The Nexframe tower is a standardized frame that is adjusted during targeting, so it does not require the overhead in time required to manufacture the STarFix frame. Also, it is comprised of disposable components thus eliminating the need to be recalibrated after repeated use like traditional frames.

The workflow follows a similar, albeit shorter, timeframe to the STarFix system as it is broken up into two stages. In Stage I, the patient undergoes implantation of 4 to 6 bone fiducial markers that are used for rigid registration. This can be performed on the day of surgery or 1 to 2 days prior. CT images with the fiducials in place are obtained and merged with the preoperative MRI imaging on the StealthStation. Target selection is performed in a standard fashion. The centers of the fiducials are then marked, and the entry point is selected. A

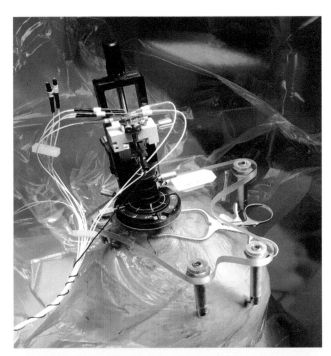

Fig. 2.3 The Microtable system. The Microtable (FHC Inc., Bowdoin, ME) is a Lexan plate that reproduces a single trajectory using variously staggered legs holding the platform.

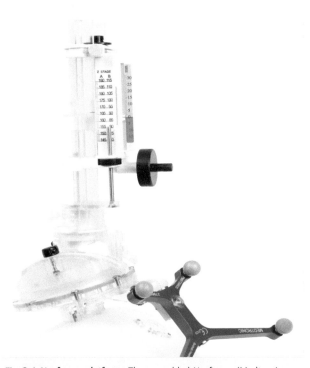

Fig. 2.4 Nexframe platform. The assembled Nexframe (Medtronic Inc., Minneapolis, MN) with the optical tracking reference shown in the bottom.

standard burr hole is created overlying the entry point and the Stimloc base is attached to the skull to act as a base for the Nexframe and the reference arc. The fiducial markers are then used to register the patient space using optical tracking. The tower is assembled and attached to the base to align with the target. The Nexdrive is then attached with light-emitting diodes to track the electrodes' location. The final tract can still be adjusted but it is limited by the excursion of the tower. The base allows for two possible movements: 360 degree of rotation and 25 degree of angling in any two directions.

The largest case series using the Nexframe included 60 patients with 119 electrode implantations over an 18-month period.[7] In this case series, both stages were done in the same setting and under general anesthesia. The mean targeting error was 1.24 ± 0.87 mm across all targets (subthalamic nucleus, globus pallidus pars interna, and ventralis intermedius nucleus) and was correlated with the distance from the ventricle. No frame-related complications were reported.

The Nexframe has advantages similar to the STarFix system in terms of patient comfort and bilateral simultaneous trajectories. In addition, it does not require the manufacturing time that is required for the STarFix system, with a significantly shorter workflow than can be done in the same day. Although accuracy in experienced hands is comparable to other framed and frameless systems, there is a learning curve to pointing and tightening the frame to secure the trajectory. This can lead to a lack of reproducible precision in less-experienced hands.

2.2.3 Robotic Assisted Placement

Another approach to stereotaxis was marked by the advent of robotic systems in neurosurgery.[8] They offer in vivo submillimetric accuracy in a reproducible fashion. Robotic systems have been more widely adopted for stereoelectroencephalography,[9] but there are only a few reports about their use for DBS.[10,11,12] Several robotic systems are currently available that have been reportedly used in DBS implantation, such as The Robotic Stereotactic Assistance (ROSA) (Medtech Surgical/Zimmer Biomet, New York, NY) and NeuroMate (Renishaw-Mayfield, Renishaw plc, Wotton-Under-Edge, Gloucestershire, UK). Another system, Renaissance (Mazor Robotics Ltd.), has been used for stereotaxis[13] but not for DBS use. However, it is FDA approved only for spine applications.

Both systems consist of a robotic manipulator and proprietary surgical planning software. The manipulator is a robotic arm, with varying movement degrees of freedom (6 for ROSA and 5 for NeuroMate), that automatically moves into the planned trajectory. The two systems share a similar workflow. The robotic system is registered to preoperative surgical planning MRI through either frameless or frame-based rigid registration. While both are applicable, only rigid frame-based registration has been reported for DBS using CT imaging and bone fiducial. Even if using frameless registration, the patient's head must remain in rigid fixation with a head clamp to attach to the robotic arm. The trajectories are calculated automatically using the planning software and the robotic arm moves into the trajectory. The entry point is marked using a laser beam. After the skin incision and burr hole, the microdrive is mounted on the robotic arm. The mapping portion is performed in a standard fashion and can be controlled manually or automatically by the robotic arm. The automatic targeting and delivery of the electrodes eliminates any errors from manually entering coordinates through a rigid, tremorless applicator.

The reported experience for DBS remains limited for both systems. Only two case reports exist on the use of the ROSA system. On the other hand, a small case series of 17 patients (30 electrodes) using NeuroMate demonstrated an in vivo accuracy of 0.86 ± 0.32 mm. This limited adoption is likely due to the current high pricing of each system.

2.3 System Comparison

The aim of stereotaxis is to reach the intended target with minimal error that is usually measured by accuracy and precision. Accuracy measures how far the trajectory was from the intended target, while precision measures how wide is the variation in the trajectories. Accuracy can be measured through the targeting error while precision relates to the standard deviation of that targeting error. All three systems show comparable accuracy to each other and to traditional frames, with the highest accuracy seen with robotic systems (▶ Table 2.1). There is wide variation on the reported accuracy of each system but there is a clear trend in improved accuracy across time as groups become more familiar and adapt at their use.[14]

Conceptually, all three systems use the coordinate system in the patient's imaging rather than having an internal coordinate

Table 2.1 Feature comparison between traditional frame and frameless DBS systems

Category	Traditional frames (Leksell and CRW)	Nexframe	STarFix frame	Robotic-assisted
Targeting error in phantom models (mm)	1.7 ± 1, 1.8 ± 1.1[15]	1.25 ± 0.6[15]	0.42 ± 0.15	0.44 ± 0.23[11]
Targeting error in cases series (mm)	1.4,[16] 1.03 ± 0.76[17]	1.24 ± 0.87[7]	1.24 ± 0.4[5]	0.87 ± 0.32[11]
Registration method	Fixed	Fixed or deformable	Fixed	Fixed or deformable
Targeting method	Structural	Virtual	Structural	Structural
Targeting limitation	Unlimited	Adjustment limited by tower excursion	Adjustments limited	Unlimited
Multiple trajectories	Only one	Two are possible	Unlimited	Only one
Coordinate system	Inherent to the frame	Borrowed from imaging	Borrowed from imaging	Borrowed from imaging

Abbreviation: CRW, Cosman-Roberts-Wells.

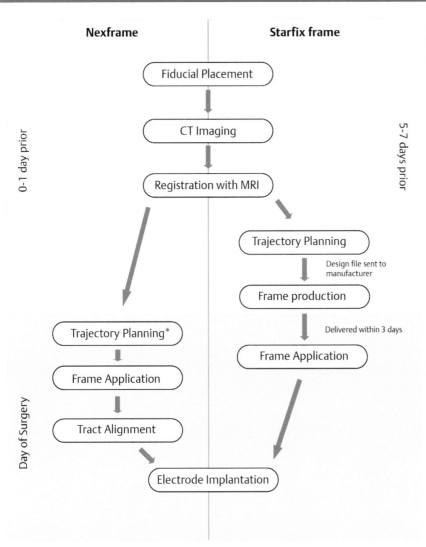

Nexframe

Starfix frame

0–1 day prior

5–7 days prior

Fiducial Placement

CT Imaging

Registration with MRI

Trajectory Planning

Design file sent to manufacturer

Frame production

Delivered within 3 days

Frame Application

Trajectory Planning*

Frame Application

Tract Alignment

Day of Surgery

Electrode Implantation

Fig. 2.5 Workflow summary and comparison between the STarFix and Nexframe systems. The Nexframe (left) and STarFix (right) systems share similar workflows with few diverging points. Of note, the Nexframe workflow can all be performed in the same day. *Can be performed on the same day or before surgery.

system, as seen in traditional frames, affording more flexibility. Both the STarFix and Nexframe systems offer better patient comfort by obviating the need for rigid fixation to the table. However, robotic systems still require the patient to remain in a rigid head clamp even if frameless registration is used. All systems use skull-mounted fiducials for registration but the Nexframe and robotic system offer the option of surface-based deformable registration. Finally, all systems except for the STarFix system can be deployed in the same day. A comparison of the workflow of the STarFix and the Nexframe is summarized here (▶ Fig. 2.5).

Overall, the advent of these novel systems has provided a variety of solutions to improve patient comfort and surgical efficiency while maintaining accuracy and precision. They have grown to comprise a substantial proportion of DBS surgeries performed nationally and their application to other stereotactic surgeries, such as laser interstitial thermal therapy and SEEG, may expand their utilization in the future.

References

[1] Kandel' EI, Shchavinskii YV. First stereotaxic apparatus created by Russian scientists in the 19th century. Biomed Eng (NY). 1973; 7(2):121–124

[2] Clarke R, Horsley V. On a method of investigating the deep ganglia and tracts of the central nervous system (cerebellum). Br Med J. 1906; 2:1799–1800

[3] Spiegel EA, Wycis HT, Marks M, Lee AJ. Stereotaxic apparatus for operations on the human brain. Science. 1947; 106(2754):349–350

[4] Leksell L, Leksell D, Schwebel J. Stereotaxis and nuclear magnetic resonance. J Neurol Neurosurg Psychiatry. 1985; 48(1):14–18

[5] Konrad PE, Neimat JS, Yu H, et al. Customized, miniature rapid-prototype stereotactic frames for use in deep brain stimulator surgery: initial clinical methodology and experience from 263 patients from 2002 to 2008. Stereotact Funct Neurosurg. 2011; 89(1):34–41

[6] Holloway KL, Gaede SE, Starr PA, Rosenow JM, Ramakrishnan V, Henderson JM. Frameless stereotaxy using bone fiducial markers for deep brain stimulation. J Neurosurg. 2005; 103(3):404–413

[7] Burchiel KJ, McCartney S, Lee A, Raslan AM. Accuracy of deep brain stimulation electrode placement using intraoperative computed tomography without microelectrode recording. J Neurosurg. 2013; 119(2):301–306

[8] McBeth PB, Louw DF, Rizun PR, Sutherland GR. Robotics in neurosurgery. Am J Surg. 2004; 188(4A) Suppl:68S–75S

[9] Serletis D, Bulacio J, Bingaman W, Najm I, González-Martínez J. The stereotactic approach for mapping epileptic networks: a prospective study of 200 patients. J Neurosurg. 2014; 121(5):1239–1246

[10] Vadera S, Chan A, Lo T, et al. Frameless stereotactic robot-assisted subthalamic nucleus deep brain stimulation: case report. World Neurosurg. 2017; 97: 762.e11–762.e14

[11] von Langsdorff D, Paquis P, Fontaine D. In vivo measurement of the frame-based application accuracy of the NeuroMate neurosurgical robot. J Neurosurg. 2015; 122(1):191–194

[12] Lefranc M, Le Gars D. Robotic implantation of deep brain stimulation leads, assisted by intra-operative, flat-panel CT. Acta Neurochir (Wien). 2012; 154 (11):2069–2074

[13] Grimm F, Naros G, Gutenberg A, Keric N, Giese A, Gharabaghi A. Blurring the boundaries between frame-based and frameless stereotaxy: feasibility study for brain biopsies performed with the use of a head-mounted robot. J Neurosurg. 2015; 123(3):737–742

[14] Li Z, Zhang J-G, Ye Y, Li X. Review on factors affecting targeting accuracy of deep brain stimulation electrode implantation between 2001 and 2015. Stereotact Funct Neurosurg. 2016; 94(6):351–362

[15] Henderson JM, Holloway KL, Gaede SE, Rosenow JM. The application accuracy of a skull-mounted trajectory guide system for image-guided functional neurosurgery. Comput Aided Surg. 2004; 9(4):155–160

[16] Starr P, Christine C, Theodosopoulos P, et al. Implantation of deep brain stimulators into the subthalamic nucleus: technical approach and magnetic resonance imaging-verified electrode locations. J Neurosurg. 2002; 97(2):370–387

[17] Pollo C, Vingerhoets F, Pralong E, et al. Localization of electrodes in the subthalamic nucleus on magnetic resonance imaging. J Neurosurg. 2007; 106(1): 36–44

3 Microelectrode Recording Methods

Michael D. Staudt, Jonathan P. Miller

Abstract

Microelectrode recording (MER) involves the use of high-impedance electrodes that allow precise identification of subcortical structures. MER is routinely employed to reconcile stereotactic targeting based on indirect and direct imaging methods prior to lesion creation or implantation of deep brain stimulator electrodes. Targeting based on anatomical landmarks or direct imaging visualization is prone to error due to individual anatomic variability and imaging distortion. The electrophysiological data generated from MER allows for the correction of stereotactic targeting error and brain shift. Each of the common targets used for neuromodulation for movement disorders demonstrate a unique signature of electrophysiological activity that can allow for detailed mapping with unparalleled precision. MER also has an invaluable role as a research tool, such as for delineating the physiology of deep brain structures in disease states and identifying new targets for deep brain stimulation. Recent advancements in imaging technology and stereotactic technique have allowed for better visualization and targeting of subcortical targets; however, excellent outcomes have been reported with and without MER, and a direct comparison of these techniques has never been performed. The role of MER in neuromodulation surgery will undoubtedly evolve as technologies for intraoperative targeting continue to improve. However, the use of MER continues to be widespread and it remains the most utilized method of target confirmation in movement disorder surgery.

Keywords: microelectrode recording, intraoperative mapping, stereotactic targeting, deep brain stimulation, neuromodulation, movement disorders, functional neurosurgery

3.1 Introduction

Microelectrode recording (MER) is an important targeting tool for stereotactic surgery and has played a critical role in the development of surgical treatment of movement disorders where clinical efficacy is critically dependent on accurate intraoperative targeting. The modern era of MER can be traced to the early the 1960s when Albe-Fessard and colleagues described the use of low-impedance bipolar electrodes to distinguish between thalamic nuclei and the internal capsule.[1,2] This was a significant breakthrough that bridged the recording of single cell action potentials from the laboratory to the clinical setting: not only was MER able to differentiate white matter from gray matter, but it could also discriminate the borders of different subcortical nuclei by resolving each structure's characteristic neural firing pattern.[1] Subsequently, microelectrode technology has been refined to allow precise physiological localization by analyzing the relationship to local field potentials, synchrony with movement or tremor activity, and response to microstimulation.[3,4,5,6]

Within a few years of its development, MER use for targeting of therapeutic lesions became widespread, but the introduction of levodopa in 1967 led to a transition away from surgery toward medical management that lasted nearly two decades.[7,8,9] Nevertheless, experimental and clinical studies using MER continued to facilitate interest in surgery as an important component of movement disorder management[10] and in the discovery of new therapeutic targets such as the subthalamic nucleus (STN).[11] Moreover, the development of deep brain stimulation (DBS) as a titratable and reversible therapeutic application reinvigorated MER as an adjunct for target localization when placing DBS electrodes.[12] Although imaging and intraoperative techniques have improved and now allow for direct anatomic targeting, MER and intraoperative stimulation continue to be widely used in functional neurosurgery.

The localization of intracranial targets via radiographic and anatomic means is the critical first step in planning stereotactic procedures, and advances in imaging technologies allow for increasingly greater visualization and identification of therapeutic targets. However, even modern imaging modalities sometimes do not clearly display the target structure due to limitations such as distortion. MER, as an intraoperative adjunct, allows for accurate target localization based on physiological criteria and correction of targeting errors. Furthermore, MER allows precise definition of the ideal physiological target which may differ in some cases from the anatomical target.[13] The potential disadvantages of MER include an elevated risk of complications (in particular, hemorrhage) and the increased cost, time, and complexity it adds to the surgical case. The goal of this chapter is to describe the utility of MER for the localization of intracranial targets in stereotactic neurosurgery and outline principles of its use for specific targets.

3.2 The Rationale for Mapping

Accurate subcortical target localization can be achieved by careful planning and skilled interpretation of anatomical and/or electrophysiological data. Indirect and direct anatomical visualization via landmarks, stereotactic atlases, and imaging remains the essential first step in planning for movement disorder surgery. However, there are multiple potential sources of error that can be introduced during planning and localization, such as imaging distortion and variability in individual patient anatomy. Furthermore, human and mechanical error must always be considered. MER has the potential to address these sources of error in order to improve target localization.

Stereotaxy is prone to small errors, even under optimal conditions, which can add up to several millimeters. These causes of error may include the distortion and spatial inaccuracy of magnetic resonance imaging (MRI), and brain shift due to intraoperative pneumocephalus from cerebrospinal fluid loss.[14,15] The passage of a stiff cannula or electrode into the soft brain parenchyma can also cause deflection from the intended target. The use of routine landmarks for the purposes of indirect targeting can be quite variable due to subtle differences in the location of subcortical nuclei.[16,17] Critical differences have also been observed in standard stereotactic atlases that are commonly used as overlays during planning.[18] MER has the potential to correct for sources of error attributable to spatial inaccuracy, brain shift, or distortion, with real-time feedback and a high degree of accuracy. When targeting is refined using MER data, postoperative imaging sometimes indicates that the corrected electrode position is within the intended target, suggesting that physiological data allowed compensation for a targeting error that would otherwise have been unrecognized.

Structure and function do not always correspond, and there may be a difference between physiologic and anatomic targets. MER has the ability to identify physiological structures directly, including structural borders and somatotopic organization. MER can also identify differences in spontaneous firing rates, patterns, and responses to movement between individual nuclei, and it does so with better spatial resolution and accuracy than many MRI sequences. Despite advances in MRI technology, intracranial targets remain challenging to identify. At standard clinical field strength, the globus pallidus is best visualized, the STN somewhat less so, and ventral thalamus least because the radiographic borders of individual thalamic nuclei are indistinct.

Precise mapping in three dimensions is possible with MER, including identifying the contours of the nuclei.[19] For example, the dorsolateral two-thirds of the STN corresponds to the sensorimotor region and its targeting is optimized with MER and stimulation techniques.[20] Precise mapping of nuclear borders can facilitate optimization of the physiological effects of stimulation and prevention of side effects or unintended injury to eloquent structures.[21,22] MER and microstimulation are very useful in identifying smaller targets and create smaller lesion tracts compared to macrostimulation, should a new trajectory be required. Furthermore, micro- or macrostimulation alone can produce variable or delayed effects, even at target. Localization via MER is essential when these discrepancies arise, and requires skilled interpretation of neuronal firing patterns.[18,23,24]

In addition to its clinical use, MER has a valuable role in research. Both historical and contemporary research has relied on MER to help delineate the pathophysiology of movement disorders, the physiology of deep brain structures, and the effect of DBS on downstream neurons. New targets for DBS are being identified with the use of MER, including Parkinson's disease (PD)-associated freezing of gait[25,26] and epilepsy.[27]

3.3 Microelectrode Technology and Technique

The methodology for target localization and use of MER varies widely between neurosurgical centers; however, the general setup and technical aspects of MER insertion and recording are standard. In general, the essential components include the microelectrode or semi-microelectrode, audio/video monitors, and an amplifier/oscilloscope. A motorized microdriver for electrode advancement is often used that must be compatible with the available stereotactic targeting system. Microdriver systems may be hydraulic or motorized, with the latter allowing electrode advancement via an electronic control. Intraoperative stimulation can be performed using a current isolation stimulator, and stimulation is either passed through the high-impedance

recording contact (microstimulation) or referential contact (macrostimulation).

The microelectrode usually consists of a tungsten or platinum-iridium bipolar electrode with a glass-insulated tapered tip having a diameter of 5 μm (or less) and a length of 10 to 15 μm for recording. Microelectrodes have high impedances (greater than 500 kΩ) that allow for single unit isolation in regions with a high density of neurons, and thus better target differentiation during recording.[28,29] Semi-microelectrodes have a larger tip diameter (25 μm or larger) with lower impedance resulting in greater sensitivity to neural activity at the expense of inability to discriminate single-cell recordings, thus providing less specific information.[30] The physical properties of the electrodes ensure durability to microstimulation, although the passage of current degrades the glass insulation and lowers the impedance, resulting in decreased noise but increased difficulty in isolation of single units.

The microelectrode is inserted within a protective stainless-steel cannula that allows for stability and retraction of the electrode tip during advancement through brain parenchyma. The MER apparatus is first positioned at a predetermined distance above the intracranial target (typically 15–25 mm) and the electrode is slowly advanced to target and a short distance beyond as recording is performed. During microelectrode advancement, the signal is filtered and amplified via isolated preamplifiers and processed through low- and high-pass filters to eliminate excess noise. An oscilloscope displays this filtered signal that is often enhanced through digital processing. Sound is also transmitted through speakers, and the signal is heard as multiple discharges. Individual neuronal firing activity can be isolated by using window discriminators.

There are many different philosophies about how MER should be used and how much electrophysiological detail is necessary. For example, electrode passage along a single trajectory can verify the presence of the target structure and define its depth along that specific trajectory. An alternative option is to employ multiple parallel passes to create detailed three-dimensional maps that define the borders of multiple subcortical structures. Multiple electrodes can be simultaneously inserted and recorded from during a single pass using a multichannel microarray. One such example, the "Ben gun," has one central channel and four side channels positioned 2 mm from the central channel. This device allows the advancement of up to five parallel microelectrodes simultaneously.[31] This technique allows the user to directly compare recordings between electrodes, and a theoretical volume of tissue can be delineated given the fixed distance between the electrodes.[32]

MER can be used alone or in conjunction with micro- or macrostimulation delivered via an isolated current stimulator. Recordings from MER are accurate to about 0.1 mm, whereas stimulation current spreads over a much wider area of up to a few millimeters. Thus, mapping by stimulation is somewhat less precise. Stimulation is performed using monopolar or bipolar biphasic charge-balanced square wave pulse trains of 0.06 to 0.3 milliseconds at 130 to 300 Hz. Depending on the position of the electrode, a variety of sensory, pyramidal, or extrapyramidal manifestations can assist in physiological mapping. It is imperative to have a trained practitioner for interpretation of these manifestations, as the physiological manifestations of stimulation can vary on the basis of location. Although documenting changes in tremor may be straightforward to quantify, tremor arrest may also be seen in areas outside of target, such as the corticospinal tract and zona incerta. Stimulation also tends to be accurate to approximately 5 mm of targeted tissue,[32] and this can produce false negatives.

3.3.1 Ventral Thalamus

The thalamus was an important early stereotactic target in the treatment of PD as thalamotomy provides significant relief of tremor, and the ventral thalamic nuclei are commonly targeted with DBS to treat movement disorders. These nuclei include: the ventral oral (Vo) or pallidal relay nucleus targeted for parkinsonism or dystonia; the ventral intermediate (Vim) or cerebellar relay nucleus targeted for tremor; and the ventral caudal (Vc) or somatic sensory nucleus targeted to aid in localization of the Vim and also to treat certain neuropathic pain syndromes.[33,34] These targets are not clearly visualized on MRI; thus, radiological determination of the anterior and posterior commissures (AC-PC line) is first performed which allows for "indirect" targeting based on standard coordinates. Targeting may be aided by using preprogrammed atlas maps which approximate the location of nuclei based on the AC-PC line or other surrounding structures. Physiological localization can then be performed with recording and/or stimulation with a micro- or macroelectrode to identify the thalamic nuclei based on their unique electrophysiological responses.

The Vim is organized somatotopically, with face medial and leg lateral. The Vim also contains "kinesthetic cells" which respond to passive joint movements and demonstrate firing synchronous with tremor activity.[35,36,37] These kinesthetic cells demonstrate variable firing rates depending on the disease pathology: tremor cells fire in rhythmic bursts with clinical tremor activity, and in essential tremor these fire at a higher frequency compared with PD or pain.[34,38] Tremor cells have been theorized to cluster approximately 2 mm anterior to the anterior border of Vc, and 3 mm above the AC-PC line.[39] The anterior Vo (Voa) nucleus has been proposed as a superior target for rigidity control, whereas the posterior Vo (Vop) is preferred for tremor.[40,41] MER of the Vop has also demonstrated rhythmic bursting activity at tremor frequencies.

Microelectrode mapping of Voa/Vop, Vim, and Vc

Vc is sometimes chosen for initial localization with MER, as it is the most easily identifiable of all the ventral thalamic nuclei, and the final electrode trajectory can then be fine-tuned based on the electrophysiological findings. Due to the frontal angle of entry, the electrode is likely to first enter the Vop, then Vim, before entering Vc.

Neuronal activity within the Vop and Voa correlates with movement in response to commands, the active phase of movement, and a state of maximal muscle contraction.[36,42,43] As such, spontaneous firing activity is lower compared with other targets. So-called voluntary cells produce the largest proportional change in firing rates in response to active movement, and tremor cells may be encountered that fire in synchrony with the patient's tremor. The execution of particular movements often preferentially relates to a specific firing pattern, and the

somatotopy is parallel to the cutaneous core of Vc.[42] Vim and Vop are readily identified by the response to stimulation of deep structures, such as tendons, or movement of joints and phasic tremor frequency. Certain cells also respond to both somatosensory stimulation and active movement. In addition, Vop is identifiable by EEG spindle activity with a 7 to 10-Hz rhythm, and increases and decreases in amplitude.[34]

Posterior to Voa and Vop and anterior to the cutaneous core in the anterior dorsal cap of Vc is the Vim which contains "kinesthetic cells" that respond primarily to passive joint movement, deep pressure, and squeezing of muscles and tendons, but not manipulation of skin deformed by these movements. Although there is some activation with voluntary movement, the amplitude is often equal or less than that produced by passive movement. Kinesthetic cells may fire concurrently with tremor if the receptive fields overlap.[44] Vim and Vc share a similar somatotopy, with deep sensory cells of the wrist anterior to the cutaneous representation of digits.[45,46] The border between Vim and Vc can be difficult to identify, as macrostimulation produces paresthesias within similar parts of the body. However, threshold for activation tends to be higher in Vim.

Initial entry from the Vim is into the dorsal shell of Vc where proprioceptive receptor fields are located. Further progression caudally reveals "tactile cells" that readily demonstrate rate changes in response to sensory stimulation in well-defined receptive fields with mediolateral somatotopy,[45] and this somatotopy can provide information for choosing an appropriate Vim trajectory. Stimulation of tactile cells produces paresthesias within the region of the corresponding receptive field. As the microelectrode passes through the bottom of the thalamus, there tends to be a distinct reduction in background noise and unit recordings. Stimulation in this region may continue to produce paresthesias due to activation of the medial lemniscus, although requiring higher thresholds than those in Vc, and muscle contractions may be elicited if the electrode is too close to the internal capsule.

3.3.2 Globus Pallidus

The globus pallidus is divided into two segments: the medial internal segment (GPi) and lateral external segment (GPe). The distribution of pallidal tremor cells is primarily within the ventral portion of GPi[47] which corresponds to the sensorimotor component located laterally, ventrally, and posteriorly.[10] The target location for DBS is approximately 1 to 2 mm from the external segment of GPe and 3 to 5 mm from the pallidocapsular border.[48] Ideally, this target is posterior and ventral within the GPi, although not positioned too posteriorly to avoid inducing muscle contractions with stimulation.[49] Compared to the thalamus, the GPi is relatively easy to visualize on MRI.

GPi is the preferred target for the treatment of primary dystonia[50,51] and for certain forms of secondary dystonia including tardive dyskinesia.[52,53] It is also the target for effective treatment for parkinsonian symptoms.[54,55] Different firing patterns are present depending on movement disorder pathology. In PD patients, the GPi firing rate is significantly amplified due to dopamine depletion.[56] The responses to kinesthetic movements are exaggerated and lack specificity, and there is a greater spread of response across multiple joints. Both contralateral and ipsilateral activation may be observed. The firing pattern may also be synchronous with tremor.[55,57] In contrast to PD where GPi firing is dramatically increased compared to GPe, dystonia is associated with a less pronounced increase in GPi firing compared to GPe, which can make discrimination of the nuclei challenging.[58] Furthermore, dystonia is associated with an increased tendency for group discharges because of changes in the specificity of receptive fields.[59] Some of these effects may actually be artifact of anesthesia, since many patients with dystonia require deeper anesthesia to facilitate implantation.[60]

Microelectrode mapping of GPi

The electrode must first traverse the putamen and GPe before entering the GPi. Minimal activity is seen during passage through the striatum, with rare discharges related to injury and occasional tonically active cells at 4 to 6 Hz.[55] The GPe has distinct firing patterns compared to GPi and is characterized by large spontaneously active units. There are units which demonstrate intermediate-frequency discharges (60 Hz) with occasional pauses ("pauser" cells), and those demonstrating low-frequency discharges (10–20 Hz) punctuated by rapid bursts ("burster" cells). Upon exiting the GPe ventrally, the medial pallidal lamina is entered which is an area with minimal activity due to a 1 to 2 mm band of white matter fibers. Cholinergic "border cells" are sometimes encountered at the border of the nuclei. These are cells with diffuse cortical inputs that produce a regular, slow steady tonic discharge (20–40 Hz) of wide action potentials at a nearly constant interspike interval. These cells will occasionally fire in response to movement or in a spontaneous bursting pattern.

The internal and external segments of the GPi are separated by an incomplete pallidal lamina. As the GPi is entered, discharges become more rapid and regular compared to GPe; the frequency can approach 80 to 90 Hz in patients with PD. Approximately 25% of cells within the GPi respond to kinesthetic movements, with representation of the face, extraocular muscles, and upper and lower limbs.[55] This response is variable and the firing rate may increase, decrease, or reciprocally increase/decrease. Appropriate sensorimotor responses and identification of both the optic tract and internal capsule are essential for appropriate electrode placement.

Once the GPi has been exited, there is a reduction in background noise as white matter is encountered, with the optic and corticospinal tracts in close proximity. Microstimulation within the optic tract as low as 1 µA at 300 Hz will cause the patient to perceive phosphenes of light in the contralateral visual field.[18] Flashes of light into the patient's eyes will also produce evoked potentials that can be recorded from the optic tract. The corticospinal tract is identified by contralateral muscle tetanus with stimulation. The threshold of muscle contractions in relation to stimulation can indirectly identify electrode position relative to the internal capsule. The corresponding somatotopy may also provide information regarding laterality (face represented medially, then upper extremities, then lower extremities most lateral).[55]

3.3.3 Subthalamic Nucleus

The STN has extensive cortical and thalamic connections, thus playing an important role in movement disorder pathophysiology.

As part of the indirect pathway that inhibits movement, the STN receives striatal input via the GPe, and projects to GPi and substantia nigra pars reticulata (SNr).[61] It also receives extensive direct excitatory cortical input via the hyperdirect pathway.[62] There is extensive preclinical data emphasizing the importance of the STN in motor circuitry and the pathophysiology of PD. Selective lesioning in rhesus monkeys has been demonstrated to cause hemiballismus,[63] but parkinsonian symptoms have also improved in primate models of PD.[11,64] Thereafter, high-frequency stimulation was shown to improve tremor, akinesia, and rigidity in both primate models[65,66] and humans with PD.[31,67] The STN is organized into sensorimotor, limbic, and associative regions.[68] The sensorimotor region is located dorsally within the posterolateral region of the STN[69,70] and is the most common target for the surgical treatment of PD.[71]

Due to nigrostriatal dopamine depletion in PD, STN undergoes a change in firing pattern and increase in the firing rate.[72,73] STN cells typically fire at 20 Hz in nonpathological states but in patients with PD, they fire at greater than 40 Hz. Moreover, up to 20% of cells demonstrate oscillatory activity in case of PD, which is otherwise rare.[74,75] Both augmented synchrony and a loss of center-surround inhibition is observed. As a result, receptive fields are less specific and spread can be observed through multiple joints. There is also increased bursting activity and change in firing in response to active or passive contralateral joint activation, with an ipsilateral response seen in up to 25% of cells.

Microelectrode mapping of STN

Initial MER activity depends on the laterality of entry. A more medial trajectory passes through the striatum and thalamus, whereas a lateral trajectory may exclusively traverse the corona radiata and internal capsule.[71] The striatum is relatively quiet with occasional injury discharges and tonically active cells at 4 to 6 Hz. The reticular shell of the thalamus demonstrates relatively slow, regular discharges.[23] Deeper in the thalamus, cells are more tonically active and can be distinguished from the STN on the basis of a lower firing rate and quieter background. The cell-poor zona incerta is then encountered upon exiting the thalamus which is characterized by infrequent activity.

Upon entering the dorsal border of the STN, there is a dramatic increase in cellularity and the number of action potentials. Spikes generally have a negative wave followed by a smaller and narrower positive deflection. There are two different extracellular spike waveforms which demonstrate both monophasic and biphasic behavior. The first waveform pattern is a mixed pattern characterized by tonic activity and an irregular discharge pattern with occasional bursts, whereas the second is a burst pattern with periodic oscillatory bursts that are synchronous with the rest tremor.[76] Electrode placement within the dorsolateral STN is confirmed by movement-related activity, with arm-related activity predominantly in the lateral region. Approximately 40 to 50% of cells will respond to passive movement. Microelectrode stimulation in these regions aids in localization, as bulbar responses indicate a lateral proximity to the corticobulbar tract, whereas ipsilateral eye deviation may indicate proximity to the oculomotor nerve or nucleus located medially.[77] With macrostimulation, facial contraction or dysarthria may be observed with corticobulbar activation and contralateral paresthesias with leminiscal activation.[77]

The SNr is encountered ventral to the STN. The cellularity and activity in SNR is less rich and sparser compared to the STN, but the irregular firing produces a continuous melodic hum that is readily appreciated through a speaker. Spikes in this region are symmetrical and biphasic with large amplitudes and rates of approximately 30 Hz (wide range of 8–80 Hz),[76] although higher firing rates have also been described.[23] An important distinction between these STN and SNr cells is that neurons within the SNr are always irregularly tonic and never burst.

3.4 Controversies and Complications

It has been suggested that exclusively anatomic targeting may confer the same clinical benefits as physiological targeting with MER and stimulation. There is precedence for this approach, as a survey of functional neurosurgeons published in 1985 reported similarly excellent results, despite variability among their preferred thalamic surgical target for PD.[78] Two previous non-MER pallidotomy studies have also described excellent clinical results with no mortality and low morbidity.[79,80] However, these results should be interpreted with caution, as the GP is a larger target than the STN, and thus the margin of error for complications may be higher.

Advances in MRI have allowed for improved preoperative visualization of subcortical targets and white matter tracts.[81] Imaging modalities have also been developed that allow intraoperative image-guided DBS, which integrate planning, targeting, and confirmation of DBS lead placement. Recent studies have reported clinical efficacy, with comparable lead placement accuracy to MER,[82,83,84,85] and decreased procedure time with little to no complications.[86,87,88] MER also significantly increases the cost and complexity of stereotactic cases requiring skilled interpretation of physiological recordings, and both specialized equipment and personnel are necessary. The use of MER increases overall operative time and is associated with increased costs.[89] In comparison, performing image-guided DBS surgeries with patients asleep has been reported to lower costs relative to surgeries where patients are awake.[90]

There is also evidence to suggest that MER is associated with an increased risk of complications, particularly hemorrhage,[91,92,93,94,95] which is correlated with the number of microelectrode passes.[96,97,98] Recent studies of image-guided DBS have reported lower hemorrhage risk compared with MER.[99,100] However, confirmation that MER is either less safe or more efficacious than other techniques would require a controlled clinical trial and no such study has been performed.

3.5 Summary

Since its earliest clinical use more than half a century ago, MER has been a cornerstone in the experimental study and clinical treatment of movement disorders. Despite continued advancement in imaging technology allowing better visualization of subcortical targets, the use of MER continues to be widespread. MER offers an unparalleled degree of precision with the ability to delineate the anatomic and electrophysiological relationships of target nuclei. Furthermore, MER allows for both target

confirmation and stereotactic error correction. Although excellent clinical outcomes have been reported with and without MER, a comprehensive, controlled clinical trial to address this direct comparison has never been performed. The role of MER in the stereotactic implantation of DBS electrodes will undoubtedly continue to evolve in clinical practice with the advent of new technologies for intraoperative targeting.

References

[1] Albe-Fessard D, Arfel G, Guiot G, et al. [Identification and precide delimitation of certain subcortical structures in man by electrophysiology. Its importance in stereotaxic surgery of dyskinesia]. C R Hebd Seances Acad Sci. 1961; 253:2412–2414

[2] Albe Fessard D, Arfel G, Guiot G, et al. [Characteristic electric activities of some cerebral structures in man]. Ann Chir. 1963; 17:1185–1214

[3] Albe-Fessard D, Arfel G, Guiot G, et al. Electrophysiological studies of some deep cerebral structures in man. J Neurol Sci. 1966; 3(1):37–51

[4] Albe-Fessard D, Arfel G, Guiot G, Derome P, Guilbaud G. Thalamic unit activity in man. Electroencephalogr Clin Neurophysiol. 1967; (suppl 25):132

[5] Gaze RM, Gillingham FJ, Kalyanaraman S, Porter RW, Donaldson AA, Donaldson IM. Microelectrode recordings from the human thalamus. Brain. 1964; 87:691–706

[6] Hardy J. Electrophysiological localization and identification of subcortical structures as an aid to stereotaxic surgery: a preliminary report. Can Med Assoc J. 1962; 86:498–499

[7] Rascol O, Lozano A, Stern M, Poewe W. Milestones in Parkinson's disease therapeutics. Mov Disord. 2011; 26(6):1072–1082

[8] Tasker RR, Siqueira J, Hawrylyshyn P, Organ LW. What happened to VIM thalamotomy for Parkinson's disease? Appl Neurophysiol. 1983; 46(1–4):68–83

[9] Narabayashi H, Maeda T, Yokochi F. Long-term follow-up study of nucleus ventralis intermedius and ventrolateralis thalamotomy using a microelectrode technique in parkinsonism. Appl Neurophysiol. 1987; 50(1–6):330–337

[10] Laitinen LV, Bergenheim AT, Hariz MI. Leksell's posteroventral pallidotomy in the treatment of Parkinson's disease. J Neurosurg. 1992; 76(1):53–61

[11] Bergman H, Wichmann T, DeLong MR. Reversal of experimental parkinsonism by lesions of the subthalamic nucleus. Science. 1990; 249(4975):1436–1438

[12] Hariz MI, Blomstedt P, Zrinzo L. Deep brain stimulation between 1947 and 1987: the untold story. Neurosurg Focus. 2010; 29(2):E1

[13] Schlaier JR, Habermeyer C, Warnat J, et al. Discrepancies between the MRI- and the electrophysiologically defined subthalamic nucleus. Acta Neurochir (Wien). 2011; 153(12):2307–2318

[14] Kondziolka D, Dempsey PK, Lunsford LD, et al. A comparison between magnetic resonance imaging and computed tomography for stereotactic coordinate determination. Neurosurgery. 1992; 30(3):402–406, discussion 406–407

[15] Sumanaweera TS, Adler JR, Jr, Napel S, Glover GH. Characterization of spatial distortion in magnetic resonance imaging and its implications for stereotactic surgery. Neurosurgery. 1994; 35(4):696–703, discussion 703–704

[16] Kelly PJ, Derome P, Guiot G. Thalamic spatial variability and the surgical results of lesions placed with neurophysiologic control. Surg Neurol. 1978; 9(5):307–315

[17] Brierley JB, Beck E. The significance in human stereotactic brain surgery of individual variation in the diencephalon and globus pallidus. J Neurol Neurosurg Psychiatry. 1959; 22:287–298

[18] Lozano A, Hutchison W, Kiss Z, Tasker R, Davis K, Dostrovsky J. Methods for microelectrode-guided posteroventral pallidotomy. J Neurosurg. 1996; 84(2):194–202

[19] Bejjani BP, Dormont D, Pidoux B, et al. Bilateral subthalamic stimulation for Parkinson's disease by using three-dimensional stereotactic magnetic resonance imaging and electrophysiological guidance. J Neurosurg. 2000; 92(4):615–625

[20] Rodriguez-Oroz MC, Rodriguez M, Guridi J, et al. The subthalamic nucleus in Parkinson's disease: somatotopic organization and physiological characteristics. Brain. 2001; 124(Pt 9):1777–1790

[21] Lozano AM, Hutchison WD, Tasker RR, Lang AE, Junn F, Dostrovsky JO. Microelectrode recordings define the ventral posteromedial pallidotomy target. Stereotact Funct Neurosurg. 1998; 71(4):153–163

[22] Giller CA, Dewey RB, Ginsburg MI, Mendelsohn DB, Berk AM. Stereotactic pallidotomy and thalamotomy using individual variations of anatomic landmarks for localization. Neurosurgery. 1998; 42(1):56–62, discussion 62–65

[23] Hutchison WD, Allan RJ, Opitz H, et al. Neurophysiological identification of the subthalamic nucleus in surgery for Parkinson's disease. Ann Neurol. 1998; 44(4):622–628

[24] Reck C, Maarouf M, Wojtecki L, et al. Clinical outcome of subthalamic stimulation in Parkinson's disease is improved by intraoperative multiple trajectories microelectrode recording. J Neurol Surg A Cent Eur Neurosurg. 2012; 73 (6):377–386

[25] Stefani A, Lozano AM, Peppe A, et al. Bilateral deep brain stimulation of the pedunculopontine and subthalamic nuclei in severe Parkinson's disease. Brain. 2007; 130(Pt 6):1596–1607

[26] Morita H, Hass CJ, Moro E, Sudhyadhom A, Kumar R, Okun MS. Pedunculopontine nucleus stimulation: where are we now and what needs to be done to move the field forward? Front Neurol. 2014; 5:243

[27] Möttönen T, Katisko J, Haapasalo J, et al. Defining the anterior nucleus of the thalamus (ANT) as a deep brain stimulation target in refractory epilepsy: delineation using 3 T MRI and intraoperative microelectrode recording. Neuroimage Clin. 2015; 7:823–829

[28] Lenz FA, Dostrovsky JO, Kwan HC, Tasker RR, Yamashiro K, Murphy JT. Methods for microstimulation and recording of single neurons and evoked potentials in the human central nervous system. J Neurosurg. 1988; 68(4): 630–634

[29] Bertrand G, Jasper H, Wong A, Mathews G. Microelectrode recording during stereotactic surgery. Clin Neurosurg. 1969; 16:328–355

[30] Favre J, Taha JM, Nguyen TT, Gildenberg PL, Burchiel KJ. Pallidotomy: a survey of current practice in North America. Neurosurgery. 1996; 39(4):883–890, discussion 890–892

[31] Limousin P, Krack P, Pollak P, et al. Electrical stimulation of the subthalamic nucleus in advanced Parkinson's disease. N Engl J Med. 1998; 339(16):1105–1111

[32] Pollak P, Krack P, Fraix V, et al. Intraoperative micro- and macrostimulation of the subthalamic nucleus in Parkinson's disease. Mov Disord. 2002; 17 Suppl 3:S155–S161

[33] Hassler R. Architectonic organization of the thalamic nuclei. In: Schaltenbrand G, Walker AE, eds. Stereotaxy of the human brain. Stuttgart: Thieme; 1982:140–180

[34] Garonzik IM, Hua SE, Ohara S, Lenz FA. Intraoperative microelectrode and semi-microelectrode recording during the physiological localization of the thalamic nucleus ventral intermediate. Mov Disord. 2002; 17 Suppl 3:S135–S144

[35] Narabayashi H, Ohye C. Nucleus ventralis intermedius of human thalamus. Trans Am Neurol Assoc. 1974; 99:232–233

[36] Crowell RM, Perret E, Siegfried J, Villoz JP. 'Movement units' and 'tremor phasic units' in the human thalamus. Brain Res. 1968; 11(3):481–488

[37] Ohye C, Shibazaki T, Hirai T, Wada H, Hirato M, Kawashima Y. Further physiological observations on the ventralis intermedius neurons in the human thalamus. J Neurophysiol. 1989; 61(3):488–500

[38] Tasker RR, Kiss ZH. The role of the thalamus in functional neurosurgery. Neurosurg Clin N Am. 1995; 6(1):73–104

[39] Lenz FA, Normand SL, Kwan HC, et al. Statistical prediction of the optimal site for thalamotomy in parkinsonian tremor. Mov Disord. 1995; 10(3):318–328

[40] Ohye C, Fukamachi A, Miyazaki M, Isobe I, Nakajima H, Shibazaki T. Physiologically controlled selective thalamotomy for the treatment of abnormal movement by Leksell's open system. Acta Neurochir (Wien). 1977; 37(1–2): 93–104

[41] Hassler R, Schmidt K, Riechert T, Mundinger F. Stereotactic treatment of action myoclonus in a case of combined status marmoratus and multiple sclerosis. A contribution to the pathophysiology of basal ganglia with multiple lesions in both the striatum and the substantia nigra. Confin Neurol. 1975; 37(4):329–356

[42] Lenz FA, Kwan HC, Dostrovsky JO, Tasker RR, Murphy JT, Lenz YE. Single unit analysis of the human ventral thalamic nuclear group. Activity correlated with movement. Brain. 1990; 113(Pt 6):1795–1821

[43] Raeva SN, Vainberg NA, Dubynin VA, Tsetlin IM, Tikhonov YN, Lashin AP. Changes in the spike activity of neurons in the ventrolateral nucleus of the thalamus in humans during performance of a voluntary movement. Neurosci Behav Physiol. 1999; 29(5):505–513

[44] Lenz FA, Tasker RR, Kwan HC, et al. Single unit analysis of the human ventral thalamic nuclear group: correlation of thalamic "tremor cells" with the 3–6 Hz component of parkinsonian tremor. J Neurosci. 1988; 8(3):754–764

[45] Lenz FA, Dostrovsky JO, Tasker RR, Yamashiro K, Kwan HC, Murphy JT. Single-unit analysis of the human ventral thalamic nuclear group: somatosensory responses. J Neurophysiol. 1988; 59(2):299–316

[46] McClean MD, Dostrovsky JO, Lee L, Tasker RR. Somatosensory neurons in human thalamus respond to speech-induced orofacial movements. Brain Res. 1990; 513(2):343–347

[47] Hutchison WD, Lozano AM, Tasker RR, Lang AE, Dostrovsky JO. Identification and characterization of neurons with tremor-frequency activity in human globus pallidus. Exp Brain Res. 1997; 113(3):557–563

[48] Starr PA, Turner RS, Rau G, et al. Microelectrode-guided implantation of deep brain stimulators into the globus pallidus internus for dystonia: techniques, electrode locations, and outcomes. J Neurosurg. 2006; 104(4):488–501

[49] Tisch S, Zrinzo L, Limousin P, et al. Effect of electrode contact location on clinical efficacy of pallidal deep brain stimulation in primary generalised dystonia. J Neurol Neurosurg Psychiatry. 2007; 78(12):1314–1319

[50] Kupsch A, Benecke R, Müller J, et al. Deep-Brain Stimulation for Dystonia Study Group. Pallidal deep-brain stimulation in primary generalized or segmental dystonia. N Engl J Med. 2006; 355(19):1978–1990

[51] Vidailhet M, Vercueil L, Houeto JL, et al. French Stimulation du Pallidum Interne dans la Dystonie (SPIDY) Study Group. Bilateral deep-brain stimulation of the globus pallidus in primary generalized dystonia. N Engl J Med. 2005; 352(5):459–467

[52] Vitek JL, Delong MR, Starr PA, Hariz MI, Metman LV. Intraoperative neurophysiology in DBS for dystonia. Mov Disord. 2011; 26 Suppl 1:S31–S36

[53] Trottenberg T, Paul G, Meissner W, Maier-Hauff K, Taschner C, Kupsch A. Pallidal and thalamic neurostimulation in severe tardive dystonia. J Neurol Neurosurg Psychiatry. 2001; 70(4):557–559

[54] Gross RE, Lombardi WJ, Lang AE, et al. Relationship of lesion location to clinical outcome following microelectrode-guided pallidotomy for Parkinson's disease. Brain. 1999; 122(Pt 3):405–416

[55] Lozano AM, Hutchison WD. Microelectrode recordings in the pallidum. Mov Disord. 2002; 17 Suppl 3:S150–S154

[56] Hutchinson WD, Levy R, Dostrovsky JO, Lozano AM, Lang AE. Effects of apomorphine on globus pallidus neurons in parkinsonian patients. Ann Neurol. 1997; 42(5):767–775

[57] Hutchison WD, Lozano AM, Davis KD, Saint-Cyr JA, Lang AE, Dostrovsky JO. Differential neuronal activity in segments of globus pallidus in Parkinson's disease patients. Neuroreport. 1994; 5(12):1533–1537

[58] Vitek JL. Pathophysiology of dystonia: a neuronal model. Mov Disord. 2002; 17 Suppl 3:S49–S62

[59] Vitek JL, Chockkan V, Zhang JY, et al. Neuronal activity in the basal ganglia in patients with generalized dystonia and hemiballismus. Ann Neurol. 1999; 46(1):22–35

[60] Lozano AM, Kumar R, Gross RE, et al. Globus pallidus internus pallidotomy for generalized dystonia. Mov Disord. 1997; 12(6):865–870

[61] DeLong MR. Primate models of movement disorders of basal ganglia origin. Trends Neurosci. 1990; 13(7):281–285

[62] Smith Y, Bevan MD, Shink E, Bolam JP. Microcircuitry of the direct and indirect pathways of the basal ganglia. Neuroscience. 1998; 86(2):353–387

[63] Carpenter MB, Whittier JR, Mettler FA. Analysis of choreoid hyperkinesia in the Rhesus monkey; surgical and pharmacological analysis of hyperkinesia resulting from lesions in the subthalamic nucleus of Luys. J Comp Neurol. 1950; 92(3):293–331

[64] Aziz TZ, Peggs D, Sambrook MA, Crossman AR. Lesion of the subthalamic nucleus for the alleviation of 1-methyl-4-phenyl-1,2,3,6-tetrahydropyridine (MPTP)-induced parkinsonism in the primate. Mov Disord. 1991; 6(4):288–292

[65] Benazzouz A, Boraud T, Féger J, Burbaud P, Bioulac B, Gross C. Alleviation of experimental hemiparkinsonism by high-frequency stimulation of the subthalamic nucleus in primates: a comparison with L-Dopa treatment. Mov Disord. 1996; 11(6):627–632

[66] Gao DM, Benazzouz A, Piallat B, et al. High-frequency stimulation of the subthalamic nucleus suppresses experimental resting tremor in the monkey. Neuroscience. 1999; 88(1):201–212

[67] Limousin P, Pollak P, Benazzouz A, et al. Effect of parkinsonian signs and symptoms of bilateral subthalamic nucleus stimulation. Lancet. 1995; 345 (8942):91–95

[68] Alexander GE, Crutcher MD, DeLong MR. Basal ganglia-thalamocortical circuits: parallel substrates for motor, oculomotor, "prefrontal" and "limbic" functions. Prog Brain Res. 1990; 85:119–146

[69] Parent A, Hazrati LN. Functional anatomy of the basal ganglia. II. The place of subthalamic nucleus and external pallidum in basal ganglia circuitry. Brain Res Brain Res Rev. 1995; 20(1):128–154

[70] Monakow KH, Akert K, Künzle H. Projections of the precentral motor cortex and other cortical areas of the frontal lobe to the subthalamic nucleus in the monkey. Exp Brain Res. 1978; 33(3–4):395–403

[71] Gross RE, Krack P, Rodriguez-Oroz MC, Rezai AR, Benabid AL. Electrophysiological mapping for the implantation of deep brain stimulators for Parkinson's disease and tremor. Mov Disord. 2006; 21 Suppl 14:S259–S283

[72] Bergman H, Wichmann T, Karmon B, DeLong MR. The primate subthalamic nucleus. II. Neuronal activity in the MPTP model of parkinsonism. J Neurophysiol. 1994; 72(2):507–520

[73] Bezard E, Boraud T, Bioulac B, Gross CE. Involvement of the subthalamic nucleus in glutamatergic compensatory mechanisms. Eur J Neurosci. 1999; 11 (6):2167–2170

[74] Wichmann T, Bergman H, DeLong MR. The primate subthalamic nucleus. I. Functional properties in intact animals. J Neurophysiol. 1994; 72(2):494–506

[75] Levy R, Hutchison WD, Lozano AM, Dostrovsky JO. High-frequency synchronization of neuronal activity in the subthalamic nucleus of parkinsonian patients with limb tremor. J Neurosci. 2000; 20(20):7766–7775

[76] Benazzouz A, Breit S, Koudsie A, Pollak P, Krack P, Benabid AL. Intraoperative microrecordings of the subthalamic nucleus in Parkinson's disease. Mov Disord. 2002; 17 Suppl 3:S145–S149

[77] Starr PA, Christine CW, Theodosopoulos PV, et al. Implantation of deep brain stimulators into the subthalamic nucleus: technical approach and magnetic resonance imaging-verified lead locations. J Neurosurg. 2002; 97(2):370–387

[78] Laitinen LV. Brain targets in surgery for Parkinson's disease. Results of a survey of neurosurgeons. J Neurosurg. 1985; 62(3):349–351

[79] Svennilson E, Torvik A, Lowe R, Leksell L. Treatment of parkinsonism by stereotatic thermolesions in the pallidal region. A clinical evaluation of 81 cases. Acta Psychiatr Scand. 1960; 35(3):358–377

[80] Laitinen LV. Pallidotomy for Parkinson's disease. Neurosurg Clin N Am. 1995; 6(1):105–112

[81] Maiti TK, Konar S, Bir S, Kalakoti P, Nanda A. Intra-operative micro-electrode recording in functional neurosurgery: Past, present, future. J Clin Neurosci. 2016; 32:166–172

[82] Larson PS, Starr PA, Bates G, Tansey L, Richardson RM, Martin AJ. An optimized system for interventional magnetic resonance imaging-guided stereotactic surgery: preliminary evaluation of targeting accuracy. Neurosurgery. 2012; 70(1) Suppl Operative:95–103, discussion 103

[83] Burchiel KJ, McCartney S, Lee A, Raslan AM. Accuracy of deep brain stimulation electrode placement using intraoperative computed tomography without microelectrode recording. J Neurosurg. 2013; 119(2):301–306

[84] Starr PA, Markun LC, Larson PS, Volz MM, Martin AJ, Ostrem JL. Interventional MRI-guided deep brain stimulation in pediatric dystonia: first experience with the ClearPoint system. J Neurosurg Pediatr. 2014; 14(4):400–408

[85] Mirzadeh Z, Chapple K, Lambert M, et al. Parkinson's disease outcomes after intraoperative CT-guided "asleep" deep brain stimulation in the globus pallidus internus. J Neurosurg. 2016; 124(4):902–907

[86] Starr PA, Martin AJ, Ostrem JL, Talke P, Levesque N, Larson PS. Subthalamic nucleus deep brain stimulator placement using high-field interventional magnetic resonance imaging and a skull-mounted aiming device: technique and application accuracy. J Neurosurg. 2010; 112(3):479–490

[87] Ostrem JL, Galifianakis NB, Markun LC, et al. Clinical outcomes of PD patients having bilateral STN DBS using high-field interventional MR-imaging for lead placement. Clin Neurol Neurosurg. 2013; 115(6):708–712

[88] Ostrem JL, Ziman N, Galifianakis NB, et al. Clinical outcomes using ClearPoint interventional MRI for deep brain stimulation lead placement in Parkinson's disease. J Neurosurg. 2016; 124(4):908–916

[89] McClelland S, III. A cost analysis of intraoperative microelectrode recording during subthalamic stimulation for Parkinson's disease. Mov Disord. 2011; 26(8):1422–1427

[90] Jacob RL, Geddes J, McCartney S, Burchiel KJ. Cost analysis of awake versus asleep deep brain stimulation: a single academic health center experience. J Neurosurg. 2016; 124(5):1517–1523

[91] Alkhani A, Lozano AM. Pallidotomy for parkinson disease: a review of contemporary literature. J Neurosurg. 2001; 94(1):43–49

[92] Palur RS, Berk C, Schulzer M, Honey CR. A meta-analysis comparing the results of pallidotomy performed using microelectrode recording or macroelectrode stimulation. J Neurosurg. 2002; 96(6):1058–1062

[93] de Bie RM, de Haan RJ, Schuurman PR, Esselink RA, Bosch DA, Speelman JD. Morbidity and mortality following pallidotomy in Parkinson's disease: a systematic review. Neurology. 2002; 58(7):1008–1012

[94] Higuchi Y, Iacono RP. Surgical complications in patients with Parkinson's disease after posteroventral pallidotomy. Neurosurgery. 2003; 52(3):558–571, discussion 568–571

[95] Zrinzo L, Foltynie T, Limousin P, Hariz MI. Reducing hemorrhagic complications in functional neurosurgery: a large case series and systematic literature review. J Neurosurg. 2012; 116(1):84–94

[96] Gorgulho A, De Salles AA, Frighetto L, Behnke E. Incidence of hemorrhage associated with electrophysiological studies performed using macroelectrodes and microelectrodes in functional neurosurgery. J Neurosurg. 2005; 102 (5):888–896

[97] Obeso JA, Olanow CW, Rodriguez-Oroz MC, Krack P, Kumar R, Lang AE, Deep-Brain Stimulation for Parkinson's Disease Study Group. Deep-brain stimulation of the subthalamic nucleus or the pars interna of the globus pallidus in Parkinson's disease. N Engl J Med. 2001; 345(13):956–963

[98] Binder DK, Rau GM, Starr PA. Risk factors for hemorrhage during microelectrode-guided deep brain stimulator implantation for movement disorders. Neurosurgery. 2005; 56(4):722–732, discussion 722–732

[99] Saleh S, Swanson KI, Lake WB, Sillay KA. Awake neurophysiologically guided versus asleep MRI-guided STN DBS for Parkinson disease: a comparison of outcomes using levodopa equivalents. Stereotact Funct Neurosurg. 2015; 93 (6):419–426

[100] Jimenez-Shahed J, York M, Smith-Gloyd EM, Jankovic J, Viswanathan A. MER vs. MRI guidance in placement of DBS electrodes for Parkinson's disease. Mov Disord. 2014; 29 Suppl 1:68:1–687

4 Intraoperative Imaging-Based Lead Implantation

R. Mark Richardson

Abstract

This chapter outlines the evolution of intraoperative imaging-based deep brain stimulation (DBS) lead implantation. Current outcome data following DBS lead placement via intraoperative computed tomography and intraoperative or interventional magnetic resonance imaging (iMRI) are reviewed. A practical description of the workflow for iMRI-DBS is included along with remarks on the potential future evolution of this technique.

Keywords: deep brain stimulation, movement disorders, interventional MRI, intraoperative MRI, intraoperative CT, stereotactic neurosurgery

4.1 Introduction

Multiple randomized controlled studies have established deep brain stimulation (DBS) as the current standard of care for Parkinson's disease (PD) with motor fluctuations due to increase in off-time, improvements in quality of life, and reduction in medication compared to medical management alone.[1,2,3] DBS for PD, therefore, has provided a model indication for the development of intraoperative imaging-based lead implantation in patients under general anesthesia as an alternative to neurophysiology-guided placement. The primary question is no longer whether DBS helps patients with PD, but rather to what extent the method of lead implantation affects the efficacy of DBS. The use of intraoperative imaging for DBS lead implantation in dystonia and essential tremor is evolving in similar fashion. This chapter discusses the evolution of the subfield of intraoperative imaging-based DBS lead implantation.

4.2 Evolution of Lead Implantation in the Asleep Patient

The fundamental basis for the recent shift to "asleep" DBS, i.e., DBS under general anesthesia in the absence of microelectrode recording (MER), is the cumulative experience of the field in verifying effective DBS lead locations using postoperative magnetic resonance imaging (MRI). Other important factors include the desire of some patients to avoid an awake brain-mapping procedure and the desire of patients with severe symptoms to avoid potential discomfort that would come with awake surgery. Two general methods currently predominate for DBS lead implantation in patients under general anesthesia: intraoperative MRI (iMRI)-based DBS with real-time imaging, and intraoperative computed tomography (iCT)-based DBS with immediate postimplantation imaging. Prior to the advent of these techniques, however, some centers had already adopted DBS without MER on a regular basis, often under general anesthesia, using immediate postoperative MRI for lead location confirmation.

In the early 2000s, Gill and colleagues developed a method for implanting guide tubes and radiopaque stylets into the STN and verifying target accuracy with MRI, prior to lead implantation.[4] This method can be carried out with the patient under general anesthesia, although this group initially used macrostimulation through the DBS lead to evaluate the need for trajectory adjustment,[5] reporting a 61% improvement in off-medication Unified Parkinson's Disease Rating Scale (UPDRS) III scores at 1 year.

For many years, Hariz and colleagues have advocated that MER is not necessary for successful DBS implantation in PD, relying instead on dynamic impedance monitoring, including patients under general anesthesia.[6] In this method, a smooth-tip radiofrequency electrode is advanced to the target, prior to inserting the DBS lead. Immediately following implantation of the DBS leads, all patients undergo a stereotactic MRI scan to confirm the lead positions before implantation of the pulse generator. The surgery is not considered to be complete until acceptable lead placement is confirmed. This approach was shown to be both safe and efficacious with 52% improvement in off-medication UPDRS III scores at 1 year.

It should be noted that Machado and colleagues have reported an approach to MRI-verified DBS that is specific to iMRI. This group studied 33 patients with movement disorders (64 total leads, 27 PD patients). All the patients underwent implantation with standard frame-based techniques under general anesthesia and without MER.[7] MR images were acquired immediately after lead implantation and fused to the preoperative plan to verify accuracy. The authors reported 27 iMRI globus pallidus interna (GPi) implantations for PD with an average reduction of 46% in UPDRS III scores.

4.3 Intraoperative-CT-verified DBS

Ponce and colleagues[8,9,10] have pioneered the use of iCT to perform immediate verification of DBS lead locations (iCT-DBS) in patients under general anesthesia. Using this method, asleep Vim DBS for essential tremor without intraoperative test stimulation was reported to be as safe and effective as awake lead implantation (N=17).[9] In a prospective follow-up study, outcomes also did not differ between subjects implanted while awake (16) versus asleep (40).[10] This is quite notable, given that the Vim cannot be visualized at 1.5 T or 3 T, requiring a type of direct targeting based solely on other landmarks.

For PD DBS, 6-month outcome data was reported from a study of 78 GPi (16 awake, 62 asleep) and 55 STN (14 awake, 41 asleep) subjects.[8] UPDRS-III score improvement with stimulation did not differ between awake and asleep groups for GPi (awake, 38.5%; asleep, 37.5%) or STN (awake, 40.3%; asleep, 48.8%) targets. A separate study by Burchiel and colleagues[11] similarly showed no difference in UPDRS II or III score improvements between subjects who underwent DBS asleep (N = 30) versus awake (N=39), although the awake cohort represented a historical rather than prospective control. Interestingly, outcomes from asleep DBS in that study were superior with regard to speech fluency and quality of life.

On comparing DBS lead implantation awake versus iCT-DBS, no significant differences in complications, length of stay, and

30-day readmissions have been reported,[12] while iCT-DBS performed asleep may be associated with a lower cost variation relative to awake procedures.[13]

4.4 Intraoperative-MRI or Interventional-MRI-guided DBS

iMRI-guided DBS lead implantation (iMRI-DBS) relies on real-time confirmation of accurate trajectory alignment and lead placement. The benefit of iMRI over other anatomic verification approaches lies in the fact that it allows the surgeon to correct for inaccuracy in trajectory planning prior to electrode placement, almost always resulting in a single brain penetration for electrode placement. The precision achieved by functional verification of electrode location with MER enabled the iMRI-DBS field. Imaging electrode locations after MER-guided placement has demonstrated that the sensorimotor territory lies in the dorsolateral portion of the STN,[14,15] and within the ventral posterior lateral portion of the GPi,[16] allowing the identification of the functional territory of these nuclei by direct visualization on MRI.

Currently, the ClearPoint system is the sole Food and Drug Administration (FDA)-approved platform for iMRI-based stereological procedures. The platform, pioneered by the group at the University of California San Francisco (UCSF), is based on the concept of prospective stereotaxy, the alignment of a skull-mounted trajectory guide within an MRI system.[17] This approach provides immediate detection of complications, eliminates the need for microelectrode mapping, and reduces brain penetrations. The key features of this strategy are: (1) patient positioning supine on the MRI gantry under general anesthesia; (2) integration of planning, insertion, and real-time MRI confirmation of DBS lead placement during a single procedure; (3) trajectory alignment and DBS lead insertion via a burr hole-mounted trajectory guide in place of a traditional stereotactic frame and arc system; (4) definition of target coordinates with respect to the MRI isocenter rather than to a separate stereotactic space using fiducial markers. Depending on preference for how the dura is opened, acquisition of target images also can occur after burr hole creation and intracranial air entry, to account for brain shift.

The first validation of the accuracy of the ClearPoint system occurred in nonhuman primates,[18] followed by workflow simulation in the postmortem human brain,[19] both of which demonstrated an average targeting error of less than 1 mm.

Subsequent to FDA approval in 2012, the UCSF group reported 1-year outcomes following iMRI-DBS for PD of 40% UPDRS III score improvement.[20] Other groups have reported various outcome measures of iMRI-DBS for PD, all of which are similar to those reported from outcome studies of MER-based-DBS for PD (▶ Table 4.1), with similar low complication rates. A classic argument against asleep DBS lead placement has been that a lack of functional verification of lead location increases the risk for side effects from stimulation. On the contrary, our retrospective study of a contemporaneous cohort of 45 consecutive patients who underwent either iMRI- or MER-guided DBS lead implantation showed that side effect thresholds during initial programming were slightly lower in the MER group, with similar thresholds for clinical benefit and no significant difference in the reduction of symptoms or levodopa equivalent doses.[21] These findings bolstered previous work indicating that iMRI-DBS lead implantation occurs with greater anatomic accuracy, in locations demonstrated to be the appropriate functional region of the STN by the production of equivalent clinical outcomes.[7,20,22,23]

Importantly, in a 10-year study period, the UCSF group reported 272 electrode implantations in 164 iMRI-guided surgical procedures, with an overall infection rate of 3.6%.[24] A modification of sterile practice occurred after the first 10 patients, reducing the infection rate to 2.6%, all of which occurred at the internal pulse generator (IPG) site. This author has experienced one scalp infection in 70 iMRI-DBS cases, which was successfully treated with intravenous plus oral antibiotics without hardware removal.

4.4.1 iMRI Environment

Depending on the resources of an institution, iMRI procedures can be performed in either iMRI or standard diagnostic MRI suites. In either case, there are several other factors to consider in the iMRI environment. First, there must be adequate space for the anesthetists to perform their duties. This includes a separate area outside of the MRI suite where patients can be intubated and lines can be placed. Most diagnostic scanner rooms in large hospitals are capable of accommodating ventilators to handle intubated patients (▶ Fig. 4.1a), but not all have adequate space for an anesthesia machine, in which case anesthesiologists may need to monitor the patient outside of the scanner room. In addition, the scanner room must have adequate space on the opposite end of the MRI bore for the sterile

Table 4.1 Clinical outcomes from published iMRI studies

Study	Method	Number of subjects (target)	UPDRS off-medication improvement	Months postop	LED reduction (%)
Ostrem et al.[25]	Nexframe	17 (STN)	49%	6	25
Sidiropoulos et al.[23]	ClearPoint	12; 6 (STN), 6 (GPi)	46% (STN), 41% (GPi)	14 (± 4)	0
Saleh et al.[22]	ClearPoint	14 (STN)	NR	6	49
Ostrem et al.[20]	ClearPoint	20; 16 (STN), 4 (GPi)	40%	12	21
Lee et al.[21]	ClearPoint	21 (STN)	a	8 (± 4)	35

Abbreviations: GPi, globus pallidus interna; NR, not reported; STN, subthalamic nucleus.
a pre-op off-med versus postop off-med/on-stim data not collected; preop on-med versus postop on-med/on-stim improvement was 21%.

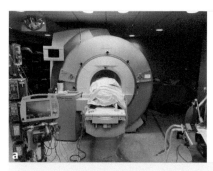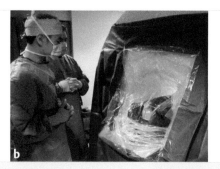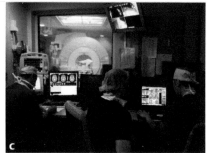

Fig. 4.1 Diagnostic imaging suite during iMRI-DBS. A view through the window of the MRI control room shows how anesthesia is positioned at the foot of the gantry **(a)**. Surgery takes place at the opposite end of the bore **(b)**. The surgeon moves to the MRI control room for planning and evaluation steps **(c)**.

table and space for the surgeon to operate (▶ Fig. 4.1b). The scanner room must also be outfitted with adequate lighting, and proper connections for suction and a pneumatic powered MRI-compatible drill. Finally, a large bore scanner is highly desired to allow for adequate clearance of the stereotactic frame during the alignment procedure.

We use the ClearPoint system in a 1.5 T Siemens Magnetom scanner for all of our iMRI procedures. Although the ClearPoint platform is approved for use in 3 T scanners, at this field strength the potential for image distortion should be carefully evaluated. The UCSF group has been the first to directly compare lead placement in 1.5 T and 3 T scanners, reporting no difference in radial error, number of additional trajectories, or procedure duration.[26] The contribution of an MR physicist to the initial establishment of scan parameters on a site's specific 3 T scanner is recommended.

4.4.2 MRI Sequences for Anatomic Targeting

MRI sequences for iMRI procedures ideally provide clear visualization of the target of interest. The STN and GPi accumulate iron deposition as one ages, and this creates a visible artifact on MR imaging. Traditionally, the GPi was targeted using a proton density-weighted T1 image.[27] We have found that the newer T1-weighted spoiled gradient echo sequences (BRAVO on GE consoles, MPRAGE on Siemens consoles) also provide good tissue contrast for identification of the GPi. The 3T-MRI fast gray matter acquisition T1 inversion recovery (FGATIR) sequence is a popular choice for visualizing the pallidum, given its delineation of the internal lamina.[28] We continue to use a volumetric T2-weighted fast-spin echo image visualizing the STN.[29] This scan is also often helpful for visualizing the GPi in conjunction with an inversion recovery sequence. Susceptibility-weighted imaging is highly sensitive to the iron deposition found in the STN and can offer better definition of the STN relative to standard T2-weighted imaging.[30] It can result in distortion at higher field strengths, however, that must be corrected with susceptibility maps to avoid targeting errors. In contrast to STN and GPi targets, which are visible due to their iron deposition, the Vim target is not distinguishable from adjacent thalamic regions at 1.5 T. Higher field strength MRI[31] and/or the addition of tractography[32] may allow for more precise image-based targeting of intrathalamic nuclei in the future.

4.4.3 ClearPoint Workflow

The ClearPoint system has a specially designed trajectory guide (SmartFrame) and integrated planning software which enables imaging to guide each of these steps in the procedure: (1) acquisition of an initial volumetric MRI and trajectory planning; (2) placement of the skull-mounted SmartFrame and burr hole creation; (3) definition of target coordinates with respect to the MRI isocenter; (4) trajectory alignment, dural puncture, and DBS electrode insertion; and (5) confirmation of DBS electrode placement.

After intubation and arterial line placement, the procedure begins with shaving the head and infiltration of an epinephrine-containing local anesthetic into the scalp at the level of the coronal suture, prior to transfer of the patient into the MRI scanner room. The head is secured in a fixation device on the MRI gantry with skull pins in a head-holder that allows positioning of two loop coils on either side of the head. The patient's head is brought through the bore of the scanner and is prepped and draped using a custom elasticized drape that allows the head to move in and out of the bore of the scanner without contaminating the operative field. Highlights and updates on this procedure are provided in the following paragraphs. Note that the detailed steps of this procedure have been described elsewhere,[33,34,35] including in the excellent iBook *Interventional MRI-Guided DBS* (https://itunes.apple.com/us/book/interventional-mri-guided-dbs/id554568402?mt=13).

The ClearPoint planning software exists on a standalone workstation in the MRI control room and communicates with the MR console via a network link (▶ Fig. 4.1c). The general workflow is divided into four different stages in the software: burr hole planning (entry), target selection and trajectory visualization (target), alignment of trajectory guide (navigate), and insertion monitoring (evaluate). The software provides the grid coordinates at which the burr holes should be created for the planned entry sites. Two options exist for mounting of the SmartFrame: (1) a base that mounts directly to the skull following retraction of a larger incision, or (2) a frame that mounts to the skull through percutaneous screws with additional screws countersunk into the scalp to maximize stability. The author's practice has evolved to prefer the percutaneously mounted base which uses two small incisions retracted with suture (▶ Fig. 4.2). In comparison to traditional frame-based surgery, lateral entry points may be limited by the presence of the

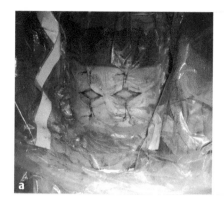

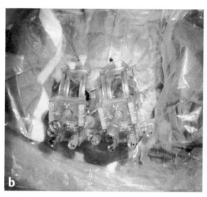

Fig. 4.2 Scalp-mounted SmartFrames. Bilateral incisions are retracted using temporary sutures **(a)**. SmartFrames are then attached side by side **(b)**. In this image, burr holes were made after affixing the SmartFrame bases and the deep brain stimulation manufacturer's lead-locking base was attached prior to mounting the SmartFrame towers. In current practice, we attach a titanium dogbone at this stage but defer the burr holes until after alignment is completed, to be made with a hand drill.

imaging coils. Likewise, although simultaneous GPi targeting is possible if the chosen trajectories are planned lateral to medial, traditional parasagittal trajectories often require unilateral, sequential implantation of GPi due to an inability to mount two SmartFrame bases with less than ~ 4.5 cm distance between burr holes.

Once the scalp is opened, the SmartFrames are mounted over the marks previously made by the awl. A pneumatic drill may be used to make bur holes centered on these awl marks, or if the scalp-mount frame is used, the burr hole may be deferred until after frame alignment and made with a hand drill. We have recently stopped using the DBS-manufacturer-provided lead lock and base, instead we use a small titanium plate to secure the lead which is secured with one screw at this time, in order to be available once the lead is in place. We also prefer to leave the dura closed at this step and puncture it later with a sharp ceramic probe just prior to DBS lead insertion. The author's current preferred workflow is shown in ▸ Fig. 4.3. Some surgeons prefer to see the cortical surface during probe penetration, especially if there is any question about the proximity of cortical vasculature to the pial entry point. If the dura is to be opened widely, these openings should be completed at this stage to allow any potential brain shift to occur prior to repeating the anatomic targeting scans.

Once targeting scans are obtained and transferred to the ClearPoint software, the target is selected based on direct anatomic visualization. The final trajectory at this stage is dependent on the mounted position of the trajectory guide, therefore one must confirm that the trajectory matches the one that was originally intended. If the SmartFrame was not mounted ideally with respect to the intended cortical entry point, the software allows the surgeon to offset the tip of the target cannula using the X-Y stage, up to 2.5 mm. If this maneuver is undertaken, one must anticipate having to rely on the pitch and roll adjustments in subsequent steps, since little room may remain on the X-Y stage. Following subsequent serial MRI-based instructions for aligning the SmartFrame, a predicted vector error of less than 0.5 mm should be achieved.

Once both SmartFrames are aligned, prior to inserting the DBS leads, we insert a fine-pointed ceramic probe to sharply pierce the dura and pia in one maneuver. A separate probe is used on each side, to avoid any issues that might occur from reuse (e.g., retraction or damage to the plastic sheath), inserting approximately 1 to 2 cm into the brain parenchyma to ensure subsequent smooth entry of the blunt ceramic probe. When

using this method, the surgeon should plan the entry such that the probe does not pass too close to cortical vessels. Then the blunt ceramic probe is inserted to target and scans are obtained to verify correct targeting and absence of complications, prior to lead implantation. Note that if the dura was opened in a previous stage, it is critical that the surgeon confirms that the pia is sufficiently opened prior to insertion of the blunt probe, and that the blunt probe is visualized to enter the pia with minimal cortical deflection in order to minimize the risk of cortical hemorrhage. When passing the ceramic probe, the surgeon also should be vigilant that there is no unusual resistance that would indicate potential deflection off of bone at the edge of the burr hole. If a complication is suspected, imaging can be obtained without fully inserting the probe and a decision can be made whether to continue, modify, or abort the procedure.

Once the probe has been placed to the target depth, a final evaluation step is used to determine the targeting error by comparing the distance from the probe artifact to the intended target (▸ Fig. 4.4). If targeting accuracy is unacceptable, the software can calculate the adjustment necessary on the X-Y stage and the surgeon can remove the probe and sheath, make the adjustment, and reinsert. When measuring the length of insertion on the DBS electrode, we typically add 2 mm when targeting the STN (target plane typically 4 mm below the AC-PC line) and 4 mm when targeting the GPi (target plane typically at the level of the AC-PC line). This maneuver attempts to consider the intention to leave the bottom of the deepest contact at the ventral border of the STN or just superiolateral to the optic tract when targeting GPi, and these distances are consistent with our typical MER-guided implantation depths.

4.5 Patient Selection for DBS Under General Anesthesia

Generally speaking, asleep DBS lead placement is appropriate for all patients who are candidates for awake DBS procedures. However, in many institutions the lack of availability of MRI scanner time (or iCT) limits asleep DBS to patients who strongly prefer to be asleep or who cannot tolerate the awake procedure. There are some patients who are not suited for traditional procedure under sedation because of less reliable airway control, such as those with severe torticollis or other anatomic considerations that increase the likelihood of airway obstruction. Clearly, performing the procedure under general anesthesia

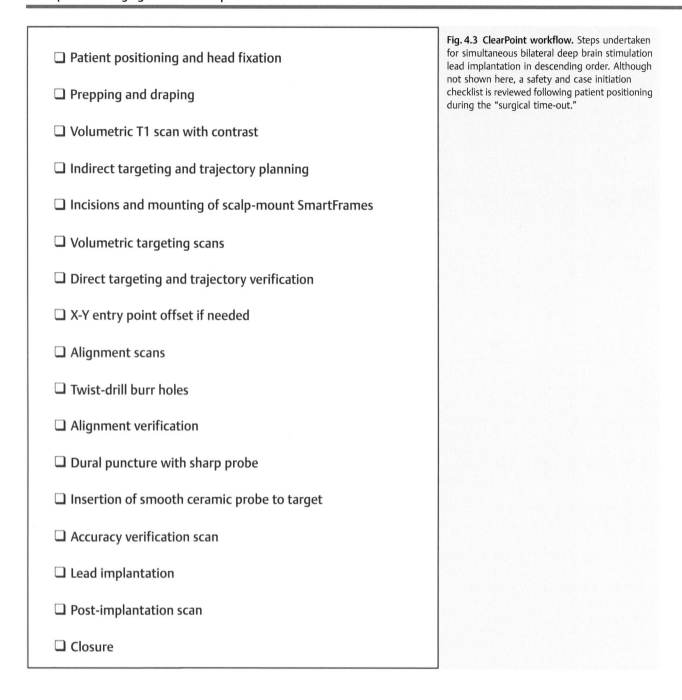

- ❑ Patient positioning and head fixation
- ❑ Prepping and draping
- ❑ Volumetric T1 scan with contrast
- ❑ Indirect targeting and trajectory planning
- ❑ Incisions and mounting of scalp-mount SmartFrames
- ❑ Volumetric targeting scans
- ❑ Direct targeting and trajectory verification
- ❑ X-Y entry point offset if needed
- ❑ Alignment scans
- ❑ Twist-drill burr holes
- ❑ Alignment verification
- ❑ Dural puncture with sharp probe
- ❑ Insertion of smooth ceramic probe to target
- ❑ Accuracy verification scan
- ❑ Lead implantation
- ❑ Post-implantation scan
- ❑ Closure

Fig. 4.3 ClearPoint workflow. Steps undertaken for simultaneous bilateral deep brain stimulation lead implantation in descending order. Although not shown here, a safety and case initiation checklist is reviewed following patient positioning during the "surgical time-out."

removes concerns about significant anxiety that might compromise a patient's ability to cooperate with an awake procedure. Since patients are not required to hold medications in order to be symptomatic for intraoperative testing, this source of discomfort is also removed. Patients with communication difficulties, such as those who have severe dysarthria, hearing loss, or who are not fluent native-language speakers, are also excellent candidates for asleep DBS. In our program, some patients are directed primarily toward iMRI surgery with significant anxiety being the most common indication followed by physical discomfort secondary to symptoms of advanced disease. iMRI and awake procedures are both offered to remaining patients and they are allowed to choose their preference.

4.6 Future Directions

If one accepts that asleep DBS is currently returning clinical outcomes equivalent to historical ones that were obtained with MER-guided lead implantation, the question arises how to obtain better outcomes. Improving and standardizing visualization of the target is the key step. Methods have recently been developed to accurately visualize the STN and GPi on a standard clinical MRI by transforming information available in a 7 T MRI dataset, and furthermore to identify the motor territory of each nucleus using individualized tractography-based parcellation.[36,37,38] Incorporating advances such as these into asleep DBS workflows may lead to improved clinical outcomes by enabling individualized and highly specific target planning.

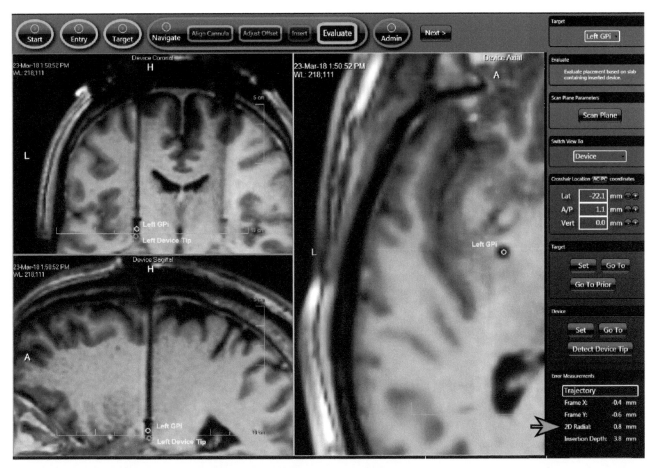

Fig. 4.4 Evaluation step during ClearPoint iMRI-DBS. Three MRI planes showing the final lead location (Left Device Tip) in relation to the target location (Left GPi). A 2-D radial error of 0.8 mm is indicated in this example (*blue arrow*).

Given that the DBS field is entering the era of closed-loop or adaptive DBS,[39] it is reasonable to consider how the placement of potential cortical sensors might be accomplished in asleep DBS. For instance, will physiological confirmation of engagement of a network target be required? or can these networks be mapped noninvasively prior to surgery in each individual and targeted based on patient-specific anatomic location? In latter case, imaging methods for real-time verification of cortical electrode locations will need to be developed.

In conclusion, recent increase in asleep DBS likely has helped to bring DBS therapy to a large and significant number of patients who otherwise might not have considered undergoing awake surgery, translating into a gain of many years of improved quality of life for these patients and downstream benefits to society. As technological improvements continue to improve outcomes of asleep DBS that already appear to be equivalent to those obtained with traditional awake DBS, a new challenge for the field is identifying the indications and conditions for which awake surgery will be necessary in the future.

References

[1] Weaver FM, Follett K, Stern M, et al. CSP 468 Study Group. Bilateral deep brain stimulation vs best medical therapy for patients with advanced Parkinson disease: a randomized controlled trial. JAMA. 2009; 301(1):63–73

[2] Schuepbach WM, Rau J, Knudsen K, et al. EARLYSTIM Study Group. Neurostimulation for Parkinson's disease with early motor complications. N Engl J Med. 2013; 368(7):610–622

[3] Deuschl G, Schade-Brittinger C, Krack P, et al. German Parkinson Study Group, Neurostimulation Section. A randomized trial of deep-brain stimulation for Parkinson's disease. N Engl J Med. 2006; 355(9):896–908

[4] Patel NK, Plaha P, Gill SS. Magnetic resonance imaging-directed method for functional neurosurgery using implantable guide tubes. Neurosurgery. 2007; 61(5) Suppl 2:358–365, discussion 365–366

[5] Patel NK, Heywood P, O'Sullivan K, Love S, Gill SS. MRI-directed subthalamic nucleus surgery for Parkinson's disease. Stereotact Funct Neurosurg. 2002; 78 (3–4):132–145

[6] Foltynie T, Zrinzo L, Martinez-Torres I, et al. MRI-guided STN DBS in Parkinson's disease without microelectrode recording: efficacy and safety. J Neurol Neurosurg Psychiatry. 2011; 82(4):358–363

[7] Matias CM, Frizon LA, Nagel SJ, Lobel DA, Machado AG. Deep brain stimulation outcomes in patients implanted under general anesthesia with frame-based stereotaxy and intraoperative MRI. J Neurosurg. 2018:1–7

[8] Chen T, Mirzadeh Z, Chapple KM, et al. Clinical outcomes following awake and asleep deep brain stimulation for Parkinson disease. J Neurosurg. 2018: 1–12

[9] Chen T, Mirzadeh Z, Chapple K, Lambert M, Dhall R, Ponce FA. "Asleep" deep brain stimulation for essential tremor. J Neurosurg. 2016; 124:1842–1849

[10] Chen T, Mirzadeh Z, Chapple KM, et al. Intraoperative test stimulation versus stereotactic accuracy as a surgical end point: a comparison of essential tremor outcomes after ventral intermediate nucleus deep brain stimulation. J Neurosurg. 2018; 129:290–298

[11] Brodsky MA, Anderson S, Murchison C, et al. Clinical outcomes of asleep vs awake deep brain stimulation for Parkinson disease. Neurology. 2017; 89 (19):1944–1950

[12] Chen T, Mirzadeh Z, Chapple K, Lambert M, Ponce FA. Complication rates, lengths of stay, and readmission rates in "awake" and "asleep" deep brain simulation. J Neurosurg. 2017; 127(2):360–369

[13] Jacob RL, Geddes J, McCartney S, Burchiel KJ. Cost analysis of awake versus asleep deep brain stimulation: a single academic health center experience. J Neurosurg. 2016; 124(5):1517–1523

[14] Theodosopoulos PV, Marks WJ, Jr, Christine C, Starr PA. Locations of movement-related cells in the human subthalamic nucleus in Parkinson's disease. Mov Disord. 2003; 18(7):791–798

[15] Starr PA, Christine CW, Theodosopoulos PV, et al. Implantation of deep brain stimulators into the subthalamic nucleus: technical approach and magnetic resonance imaging-verified lead locations. J Neurosurg. 2002; 97(2):370–387

[16] Schönecker T, Gruber D, Kivi A, et al. Postoperative MRI localisation of electrodes and clinical efficacy of pallidal deep brain stimulation in cervical dystonia. J Neurol Neurosurg Psychiatry. 2015; 86(8):833–839

[17] Truwit CL, Liu H. Prospective stereotaxy: a novel method of trajectory alignment using real-time image guidance. J Magn Reson Imaging. 2001; 13(3):452–457

[18] Richardson RM, Kells AP, Martin AJ, et al. Novel platform for MRI-guided convection-enhanced delivery of therapeutics: preclinical validation in non-human primate brain. Stereotact Funct Neurosurg. 2011; 89(3):141–151

[19] Larson PS, Starr PA, Bates G, Tansey L, Richardson RM, Martin AJ. An optimized system for interventional magnetic resonance imaging-guided stereotactic surgery: preliminary evaluation of targeting accuracy. Neurosurgery. 2012; 70(1) Suppl Operative:95–103, discussion 103

[20] Ostrem JL, Ziman N, Galifianakis NB, et al. Clinical outcomes using ClearPoint interventional MRI for deep brain stimulation lead placement in Parkinson's disease. J Neurosurg. 2016; 124(4):908–916

[21] Lee PS, Weiner GM, Corson D, et al. Outcomes of interventional-MRI versus microelectrode recording-guided subthalamic deep brain stimulation. Front Neurol. 2018; 9:241

[22] Saleh S, Swanson KI, Lake WB, Sillay KA. Awake neurophysiologically guided versus asleep MRI-guided STN DBS for Parkinson disease: a comparison of outcomes using levodopa equivalents. Stereotact Funct Neurosurg. 2015; 93(6):419–426

[23] Sidiropoulos C, Rammo R, Merker B, et al. Intraoperative MRI for deep brain stimulation lead placement in Parkinson's disease: 1 year motor and neuropsychological outcomes. J Neurol. 2016; 263(6):1226–1231

[24] Martin AJ, Larson PS, Ziman N, et al. Deep brain stimulator implantation in a diagnostic MRI suite: infection history over a 10-year period. J Neurosurg. 2017; 126(1):108–113

[25] Ostrem JL, Galifianakis NB, Markun LC, et al. Clinical outcomes of PD patients having bilateral STN DBS using high-field interventional MR-imaging for lead placement. Clin Neurol Neurosurg. 2013; 115(6):708-712

[26] Southwell DG, Narvid JA, Martin AJ, Qasim SE, Starr PA, Larson PS. Comparison of deep brain stimulation lead targeting accuracy and procedure duration between 1.5- and 3-Tesla Interventional Magnetic Resonance Imaging Systems: an initial 12-month experience. Stereotact Funct Neurosurg. 2016; 94(2):102–107

[27] Hirabayashi H, Tengvar M, Hariz MI. Stereotactic imaging of the pallidal target. Mov Disord. 2002; 17 Suppl 3:S130–S134

[28] Sudhyadhom A, Haq IU, Foote KD, Okun MS, Bova FJ. A high resolution and high contrast MRI for differentiation of subcortical structures for DBS targeting: the Fast Gray Matter Acquisition T1 Inversion Recovery (FGATIR). Neuroimage. 2009; 47 Suppl 2:T44–T52

[29] Starr PA, Vitek JL, DeLong M, Bakay RA. Magnetic resonance imaging-based stereotactic localization of the globus pallidus and subthalamic nucleus. Neurosurgery. 1999; 44(2):303–313, discussion 313–314

[30] O'Gorman RL, Shmueli K, Ashkan K, et al. Optimal MRI methods for direct stereotactic targeting of the subthalamic nucleus and globus pallidus. Eur Radiol. 2011; 21(1):130–136

[31] Tourdias T, Saranathan M, Levesque IR, Su J, Rutt BK. Visualization of intrathalamic nuclei with optimized white-matter-nulled MPRAGE at 7T. Neuroimage. 2014; 84:534–545

[32] Sammartino F, Krishna V, King NK, et al. Tractography-based ventral intermediate nucleus targeting: novel methodology and intraoperative validation. Mov Disord. 2016; 31(8):1217–1225

[33] Richardson RM, Golby AJ. Chapter 13—Functional Neurosurgery: Deep Brain Stimulation and Gene Therapy. In: Chapter 13—Functional Neurosurgery: Deep Brain Stimulation and Gene Therapy. Academic Press; 2015:297–323

[34] Lee PS, Richardson RM. Interventional MRI-guided deep brain stimulation lead implantation. Neurosurg Clin N Am. 2017; 28(4):535–544

[35] Larson PS, Starr PA, Martin AJ. Deep brain stimulation: interventional and intraoperative MRI approaches. Prog Neurol Surg. 2018; 33:187–197

[36] Plantinga BR, Temel Y, Duchin Y, et al. Individualized parcellation of the subthalamic nucleus in patients with Parkinson's disease with 7T MRI. Neuroimage. 2018; 168:403–411

[37] Patriat R, Cooper SE, Duchin Y, et al. Individualized tractography-based parcellation of the globus pallidus pars interna using 7T MRI in movement disorder patients prior to DBS surgery. Neuroimage. 2018; 178:198–209

[38] Shamir RR, Duchin Y, Kim J, et al. Microelectrode recordings validate the clinical visualization of subthalamic nucleus based on 7T magnetic resonance imaging and machine learning for deep brain stimulation surgery. Neurosurgery. 2018

[39] Beudel M, Cagnan H, Little S. Adaptive brain stimulation for movement disorders. Prog Neurol Surg. 2018; 33:230–242

5 Lesioning Methods for Movement Disorders

Shayan Moosa, Travis S. Tierney, Fred A. Lenz, William S. Anderson, W. Jeffrey Elias

Abstract

Lesioning techniques, the primary surgical procedures for the treatment of movement disorders, continue to remain important therapeutic procedures for neurosurgeons in the era of neuromodulation. The technology for creating high-precision brain lesions has evolved from the original stereotactic radiofrequency thalamotomies and pallidotomies and now includes minimally invasive laser interstitial therapy with magnetic resonance (MR) thermography and transcranial MRI-guided focused ultrasound lesioning.

Keywords: therapeutic brain lesion, radiofrequency thermocoagulation, laser interstitial therapy, MRI-guided focused ultrasound

5.1 Introduction

Prior to the widespread use of deep brain stimulation (DBS) techniques (beginning in mid-late 1990s) for the treatment of movement disorders, stereotactic radiofrequency (RF) thermocoagulation techniques were the most widely used surgical procedures, with a proven track record of efficacy and safety. The use of these techniques dwindled considerably over time with advances in neuromodulation, but lesioning still has an important role in cases of patients traveling from the developing world with poor local follow-up, patients who had prior neuromodulation systems implanted but later had them removed due to infections, or patients with very thin skin or poor wound healing or nutritional issues. In such cases, RF lesioning is still occasionally utilized. In addition, with the advent of magnetic resonance (MR) thermography imaging, it is now also possible to offer transcranial methods of brain lesioning via MR-guided focused ultrasound techniques (MRgFUS). Similarly, minimally invasive lesioning procedures are being performed using stereotactically applied laser interstitial thermal therapy (LITT), again with concurrent MR thermography. In this chapter, we provide a brief historical review of RF lesioning as practiced for movement disorders and describe the new less invasive MRgFUS and LITT procedures.

Prior to the reduction in use of lesioning techniques, with the advent of dopaminergic medications and subsequently DBS, reports of tissue disruption for abnormal movements date into the early 1900s. For instance, Victor Horsely was performing cortical resections for chorea in 1906,[1] and Russell Meyers began reporting transventricular fiber disruptions in the region of the basal ganglia in the 1930s.[2] Spiegel and Wycis introduced the stereotactic frame to neurosurgical procedures in the late 1940s,[3] and other authors developed stereotactic techniques for pallidotomy in Parkinson's disease (Leksell)[4] and thalamotomy for tremor (Hassler).[5] After it became clear that even with dopaminergic therapies there are considerable side effects (dyskinesias) and continued progression of Parkinson's disease (PD) with tightening therapeutic windows,[6] the pallidotomy again grew in importance clinically for treating rigidity and bradykinesia.[7] These surgical efforts then grew further with the introduction of DBS[8] and the minimally invasive lesioning techniques described below.

5.2 Pallidotomy

In the early 1990s, the posteroventral pallidotomy in a clinical series was described by Laitinen et al.[7] In this, 38 PD patients underwent stereotactic pallidotomy with a mean follow-up of 28 months. The primary indication for the surgery was bradykinesia/akinesia. Formal motor testing was performed postoperatively and significant improvements in rigidity and bradykinesia were observed in 92% of the subjects. There was also meaningful improvement in patients with tremor (81%), and reductions in drug-induced dyskinesias were also observed. The most common significant complication was a visual field defect (central homonymous) from injury to the optic tract ventrally (6 subjects).

Several subsequent studies of pallidotomy for PD were reported,[9,10,11,12,13] some of which included blinded postoperative outcomes rating via video documentation.[9,10,12] The two widely used clinical rating scales for PD (the Hoehn and Yahr Staging Scale[14] and the Unified Parkinson's Disease Rating Scale, UPDRS)[15] began to be incorporated with surgical series at this time. Patients in these series were typically those who were in Hoehn and Yahr stage III or worse, and postoperative UPDRS improvements ranged from 14 to 70% (with ranges of follow-up from 3 months to 1 year). Specific symptomatic improvements were observed in dyskinesias, on/off fluctuations, and the cardinal features of PD, including bradykinesia, cogwheel rigidity, tremor, and gait imbalance.

A later series by the Toronto group was published, presenting 11 patients undergoing pallidotomy for PD with a 2-year follow-up period.[16] UPDRS motor improvement at the end of this time period was a stable 28%, with continuing improvements in the cardinal features of PD. The first report of the use of DBS for PD was in 1994,[17] in which Siegfried and Lippitz described three subjects undergoing placement in the globus pallidus interna (GPi). These three patients had advanced PD and all three showed significant improvements in on/off fluctuations and dyskinesias.

Stereotactic pallidotomies do have an inherent risk profile. In a small series of 15 patients undergoing the procedure,[11] 2 suffered asymptomatic hemorrhages, 1 exhibited dysarthria that was transient, 1 experienced worsening of preexisting dysarthria, and 1 had a superior quadrant visual field defect that did not improve over time. There were also reports of transient likely edema-related confusion and facial weakness in this small series. In the series of 34 patients undergoing pallidotomy described by Ondo et al, 5 patients experienced transient side effects, which included aphasia and cognitive changes.[12]

Another series of 26 patients undergoing stereotactic pallidotomy reported 1 fatal hemorrhage, 3 nonfatal hemorrhages, 3 declines in cognitive function or behavioral issues postoperatively, 1 case of aphasia, 1 case of a mild but persistent hemiparesis, and 1 case of worsening dysarthria. There were other patients having neurological changes that were not persistent, such as altered mental status, facial weakness, and dysarthria. A series of 18 patients published by Dogali et al demonstrated no significant complications after a pallidotomy procedure.[9] In 1998, the Pittsburgh group published a series of 120 stereotactic pallidotomies and reported a 5% risk of postoperative dysarthria that was always transient. This series had no significant hemorrhages.[18] A large series of 126 pallidotomies was published by Iacono et al, with 68 of them being bilateral procedures.[19] These authors reported a hemorrhage frequency of 3.2% per pallidotomy.

A large series of 334 unilateral pallidotomies was described by de Bie et al covering 8 years.[20] These authors found a risk of 13.8% for permanent significant complications, including behavioral problems, dysarthria, visual field defects, and dysphagia. Significant symptomatic hemorrhages occurred in 3.9% of the patients, and there was a 1.2% mortality rate. In general, patients undergoing microelectrode recording (MER) prior to placement of the pallidotomy lesion appear to have a higher frequency of complications.[18,20]

5.3 Ventral Thalamotomy

The ventral thalamotomy, or lesioning of the cerebellar receiving nucleus of the thalamus (nucleus ventral intermediate, Vim), has been described as a treatment for tremor-predominant PD and essential tremor (ET).[21,22] For instance, Fox et al described a series of stereotactic thalamotomies performed for tremor-predominant PD involving 36 patients with preoperative mean Hoehn and Yahr Stage 2 to 4.[23] Of these, 31 patients reported complete relief of their tremors, with 2 of them suffering recurrent tremor during the follow-up period of 14 to 68 months. Diederich et al performed an interesting blinded study, comparing tremor on the contralateral side to the thalamotomy with the ipsilateral tremor in a group of 17 patients with fairly symmetric preoperative tremor. Ratings were performed from videotape assessments at a mean follow-up time of 11 years. Tremor severity was significantly less on the contralateral side.[24] MERs have also been used to identify the area to be lesioned, and the area posterior to the nucleus ventralis oralis posterior (Vop), which was identified as the cerebellar receiving zone (Vim), was later found to have rhythmic bursting activity close to the frequency of tremor.[25]

In 1995, Jankovic et al published a retrospective review of 60 patients with a variety of tremor etiologies including PD (42 patients), ET (6 patients), cerebellar tremor (6 patients), and tremor after traumatic brain injury (TBI) (6 patients).[21] After unilateral Vim thalamotomy (2 of the PD patients had bilateral procedures) and a mean follow-up of > 50 months, the PD patients demonstrated significant improvement in tremor in 86% of cases. ET patients demonstrated significant improvement in 83% of cases, with positive but less significant results for cerebellar and post-TBI tremors. A small series from Johns Hopkins in 1999 showed similar results for ET after Vim thalamotomy with significant tremor improvement in 72% of cases.[22] Two series have described specific complications associated with thalamotomy procedures[21,23] (ranging from 58–70% of patients), including contralateral weakness, dysarthria or dysphasia, sensory changes, transient confusion, and the induction of dystonic movements. Permanent

complications described in these two series were rarer, in the range of 14 to 23%, including weakness and coordination difficulties, and dysarthria. Bilateral thalamotomies are in general not recommended due to high incidences of speech problems and dysphagia in this context. In the era of neuromodulation, many authors would now implant a DBS lead contralateral to a prior lesion.[21,24,26]

5.4 Stereotactic Surgical Technique

Both preoperative MRI and/or CT imaging as well as MERs may be used to localize ablation targets for movement disorders.[10,22] The well-known atlas-based targeting procedures may be performed by identifying the anterior and posterior commissures as described elsewhere in this text, with subsequent lesion targets defined relative to the midcommissural point or the midpoint of the posterior commissure itself. MERs may then be used with single to multiple MER passes to further refine the lesioning target.[27] Other described approaches include a variety of CT/MR fusion techniques,[28] ventriculography-guided lesioning, and semi-MERs with macrostimulation to estimate lesioning effects.[29] No systematic comparison of these techniques has ever been undertaken.

RF thermocoagulation may be performed through a variety of commercially available systems, which unfortunately are becoming rarer to find as use of this technology dwindles. One popular existing electrode has a 1.1 mm outer diameter with a 3-mm exposed tip (Integra Radionics, Burlington, MA). These electrodes often house a thermistor at the tip for temperature measurements. During lesioning, enough RF power is applied to maintain a constant tip temperature of 60 °C for typically 1 minute. Stepped increases in temperature to 80 °C have also been described for an additional 1 minute of energy application.[26] These procedures are often performed on awake interactive patients so that neurological testing can be performed during the lesioning process.

5.5 Radiosurgical Lesioning Procedures

A few centers have described the use of stereotactic radiosurgery as a means of lesioning tissue to treat movement disorders.[30,31,32] This technique (similar to the use of MRgFUS) has some advantages for patients with a history of prior stimulation hardware infections, or with health conditions or skin thickness incompatible with implanted DBS systems. The therapeutic benefit appears to be similar to studies of RF thermocoagulation. The Pittsburgh group has shown that Gamma Knife thalamotomy for ET has an approximate 69% rate of meaningful tremor amplitude reduction.[30] Of note, radiosurgical lesioning does not utilize MER for target refining as it is a completely incisionless technique, although there could be higher rates of lesioning complications due to this lack of mapping ability.[33]

The specific complications that can occur with radiosurgical lesioning procedures have been delineated by Okun et al.[31] This study reported 8 cases of complications in a series of 118 patients undergoing radiosurgical lesioning. Listed complications include weakness (3 patients), visual field cut (1 patient), dysarthria (3 patients), and 1 case of aspiration with pneumonia associated with dysphagia. As described in these studies, radiosurgical lesioning is probably best used in patients whose preoperative comorbidities would preclude safe implantation of stimulation hardware or MER-guided RF thermocoagulation.

5.6 Laser Interstitial Thermal Therapy with MR Thermography

LITT (with concurrent MRI-based thermography) has been primarily used intracranially to treat epilepsy, various grade brain tumors, and other delimited lesions including hypothalamic hamartomas and radiation necrosis.[34,35] Because of the additional benefits of concurrent MRI-based thermography (including the ability to monitor the thermal lesioning temperature as well as temperature changes in surrounding and sometimes eloquent structures), and because of the relatively minimally invasive characteristics of placing the laser applicator in the brain, a few groups have begun exploring the use of LITT for treating movement disorders. For example, Gross and Stern recently described two patients with dystonia undergoing MRI-guided LITT to perform pallidotomy lesions.[36] One subject (12-year-old male) had a primary DYT1 dystonia and underwent bilateral LITT pallidotomy. This patient demonstrated right-sided improvements in dystonia symptoms, but also suffered worsening left upper extremity hypertonicity and a jaw-opening dystonia component. The second case was a 32-year-old male with generalized dystonia who underwent a right LITT pallidotomy, and demonstrated substantial improvements in his axial symptoms and speech. Efforts for treating movement disorders with LITT are in their infancy, but the adjunctive MR thermography techniques (which cannot be performed with RF lesioning) may prove useful for increases in safety.

5.7 MR-guided Focused Ultrasound

The practice of using acoustic energy to create intracranial lesions dates back to the 1950s.[37] Recent advances in transcranial acoustic energy delivery, phase correction technology, and MR thermography have allowed for the incisionless and precise ablative procedure known as MRgFUS.[38] This procedure begins with extensive planning prior to patient arrival using a head CT scan to calculate the skull density ratio (SDR), a measure of skull favorability for the procedure, and delineate regions that would impede the transmission of the acoustic wave. The CT is later fused to a volumetric MRI for accurate targeting. When the patient arrives, the hair is clipped and then head is shaved carefully prior to administration of a stereotactic frame and silicone membrane over the scalp, which is attached to the ultrasound transducer (NeuroAblate 4000; Insightec) (▶ Fig. 5.1). Chilled, degassed water is filled into the space between the scalp and ultrasound transducer. After additional T2-weighted images are obtained to reference the patient in MR space, the transducer is positioned so that its focus precisely matches the intended target. Test lesions are first created using low-energy sonications

with a goal temperature of 40 to 45 °C, followed by initial treatment lesions that can produce clinical effects at 50 to 55 °C. Adjustments are made based on clinical feedback, similar to DBS and RF localization techniques. Finally, the energy is increased to achieve temperatures of 55 to 60 °C for permanent effect. This final temperature goal yields roughly 51 °C temperature thresholds at the margins, which most closely correlates with the final lesion size of 5 mm.[39] In the treatment of ET using focused ultrasound (FUS) thalamotomy, the lesion is then enlarged dorsally by focusing an additional sonication 2 mm superiorly.[40] A postablation MRI can be performed to confirm accurate lesioning, but a higher-quality MRI is typically obtained the next day as lesion sizes are similar one day and one month postoperatively (▶ Fig. 5.2).[41]

Three uncontrolled pilot studies[42,43,44] set the stage for a multicenter, randomized, sham-controlled trial[45] demonstrating the effectiveness of MRgFUS in the treatment of medication-refractory ET. In this trial, Elias et al analyzed hand tremor and disability scores for 76 patients with medically-refractory ET who underwent either unilateral FUS thalamotomy or a sham procedure. From blinded videotape assessment at 3 months, it was observed that mean tremor and disability scores improved 47% and 59%, respectively in the thalamotomy group, with improvement sustained to 12 months. A 2-year follow-up study of 67 of these patients demonstrated clinical durability with 56% improvement in mean tremor score and 60% improvement in disability score in the thalamotomy group.[46]

Trials that have demonstrated the feasibility of using MRgFUS for the treatment of Parkinsonian tremor have targeted the Vim[47] and pallidothalamic tract.[48] In a recent clinical trial of 27 patients with medication-refractory, tremor-dominant PD randomized to unilateral FUS thalamotomy or a sham procedure, Bond et al demonstrated 62% improvement in on-medication median tremor scores in the FUS thalamotomy group, which was significantly different from the 22% improvement observed in the group controlled by sham procedures.[49] Obeso et al published a pilot study of 10 patients who underwent unilateral FUS subthalamotomy with improvement in their motor symptoms of PD, although 1 patient developed mild hemiballism that later resolved.[50] Unilateral FUS pallidotomy has also been performed for levodopa-induced dyskinesia,[51] and there is a multicenter randomized control trial currently underway to evaluate the safety and efficacy of unilateral FUS thalamotomy to manage dyskinesia symptoms in advanced PD (ClinicalTrials.gov identifier: NCT03319485). Of note, MRgFUS thalamotomy is now approved by the Food and Drug Administration for the treatment of ET and tremor-dominant PD.

There have been no reports of intracranial hemorrhage or mortality from MRgFUS procedures for movement disorders.[52] Cavitation, i.e., the formation of microbubbles from acoustic pressure, can cause unintended tissue destruction; however, cavitation monitoring is used to automatically halt sonication in this event. Patient movement is also automatically detected, and the system stops further sonication to unintended areas. The most common side effect is paresthesia, which is typically transient but has been reported to be permanent in a small number of patients. In addition, cerebellar symptoms such as disequilibrium or ataxia have been observed but often resolve within a month.[43] Treatment effect may decrease over time like

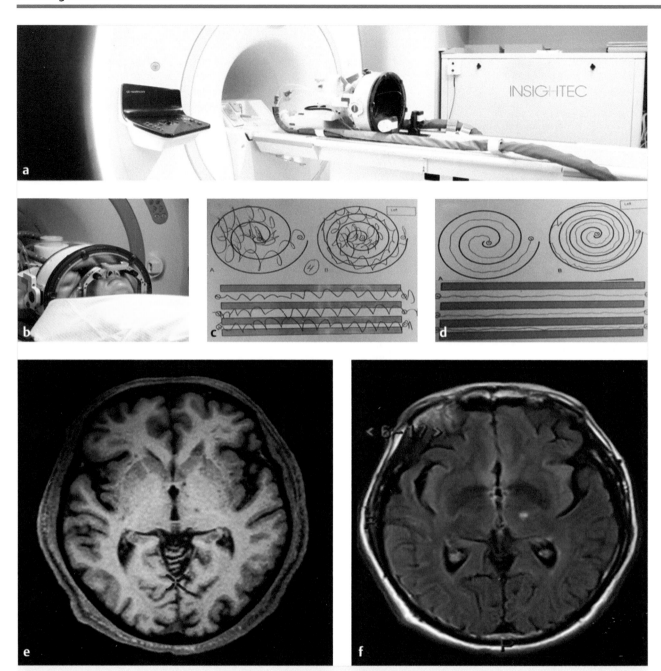

Fig. 5.1 A method for transcranial magnetic resonance image-guided focused ultrasound thermoablation surgery. A commercial FUS device that consists of a helmet affixed to a modified standard MR table incorporating a CRW frame mount. A refrigeration unit shown on the right side of the panel delivers cooled, degassed water during the sonication procedure, which is performed within the bore of the high-field strength magnet (shown on the left) to monitor the surgery in near-real time. The helmet houses acoustic microphones and the transducer array containing 1024 piezoelectric drivers capable of focusing high-intensity sound across the skull and into the brain to achieve nearly instantaneous thermocoagulation at goal peak temperatures of 56 to 60 °C **(a)**. A patient prepared for surgery. The scalp has been shaved and a modified CRW frame has been applied and mounted rigidly to the table holding the head in spatial registration with the phased array device. Note that this frame is indeed a standard commercial frame commonly used for stereotactic surgery. However, it is not being used to generate a Cartesian coordinate space, but only to stabilize the skull. A white silicone membrane surrounds the circumference of the patent's head and is attached in a water-tight fashion to the helmet. Degassed water is circulated between the phased array elements and the scalp to reduce the risk of sonic skin burn and to acoustically couple the device to the patient **(b)**. Archimedes spiral and line drawings before and after a thalamotomy of the ventral intermediate nucleus (Vim) **(c, d)**. In practice, these same drawings are also drawn during the awake procedure to monitor progression toward tremor capture. Axial FLAIR and T1-weight images at the level of the horizontal intercommissural plane demonstrating the size and location of an effective left Vim thalamic lesion 30 days after surgery **(e, f)**. Image orientations are displayed in standard radiological convention. The device images were kindly provided courtesy of Richard Schallhorn at Insightec Ltd. and used with permission.

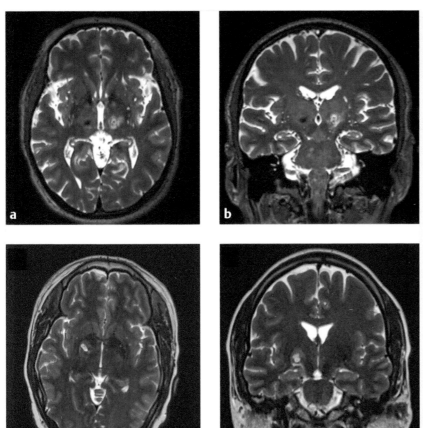

Fig. 5.2 Postoperative imaging status post transcranial magnetic resonance-guided focused ultrasound (MRgFUS) ablation. An axial T2-weighted MRI on postoperative day (POD) 1 following left-sided MRgFUS thalamotomy of the ventral intermediate nucleus for treatment of right-hand tremor in a patient diagnosed with medication-refractory essential tremor **(a)**. Coronal view **(b)**. Notice that the lesion has a hypointense core (zone I) and hyperintense rim (zone II), which are consistent with areas of coagulation necrosis. The slightly hyperintense area at the periphery of the lesion (zone III) is consistent with cytogenic edema. An axial T2-weighted MRI on POD 1 following right-sided MRgFUS pallidotomy for treatment of left-sided dyskinesia and motor fluctuation associated with Parkinson's disease **(c)**. Coronal view **(d)**.

other lesioning modalities, but salvage therapy can be performed with DBS[53] or repeat ablation. The risk of serious adverse event with MRgFUS is reported to be 1.6%,[52] making it a safe and well-tolerated procedure that can be performed on an outpatient basis. There are a few challenges with this new procedure that need to be tackled, such as optimizing lesioning parameters in patients with low SDRs, improving the durability of lesions, safely treating bilateral tremors, eliminating the need for head shaving, and reducing the overall time of the procedure for patient comfort.

5.8 Conclusion

Stereotactic RF thermocoagulation for the lesioning of specific targets in the brain declined considerably after the introduction of neuromodulation systems. However, over the past decade, there has been a resurgence of techniques of stereotactic ablation based on minimally invasive techniques. The older RF thermocoagulation literature shows rough equivalence in terms of efficacy in treating movement disorders, albeit with lack of reversibility and no opportunities for postoperative therapy tuning to enhance the efficacy relative to any induced side effects.[54] In general, lesioning, regardless of technique, may be preferred in situations where patients have had multiple prior infections due to implanted hardware or poor wound healing issues in general. Older patients with mobility and travel issues

are likely good candidates, as are patients from the developing world or from countries where postoperative support of neuromodulation devices may be difficult. In addition, neuromodulation systems are expensive to implant and maintain with eventual pulse generator depletion or other hardware complications, and eventually some public or private healthcare systems may weigh this in their decisions to support either method of treatment.

References

[1] Horsley V. The Linacre lecture on the function of the so-called motor cortex. BMJ. 1909; 2:125–132

[2] Meyers R. Surgical procedure for postencephalitic tremor, with notes on the physiology of premotor fibers. Arch Neurol Psychiatry. 1940; 44:455–459

[3] Spiegel EA, Wycis HT, Marks M, Lee AJ. Stereotaxic apparatus for operations on the human brain. Science. 1947; 106(2754):349–350

[4] Svennilson E, Torvik A, Lowe R, Leksell L. Treatment of parkinsonism by stereotatic thermolesions in the pallidal region. A clinical evaluation of 81 cases. Acta Psychiatr Scand. 1960; 35(3):358–377

[5] Hassler R, Riechert T. Indikationen und Lokalisationsmethode der gezielten Hirnoperationen. Nervenarzt. 1954; 25(11):441–447

[6] Marsden CD, Parkes JD. Success and problems of long-term levodopa therapy in Parkinson's disease. Lancet. 1977; 1(8007):345–349

[7] Laitinen LV, Bergenheim AT, Hariz MI. Leksell's posteroventral pallidotomy in the treatment of Parkinson's disease. J Neurosurg. 1992; 76(1):53–61

[8] Benabid AL, Pollak P, Gao D, et al. Chronic electrical stimulation of the ventralis intermedius nucleus of the thalamus as a treatment of movement disorders. J Neurosurg. 1996; 84(2):203–214

[9] Dogali M, Fazzini E, Kolodny E, et al. Stereotactic ventral pallidotomy for Parkinson's disease. Neurology. 1995; 45(4):753–761

[10] Lozano AM, Lang AE, Galvez-Jimenez N, et al. Effect of GPi pallidotomy on motor function in Parkinson's disease. Lancet. 1995; 346:1383–1386

[11] Baron MS, Vitek JL, Bakay RAE, et al. Treatment of advanced Parkinson's disease by posterior GPi pallidotomy: 1-year pilot study results. Ann Neurol. 1996; 40:355–366

[12] Ondo WG, Jankovic J, Lai EC, et al. Assessment of motor function after stereotactic pallidotomy. Neurology. 1998; 50(1):266–270

[13] Shannon KM, Penn RD, Kroin JS, et al. Stereotactic pallidotomy for the treatment of Parkinson's disease. Efficacy and adverse effects at 6 months in 26 patients. Neurology. 1998; 50(2):434–438

[14] Hoehn MM, Yahr MD. Parkinsonism: onset, progression and mortality. Neurology. 1967; 17(5):427–442

[15] Fahn S, Elton RL. Members of the UPDRS Development Committee. Unified Parkinson's Disease Rating S. In: Fahn S, Marsden CD, Calne DB, Goldstein M, eds. Recent Developments in Parkinson's Disease. Vol. 2. Florham Park: MacMillan Health Care Information; 1987:153–164

[16] Lang AE, Lozano AM, Montgomery E, Duff J, Tasker R, Hutchinson W. Posteroventral medial pallidotomy in advanced Parkinson's disease. N Engl J Med. 1997; 337(15):1036–1042

[17] Siegfried J, Lippitz B. Bilateral chronic electrostimulation of ventroposterolateral pallidum: a new therapeutic approach for alleviating all parkinsonian symptoms. Neurosurgery. 1994; 35(6):1126–1129, discussion 1129–1130

[18] Kondziolka D, Firlik AD, Lunsford LD. Complications of stereotactic brain surgery. Neurol Clin. 1998; 16(1):35–54

[19] Iacono RP, Shima F, Lonser RR, Kuniyoshi S, Maeda G, Yamada S. The results, indications, and physiology of posteroventral pallidotomy for patients with Parkinson's disease. Neurosurgery. 1995; 36(6):1118–1125, discussion 1125–1127

[20] de Bie RMA, de Haan RJ, Schuurman PR, Esselink RAJ, Bosch DA, Speelman JD. Morbidity and mortality following pallidotomy in Parkinson's disease: a systematic review. Neurology. 2002; 58(7):1008–1012

[21] Jankovic J, Cardoso F, Grossman RG, Hamilton WJ. Outcome after stereotactic thalamotomy for parkinsonian, essential, and other types of tremor. Neurosurgery. 1995; 37(4):680–686, discussion 686–687

[22] Zirh A, Reich SG, Dougherty PM, Lenz FA. Stereotactic thalamotomy in the treatment of essential tremor of the upper extremity: reassessment including a blinded measure of outcome. J Neurol Neurosurg Psychiatry. 1999; 66(6):772–775

[23] Fox MW, Ahlskog JE, Kelly PJ. Stereotactic ventrolateralis thalamotomy for medically refractory tremor in post-levodopa era Parkinson's disease patients. J Neurosurg. 1991; 75(5):723–730

[24] Diederich N, Goetz CG, Stebbins GT, et al. Blinded evaluation confirms long-term asymmetric effect of unilateral thalamotomy or subthalamotomy on tremor in Parkinson's disease. Neurology. 1992; 42(7):1311–1314

[25] Guiot G, Hardy J, Albe-Fessard D. [Precise delimitation of the subcortical structures and identification of thalamic nuclei in man by stereotactic electrophysiology]. Neurochirurgia (Stuttg). 1962; 5:1–18

[26] von Coelln R, Kobayashi K, Kim JH, Anderson WS, Winberry J, Lenz FA. Thalamotomy. In: Kompoliti K, Verhagen ML, eds. Encyclopedia of Movement Disorders. Vol. 3. Elsevier, Oxford: Academic Press; 2010:226–229

[27] Garonzik IM, Hua SE, Ohara S, Lenz FA. Intraoperative microelectrode and semi-microelectrode recording during the physiological localization of the thalamic nucleus ventral intermediate. Mov Disord. 2002; 17 Suppl 3:S135–S144

[28] Carlson JD, Iacono RP. Electrophysiological versus image-based targeting in the posteroventral pallidotomy. Comput Aided Surg. 1999; 4(2):93–100

[29] Burchiel KJ. Thalamotomy for movement disorders. Neurosurg Clin N Am. 1995; 6(1):55–71

[30] Kondziolka D, Ong JG, Lee JY, Moore RY, Flickinger JC, Lunsford LD. Gamma Knife thalamotomy for essential tremor. J Neurosurg. 2008; 108(1):111–117

[31] Okun MS, Stover NP, Subramanian T, et al. Complications of gamma knife surgery for Parkinson disease. Arch Neurol. 2001; 58(12):1995–2002

[32] Friedman DP, Goldman HW, Flanders AE, Gollomp SM, Curran WJ, Jr. Stereotactic radiosurgical pallidotomy and thalamotomy with the gamma knife: MR imaging findings with clinical correlation–preliminary experience. Radiology. 1999; 212(1):143–150

[33] Jankovic J. Editorial: Surgery for Parkinson disease and other movement disorders: benefits and limitations of ablation, stimulation, restoration, and radiation. Arch Neurol. 2001; 58:1970–1972

[34] Willie JT, Laxpati NG, Drane DL, et al. Real-time magnetic resonance-guided stereotactic laser amygdalohippocampectomy for mesial temporal lobe epilepsy. Neurosurgery. 2014; 74(6):569–584, discussion 584–585

[35] Barnett GH, Voigt JD, Alhuwalia MS. A systematic review and meta-analysis of studies examining the use of brain laser interstitial thermal therapy versus craniotomy for the treatment of high-grade tumors in or near areas of eloquence: An examination of the extent of resection and major complication rates associated with each type of surgery. Stereotact Funct Neurosurg. 2016; 94(3):164–173

[36] Gross RE, Stern MA. Magnetic resonance-guided stereotactic laser pallidotomy for dystonia. Mov Disord. 2018; 33(9):1502–1503

[37] Fry WJ, Mosberg WH, Jr, Barnard JW, Fry FJ. Production of focal destructive lesions in the central nervous system with ultrasound. J Neurosurg. 1954; 11(5):471–478

[38] Clement GT, White PJ, King RL, McDannold N, Hynynen K. A magnetic resonance imaging-compatible, large-scale array for trans-skull ultrasound surgery and therapy. J Ultrasound Med. 2005; 24(8):1117–1125

[39] Bond AE, Elias WJ. Predicting lesion size during focused ultrasound thalamotomy: a review of 63 lesions over 3 clinical trials. Neurosurg Focus. 2018; 44(2):E5

[40] Wang TR, Bond AE, Dallapiazza RF, et al. Transcranial magnetic resonance imaging-guided focused ultrasound thalamotomy for tremor: technical note. Neurosurg Focus. 2018; 44(2):E3

[41] Wintermark M, Druzgal J, Huss DS, et al. Imaging findings in MR imaging-guided focused ultrasound treatment for patients with essential tremor. AJNR Am J Neuroradiol. 2014; 35(5):891–896

[42] Chang WS, Jung HH, Kweon EJ, Zadicario E, Rachmilevitch I, Chang JW. Unilateral magnetic resonance guided focused ultrasound thalamotomy for essential tremor: practices and clinicoradiological outcomes. J Neurol Neurosurg Psychiatry. 2015; 86(3):257–264

[43] Elias WJ, Huss D, Voss T, et al. A pilot study of focused ultrasound thalamotomy for essential tremor. N Engl J Med. 2013; 369(7):640–648

[44] Lipsman N, Schwartz ML, Huang Y, et al. MR-guided focused ultrasound thalamotomy for essential tremor: a proof-of-concept study. Lancet Neurol. 2013; 12(5):462–468

[45] Elias WJ, Lipsman N, Ondo WG, et al. A randomized trial of focused ultrasound thalamotomy for essential tremor. N Engl J Med. 2016; 375(8):730–739

[46] Chang JW, Park CK, Lipsman N, et al. A prospective trial of magnetic resonance-guided focused ultrasound thalamotomy for essential tremor: Results at the 2-year follow-up. Ann Neurol. 2018; 83(1):107–114

[47] Schlesinger I, Eran A, Sinai A, et al. MRI guided focused ultrasound thalamotomy for moderate-to-severe tremor in Parkinson's disease. Parkinsons Dis. 2015; 2015:219149

[48] Magara A, Bühler R, Moser D, Kowalski M, Pourtehrani P, Jeanmonod D. First experience with MR-guided focused ultrasound in the treatment of Parkinson's disease. J Ther Ultrasound. 2014; 2:11

[49] Bond AE, Shah BB, Huss DS, et al. Safety and efficacy of focused ultrasound thalamotomy for patients with medication-refractory, tremor-dominant Parkinson's disease: a randomized clinical trial. JAMA Neurol. 2017; 74(12):1412–1418

[50] Martínez-Fernández R, Rodríguez-Rojas R, Del Álamo M, et al. Focused ultrasound subthalamotomy in patients with asymmetric Parkinson's disease: a pilot study. Lancet Neurol. 2018; 17(1):54–63

[51] Na YC, Chang WS, Jung HH, Kweon EJ, Chang JW. Unilateral magnetic resonance-guided focused ultrasound pallidotomy for Parkinson disease. Neurology. 2015; 85(6):549–551

[52] Fishman PS, Elias WJ, Ghanouni P, et al. Neurological adverse event profile of magnetic resonance imaging-guided focused ultrasound thalamotomy for essential tremor. Mov Disord. 2018; 33(5):843–847

[53] Wang TR, Dallapiazza RF, Moosa S, Huss D, Shah BB, Elias WJ. Thalamic deep brain stimulation salvages failed focused ultrasound thalamotomy for essential tremor: a case report. Stereotact Funct Neurosurg. 2018; 96(1):60–64

[54] Tasker RR, Munz M, Junn FSCK, et al. Deep brain stimulation and thalamotomy for tremor compared. Acta Neurochir Suppl (Wien). 1997; 68:49–53

6 Computational Modeling and Tractography for DBS Targeting

Michael D. Staudt, Sarah Ridge, Jennifer A. Sweet

Abstract

Deep brain stimulation (DBS) has an established and efficacious role in the treatment of movement disorders, with emerging indications for neuropsychiatric disorders and epilepsy. However, the underlying effects of electrical stimulation on cellular mechanisms and widespread neural networks remain unclear. Furthermore, there are little data regarding the correlation between clinical outcomes and modulation of dysfunctional neural circuitry via the direct and indirect stimulation of axonal pathways. The advent of computational modeling for DBS has been a powerful tool for better understanding of DBS and neural circuitry, including the development of surgical targets for electrode placement and refinement of stimulation parameters. Advanced imaging techniques, including tractography and high-field MRI, allow for the specific visualization of white matter tracts and individual nuclei, potentially leading to the development of patient or symptom-specific treatment models. This chapter reviews the value of computational modeling and advanced imaging technologies for DBS therapies and discusses existing and future DBS applications.

Keywords: computational modeling, deep brain stimulation, neuroimaging, targeting tractography

6.1 Introduction

Deep brain stimulation (DBS) is the delivery of electrical impulses to deep structures in the brain via surgically implanted electrodes. While DBS has proven to be an effective therapy for movement disorders, such as Parkinson's disease (PD),[1,2,3] essential tremor (ET),[4,5] and dystonia,[6,7] as well as for emerging neuropsychiatric indications including obsessive compulsive disorder,[8,9] the exact mechanism of action of DBS still remains unknown. Since many of the current intracranial DBS targets were historically lesioned producing therapeutic effects similar to DBS, stimulation was originally thought to act via the inhibition of these gray matter targets.[10] However, data suggest that DBS may also result in the excitation of surrounding white matter (WM) axons,[11,12,13] possibly contributing to the downstream effects of stimulation, seen at sites distant from the electrode target.[14,15,16,17,18,19,20,21] Prevailing theories support the notion that high-frequency DBS ultimately disrupts aberrant neuronal patterns producing global network modulation.[11,12,22]

This proposed mechanism of action, involving the stimulation of WM tracts and the propagation of widespread neuronal effects, may account for both the improvement in symptoms seen with DBS as well as many of the unwanted side effects. As such, selective activation of these complex and interconnected neural networks may further improve patient outcomes. DBS targeting can be further enhanced by using computational modeling techniques and novel imaging strategies. Such tools can improve our understanding of DBS and brain networks, and can also help in increasing accuracy, and identifying better targets for diseases that are currently treated with DBS. These tools can also aid in the discovery of new surgical targets for neurological, psychiatric, and possibly even cognitive disorders. The goal of this chapter is to review the value of computational modeling and advanced imaging technologies for DBS therapies and discuss existing and future DBS applications.

6.2 Computational Modeling Techniques

Computational modeling techniques have largely contributed to our current understanding of the mechanism of DBS in the treatment of movement disorders, allowing for more effective surgical targeting. In 1999, Grill used electrical models to demonstrate the impact of the properties of neural tissue surrounding DBS electrodes on the electric fields generated by these electrodes.[23] The models demonstrated the inhomogeneity and anisotropy of the neural tissue stimulated by DBS, reinforcing the importance of electrode lead location for generating the desired effects. On the basis of these principles, McIntyre and Grill used modeling techniques to show that axons are the most excitable neural elements with stimulation.[24,25,26] They also demonstrated that knowledge of the electrical conductivity of the tissue around the DBS lead as well as familiarity of the electrode shape and position within the brain can help to predict the electric field generated by DBS and the subsequent neural response.[25,26] Thus, understanding the influence that surrounding neural tissue has on the effects of DBS could potentially lead to improved predictions of the clinical responses to stimulation.

6.2.1 Volume of Tissue Activated

Developments in computational modeling techniques have ever since utilized this principle, allowing investigators to better understand the relationship between lead placement and the delivery of stimulation to adjacent anatomical structures, and how this relationship impacts clinical outcomes.[15,27,28,29] One method by which this has been done involves the use of models to allow the visualization of the volume of tissue activated (VTA) by DBS. VTAs are created using finite element modeling (FEM) that combines an anatomical model, based on imaging data from subjects who have undergone DBS implantation, with an electrical model using actual or theoretical DBS stimulation parameters to determine the voltage spread from stimulation.[11,15,27] The results depend on the composition of the tissue surrounding the electrode, such as gray matter versus WM, as this affects electrode capacitance and impedance as well as the type of stimulation and the parameters used.[15] The axonal activation pattern can then be predicted from the presumed electrical field created from each active DBS electrode contact, and the threshold for generating an action potential by adjacent axons.[11,15,27] Ideally, a truly "connectomic" approach will allow for identification of the differential effects of electrical stimulation on different parts of the neuron (i.e., soma, axons, dendrites) as part of a greater neural network.[30] Computational models have been developed that emulate the effects of electrical stimulation on networks of multicompartmental neurons,[31,32] although these paradigms have not yet been translated to DBS research.

Clinical applications of the VTA can be valuable for determining which structures are responsible for producing the clinical effects of DBS. In 2004, McIntyre et al, combined tissue conductivity information with an FEM to show the shape and volume of stimulation with standard DBS parameters in the subthalamic nucleus (STN) for PD, demonstrating that even subtle deviations in electrode positions would result in the stimulation of different structures, thus resulting in variable clinical effects.[12] Miocinovic et al similarly used this concept to devise a computational model integrating STN anatomical data from Parkinsonian macaques to an FEM of the electric field from DBS, while also incorporating the biophysical properties of neurons in the STN, the globus pallidus interna (GPi), and the internal capsule.[15] In this way, they predicted the axonal activation patterns of STN DBS and showed that although stimulation of this target resulted in both STN and GPi fiber activation, it was the volume of STN tissue activated that resulted in the specific therapeutic effects.[15]

Butson et al also used the VTA to study the effects of STN DBS in a PD patient by fusing the preoperative and postoperative imaging data to determine the exact location of the electrode.[27] They then created VTA models according to the different DBS programming parameters used and correlated this with clinical outcomes. The authors found that corticospinal tract symptoms correlated well with involvement of the corticospinal tract in the VTA, and improvement in bradykinesia and rigidity corresponded to VTAs that involved the zona incerta.[27] In 2009, Maks et al retrospectively studied 10 PD patients with STN DBS and determined the VTA from imaging data and reports of the active contacts used for each subject.[28] They showed that when the active contacts were near the dorsal border of the STN, the resultant VTAs produced optimal therapeutic benefits. In a similar manner, Mikos et al found that PD patients with STN DBS whose VTA included nonmotor areas of the STN had worsening verbal fluency compared to PD patients with VTA involving only motor STN.[29] Thus, the VTA can be retrospectively assessed in patients previously implanted with DBS electrodes to help ascertain what structures are being stimulated by the active contact to produce the observed effects, consequently helping to determine the optimal DBS target (▶ Fig. 6.1).[33]

Moreover, there is great interest in creating patient-specific models that can prospectively define anatomical pathways of

interest and calculate the response to DBS stimulation. Pathway activation models integrate imaging data with both tractography and the biophysics of electrical stimulation modeling to theoretically estimate pathway activation a priori.[35] These models calculate the axonal response to DBS in relation to electrode configuration, the characteristics of the applied stimuli, the tissue conduction properties, axonal geometry, and axonal membrane biophysics.[35] In comparison, conventional VTA modeling relies primarily on activation volume to generate seeds for tractography and is primarily performed retrospectively. As such, pathway activation models are much more time- and resource-intensive to develop.[35,36] They are potentially powerful tools of analysis, but lack in their current inability to quantify the effects of DBS stimulation on a network level.

6.2.2 Whole-Brain Network Models

Other computational modeling techniques have aided in our understanding of the influence of DBS on widespread, complex neural networks. In 2004, Rubin and Terman created a computational network model to determine how DBS of the STN for the treatment of the motor symptoms in PD results in the disruption of downstream pathological thalamic rhythms.[37] By simulating the molecular environment surrounding neurons in the STN, the GPi, and the thalamus under conditions of a healthy state, a parkinsonian state, and a parkinsonian state with STN DBS, the authors demonstrated that STN DBS restores abnormal oscillations within the basal ganglia, ultimately normalizing thalamic relay processes.[37] In 2010, Hahn and McIntyre evaluated the VTA of STN DBS by incorporating presumed cortical and striatal inputs to the basal ganglia into their computational model, thus allowing for investigation into the influence of networks as opposed to isolated cell-to-cell interactions.[38] These authors found that the STN VTA plays a key role in correcting pathologic GPi bursting in PD, thus influencing cortico-striatal-thalamic networks. They concluded that there may be a critical VTA required to produce the observed outcomes of DBS.

Humphries and Gurney devised a computational model of the basal ganglia to show that DBS of the STN results in a mixture of excitatory and inhibitory responses from the basal ganglia output nuclei.[39] They postulated that this diversification of responses from the basal ganglia ultimately produces far-reaching network effects accounting for the clinical effects of DBS. Thus, these studies demonstrate complexity of the widespread signaling pathways in PD, the downstream effects of

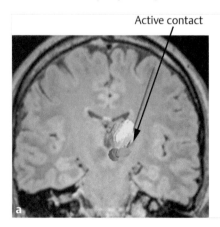
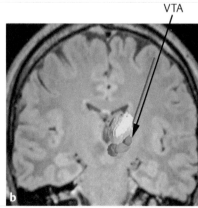

Fig. 6.1 Visualization of active electrode contact (a) in subthalamic nucleus (STN) deep brain stimulation model and volume of tissue activated (b; *dark pink*) from active electrode contact in relation to surrounding nuclei. Thalamus shown in *yellow*, STN in *green*, red nucleus in *red*. (Adapted from Sweet et al.[34])

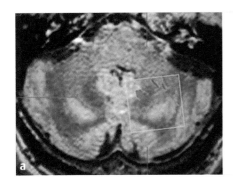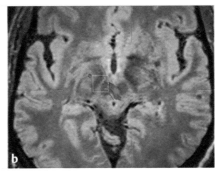

Fig. 6.2 Visualization of the dentatorubrothalamic tract traversing from dentate nucleus (**a**), to contralateral red nucleus (**b**); *yellow* boxes represent regions of interest.

DBS on these networks, and the value of computational modeling in discovering such processes.

6.2.3 Beyond Conventional Stimulation

Computational models have also been developed to determine the effects of different stimulation paradigms beyond conventional parameters such as frequency, current/voltage, and pulse width. One novel paradigm, coordinated reset, is a desynchronization technique that specifically targets pathological parkinsonian neuronal synchrony.[40] Extensively described by Tass et al, the function of coordinated reset is via the delivery of brief, high-frequency pulse trains through different DBS electrode contacts, resulting in unlearning or "resetting" of pathological neuronal synchrony and synaptic connectivity.[40,41,42] First described in computational model-based stimulations, coordinated reset has been translated to early human studies in PD patients, demonstrating promising acute and cumulative improvements in motor function.[43,44]

6.3 Advanced Imaging Techniques

6.3.1 Diffusion-Weighted Imaging and Tractography

The advent of sophisticated neuroimaging technologies has also improved our knowledge of complex neural circuitry and the role of DBS in modulating such pathways. As previously discussed, the clinical effects of DBS are at least in part due to the activation of adjacent WM fiber tracts from stimulation of the electrode. Visualization of these WM pathways is now increasingly possible using MR-based diffusion-weighted imaging (DWI) and tractography techniques.[33] DWI demonstrates the diffusion of water molecules within the brain. Since water diffuses more readily along the direction of a cellular barrier, such as an axon, rather than across it, it can be assumed that the path of water will follow axonal pathways. Thus, DWI approximates the course of WM fibers within the brain.[45,46] From the diffusion of water, a tensor model can be applied to reveal information pertaining to the directionality of the water diffusion, allowing for diffusion tensor imaging (DTI)[46]. However, while DTI may be sufficient to view large and known WM pathways, it is less helpful for visualizing smaller, more complex, and/or unknown fiber tracts. Thus, tractography techniques utilize data-driven algorithms, via various computer software platforms, to precisely identify specific WM tracts

traversing between set regions of interest (ROIs) based on the raw DWI data incorporated with structural T1 MRI data sets (▶ Fig. 6.2).[46,47]

The ability to model these axonal fibers with tractography lends itself to the application of DBS. Tractography can be used to improve understanding about anatomical networks affected by DBS, and to aid in preoperative surgical targeting as well as in postoperative assessments of outcomes. Pouratian et al used probabilistic tractography-based thalamic segmentation to evaluate the connectivity of the region of ventralis intermedius nucleus (Vim) implanted with DBS electrodes for tremor control.[48] Though the authors expected the region of Vim with the active electrode contact to have greater connectivity to the motor cortex, instead they found that there was greater connectivity to premotor cortex, thus providing insight into the connectivity networks involved in tremor control. In 2014, Rozanski et al assessed the connectivity pattern of the GPi in patients implanted with DBS electrodes for dystonia to determine why the ventral GPi is a more effective target than the dorsal region.[49] They used fiber tractography to visualize the specific WM fibers comprising the ventral and dorsal regions of the GPi, as well as their efferent projections. They found notable somatotopy within the GPi, such that the ventral region had greater connectivity to primary sensory and posterior motor cortices, whereas the dorsal region showed more connectivity to motor and premotor cortices. Therefore, these studies demonstrate the utility of tractography in furthering the understanding of connectivity and the networks affected by DBS for movement disorders.

In addition, knowledge of the location of certain WM tracts can allow for such tracts to be selectively targeted or avoided via DBS to produce the desired effects of stimulation. In 2014, Coenen et al studied 11 patients with tremor of various etiologies, who were implanted with DBS electrodes, using microelectrode recording and awake testing to localize the optimal electrode position within the Vim.[47] The authors then performed tractography from the preoperative imaging to visualize the dentatorubrothalamic tract (DRT) and computational modeling to view the electric field of the active contacts. They found that the most effective targets were within or adjacent to the DRT and the electric fields involved the DRT, thus concluding that tractography can be used to aid in surgical targeting using DBS. Similarly, Sweet et al assessed tremor outcomes in 14 tremor-predominant PD patients implanted with STN DBS electrodes.[34] They determined the active contacts from programming sessions and used computational modeling to find the VTA, which was then combined with tractography to visualize the

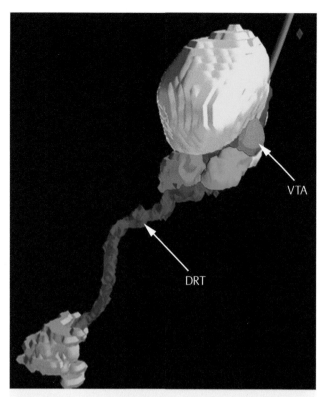

Fig. 6.3 Integration of computer modeling and tractography to demonstrate the relationship between the dentatorubrothalamic tract (*dark blue*) and volume of tissue activated of the active subthalamic nucleus contact (*dark pink*) in patients with tremor-predominant PD. Thalamus shown in *yellow*, STN in *green*, red nucleus in *red*, dentate nuclei in *light pink*. (Adapted from Sweet et al.[33])

Although DBS has demonstrated efficacy in smaller open-label studies of patients with treatment-resistant major depression and bipolar depression, larger scale randomized trials have been less successful at producing clinical improvement.[56,57] These discouraging results may be attributable to the unclear determination of targets that would effectively produce the same results seen with lesioning techniques. As psychiatric disorders are complex pathologies that are attributable to a dysfunction of networks as opposed to distinct anatomical correlates, new approaches are needed to identify more accurate targets. The convergence of multiple targeting methods, including tractography, has the potential for hypothesis-directed targeting for the treatment of specific neuropsychiatric symptoms.[58] The early results reported by Riva-Posse et al regarding their "connectomic approach" to DBS for depression provide a promising blueprint for the use of tractography in surgical targeting.[53]

An inherent limitation of computational models of network tractography is the high number of false-positive bundles that are produced when relying solely on orientation data.[59] These challenges present themselves whenever WM tracts converge or possess complex geometries.[60] Multiple methodological innovations are under development that can potentially generate better computational models, including the development of novel tractography algorithms, advances in machine learning, the optimization of signal prediction error via streamline filtering, and advanced microstructure modeling of directional vectors.[59,61] Despite these inherent limitations, the use of tractography in neuroscience will continue to expand as it is a noninvasive and powerful research tool.

6.3.2 Advancements in Anatomic Imaging

Improvements in the efficacy of neuromodulation will also be realized with advances in neuroimaging technology, allowing for better visualization of target structures. In clinical practice, DBS targets are often visualized with 1.5 or 3 T MRI, which provides adequate but indistinct localization of certain structures such as the STN.[62] Images obtained at this field strength cannot fully distinguish the STN from the substania nigra, and are unable to delineate the subdivisions of the thalamus. Higher field strength (so-called ultra-high-field MRI) using a 7 T magnet improves the identification of target structures by increasing the signal-to-noise ratio and enhancing image contrast.[63,64]

Susceptibility-weighted imaging (SWI) has also emerged as a promising modality that provides excellent delineation between gray matter and WM, especially at high field strength.[65,66] Using the combination of ultra-high-field MRI and SWI, Abosch et al reported the direct visualization and differentiation of the STN and substania nigra, and internal and external globus pallidus.[66] Impressively these technologies also allow for delineation of the internal thalamic nuclei.[66,67] The convergence of these improved anatomic imaging technologies and tractography has also been demonstrated in a preclinical model in rhesus macaque monkeys,[67] and requires further clinical study and validation. Ultimately, the combined use of imaging techniques provides an exciting new avenue of research for DBS target selection and verification.

DRT (▶ Fig. 6.3), and found that greater tremor control correlated with a closer proximity of the active electrode contact to the WM fibers of the DRT.[34] Furthermore, it is also possible to combine visualization of different tracts to maximize clinical effectiveness and minimize or avoid side effects. For example, Hana et al described the preoperative determination of the DRT in relation to the corticospinal tract for DBS planning.[50] Combination tractography has also been described in target selection for high-frequency-focused ultrasound ablation, with pre- and postoperative determination of the corticospinal tract, medial lemniscus, and DRT.[51]

Several studies have also utilized tractography to aid in DBS targeting for the treatment of psychiatric disorders.[52,53,54,55] In 2009, Gutman et al used tractography to look at two potential DBS targets, the subcallosal cingulate gyrus (SCC) and the anterior limb of the internal capsule for the treatment of depression.[52] The authors found that both targets had their own distinct connectivity patterns, but also contained overlapping WM connections. Riva-Posse et al utilized tractography for preoperative targeting of the SCC in 11 treatment-resistant depression patients, to visualize the point of convergence of four fiber bundles thought to be implicated in the pathophysiology of the disease.[53] They found that using this technique, 81.8% of patients were treatment responders at 1 year, of which six patients went into remission.

6.4 Future Applications of Computational Modeling and Advanced Imaging

With an increased understanding of neural networks and brain connectivity, and the effects of DBS in modulating these complex circuits, computational modeling and advanced imaging techniques can be used to aid in the discovery of new targets for diseases currently treated with DBS and for diseases that do not yet have effective therapies. As an example, perhaps targeting the DRT rather than the Vim or STN will become the most efficacious treatment for tremor control. Although most of the current tractography studies are performed retrospectively, there is great interest in the prospective and intraoperative determination of the ideal DBS target. Novel software research tools, such as StimVision, can provide interactive intraoperative visualization and adjustment of DBS electrode placement and VTA in relation to an individual patient's imaging and tractography data.[68]

Investigations and treatments for anorexia nervosa,[69] Alzheimer disease,[70] depression,[53,54,55] epilepsy,[71] pain,[72] and numerous other diseases could be largely improved with such technologies, with focus on a hypothesis-driven approach to target selection. The contemporary understanding of these complex disease states is likely attributable to a dysfunction of networks rather than an isolated neurotransmitter or structural abnormality, and thus an understanding of the widespread WM connections and underlying brain circuitry is essential to facilitate optimal target selection. Ultimately, patient heterogeneity may require an individualized symptom-directed or patient-directed approach. Utilizing computational modeling techniques to simulate stimulation of a given region of the brain and combining this with imaging modalities such as tractography, can provide insight into the pathophysiology of diseases and how treatment strategies influence such disease states, while also enabling more effective targeting for DBS. Understanding the potential for such tools both in everyday practice and in investigational endeavors will be a critical aspect of progress for the field and for the treatment of patients.

References

[1] Deuschl G, Schade-Brittinger C, Krack P, et al. German Parkinson Study Group, Neurostimulation Section. A randomized trial of deep-brain stimulation for Parkinson's disease. N Engl J Med. 2006; 355(9):896–908

[2] Follett KA, Weaver FM, Stern M, et al. CSP 468 Study Group. Pallidal versus subthalamic deep-brain stimulation for Parkinson's disease. N Engl J Med. 2010; 362(22):2077–2091

[3] Obeso JA, Olanow CW, Rodriguez-Oroz MC, Krack P, Kumar R, Lang AE, Deep-Brain Stimulation for Parkinson's Disease Study Group. Deep-brain stimulation of the subthalamic nucleus or the pars interna of the globus pallidus in Parkinson's disease. N Engl J Med. 2001; 345(13):956–963

[4] Limousin P, Speelman JD, Gielen F, Janssens M. Multicentre European study of thalamic stimulation in parkinsonian and essential tremor. J Neurol Neurosurg Psychiatry. 1999; 66(3):289–296

[5] Schuurman PR, Bosch DA, Bossuyt PM, et al. A comparison of continuous thalamic stimulation and thalamotomy for suppression of severe tremor. N Engl J Med. 2000; 342(7):461–468

[6] Fasano A, Lozano AM. Deep brain stimulation for movement disorders: 2015 and beyond. Curr Opin Neurol. 2015; 28(4):423–436

[7] Kupsch A, Benecke R, Müller J, et al. Deep-Brain Stimulation for Dystonia Study Group. Pallidal deep-brain stimulation in primary generalized or segmental dystonia. N Engl J Med. 2006; 355(19):1978–1990

[8] Nuttin B, Cosyns P, Demeulemeester H, Gybels J, Meyerson B. Electrical stimulation in anterior limbs of internal capsules in patients with obsessive-compulsive disorder. Lancet. 1999; 354(9189):1526

[9] Alonso P, Cuadras D, Gabriëls L, et al. Deep brain stimulation for obsessive-compulsive disorder: a meta-analysis of treatment outcome and predictors of response. PLoS One. 2015; 10(7):e0133591

[10] Kern DS, Kumar R. Deep brain stimulation. Neurologist. 2007; 13(5):237–252

[11] Butson CR, McIntyre CC. Tissue and electrode capacitance reduce neural activation volumes during deep brain stimulation. Clin Neurophysiol. 2005; 116 (10):2490–2500

[12] McIntyre CC, Savasta M, Kerkerian-Le Goff L, Vitek JL. Uncovering the mechanism(s) of action of deep brain stimulation: activation, inhibition, or both. Clin Neurophysiol. 2004; 115(6):1239–1248

[13] Lozano AM, Dostrovsky J, Chen R, Ashby P. Deep brain stimulation for Parkinson's disease: disrupting the disruption. Lancet Neurol. 2002; 1(4):225–231

[14] Grafton ST, Turner RS, Desmurget M, et al. Normalizing motor-related brain activity: subthalamic nucleus stimulation in Parkinson disease. Neurology. 2006; 66(8):1192–1199

[15] Miocinovic S, Parent M, Butson CR, et al. Computational analysis of subthalamic nucleus and lenticular fasciculus activation during therapeutic deep brain stimulation. J Neurophysiol. 2006; 96(3):1569–1580

[16] Kahan J, Mancini L, Urner M, et al. Therapeutic subthalamic nucleus deep brain stimulation reverses cortico-thalamic coupling during voluntary movements in Parkinson's disease. PLoS One. 2012; 7(12):e50270

[17] Gradinaru V, Mogri M, Thompson KR, Henderson JM, Deisseroth K. Optical deconstruction of parkinsonian neural circuitry. Science. 2009; 324(5925): 354–359

[18] Mayberg HS. Limbic-cortical dysregulation: a proposed model of depression. J Neuropsychiatry Clin Neurosci. 1997; 9(3):471–481

[19] Laxton AW, Tang-Wai DF, McAndrews MP, et al. A phase I trial of deep brain stimulation of memory circuits in Alzheimer's disease. Ann Neurol. 2010; 68 (4):521–534

[20] Figee M, Wielaard I, Mazaheri A, Denys D. Neurosurgical targets for compulsivity: what can we learn from acquired brain lesions? Neurosci Biobehav Rev. 2013; 37(3):328–339

[21] van Hartevelt TJ, Cabral J, Møller A, et al. Evidence from a rare case study for Hebbian-like changes in structural connectivity induced by long-term deep brain stimulation. Front Behav Neurosci. 2015; 9:167

[22] Grill WM, Snyder AN, Miocinovic S. Deep brain stimulation creates an informational lesion of the stimulated nucleus. Neuroreport. 2004; 15(7):1137–1140

[23] Grill WM, Jr. Modeling the effects of electric fields on nerve fibers: influence of tissue electrical properties. IEEE Trans Biomed Eng. 1999; 46(8):918–928

[24] McIntyre CC, Grill WM. Excitation of central nervous system neurons by nonuniform electric fields. Biophys J. 1999; 76(2):878–888

[25] McIntyre CC, Grill WM. Finite element analysis of the current-density and electric field generated by metal microelectrodes. Ann Biomed Eng. 2001; 29 (3):227–235

[26] McIntyre CC, Grill WM. Extracellular stimulation of central neurons: influence of stimulus waveform and frequency on neuronal output. J Neurophysiol. 2002; 88(4):1592–1604

[27] Butson CR, McIntyre CC. Current steering to control the volume of tissue activated during deep brain stimulation. Brain Stimul. 2008; 1(1):7–15

[28] Maks CB, Butson CR, Walter BL, Vitek JL, McIntyre CC. Deep brain stimulation activation volumes and their association with neurophysiological mapping and therapeutic outcomes. J Neurol Neurosurg Psychiatry. 2009; 80(6): 659–666

[29] Mikos A, Bowers D, Noecker AM, et al. Patient-specific analysis of the relationship between the volume of tissue activated during DBS and verbal fluency. Neuroimage. 2011; 54 Suppl 1:S238–S246

[30] Cazemier JL, Clascá F, Tiesinga PH. Connectomic analysis of brain networks: novel techniques and future directions. Front Neuroanat. 2016; 10:110

[31] Kudela P, Anderson WS. Computational modeling of subdural cortical stimulation: a quantitative spatiotemporal analysis of action potential initiation in a high-density multicompartment model. Neuromodulation. 2015; 18(7): 552–564, discussion 564–565

[32] Boothe DL, Yu AB, Kudela P, Anderson WS, Vettel JM, Franaszczuk PJ. Impact of neuronal membrane damage on the local field potential in a large-scale simulation of cerebral cortex. Front Neurol. 2017; 8:236

[33] Sweet JA, Pace J, Girgis F, Miller JP. Computational modeling and neuroimaging techniques for targeting during deep brain stimulation. Front Neuroanat. 2016; 10:71

[34] Sweet JA, Walter BL, Gunalan K, Chaturvedi A, McIntyre CC, Miller JP. Fiber tractography of the axonal pathways linking the basal ganglia and cerebellum in Parkinson disease: implications for targeting in deep brain stimulation. J Neurosurg. 2014; 120(4):988–996

[35] Gunalan K, Chaturvedi A, Howell B, et al. Creating and parameterizing patient-specific deep brain stimulation pathway-activation models using the hyperdirect pathway as an example. PLoS One. 2017; 12(4):e0176132

[36] Gunalan K, Howell B, McIntyre CC. Quantifying axonal responses in patient-specific models of subthalamic deep brain stimulation. Neuroimage. 2018; 172:263–277

[37] Rubin JE, Terman D. High frequency stimulation of the subthalamic nucleus eliminates pathological thalamic rhythmicity in a computational model. J Comput Neurosci. 2004; 16(3):211–235

[38] Hahn PJ, McIntyre CC. Modeling shifts in the rate and pattern of subthalamopallidal network activity during deep brain stimulation. J Comput Neurosci. 2010; 28(3):425–441

[39] Humphries MD, Gurney K. Network effects of subthalamic deep brain stimulation drive a unique mixture of responses in basal ganglia output. Eur J Neurosci. 2012; 36(2):2240–2251

[40] Tass PA. A model of desynchronizing deep brain stimulation with a demand-controlled coordinated reset of neural subpopulations. Biol Cybern. 2003; 89 (2):81–88

[41] Tass PA, Majtanik M. Long-term anti-kindling effects of desynchronizing brain stimulation: a theoretical study. Biol Cybern. 2006; 94(1):58–66

[42] Ebert M, Hauptmann C, Tass PA. Coordinated reset stimulation in a large-scale model of the STN-GPe circuit. Front Comput Neurosci. 2014; 8:154

[43] Adamchic I, Hauptmann C, Barnikol UB, et al. Coordinated reset neuromodulation for Parkinson's disease: proof-of-concept study. Mov Disord. 2014; 29 (13):1679–1684

[44] Syrkin-Nikolau J, Neuville R, O'Day J, et al. Coordinated reset vibrotactile stimulation shows prolonged improvement in Parkinson's disease. Mov Disord. 2018; 33(1):179–180

[45] Henderson JM. "Connectomic surgery": diffusion tensor imaging (DTI) tractography as a targeting modality for surgical modulation of neural networks. Front Integr Nuerosci. 2012; 6:15

[46] Klein JC, Lorenz B, Kang JS, et al. Diffusion tensor imaging of white matter involvement in essential tremor. Hum Brain Mapp. 2011; 32(6): 896–904

[47] Coenen VA, Allert N, Paus S, Kronenbürger M, Urbach H, Mädler B. Modulation of the cerebello-thalamo-cortical network in thalamic deep brain stimulation for tremor: a diffusion tensor imaging study. Neurosurgery. 2014; 75 (6):657–669, discussion 669–670

[48] Pouratian N, Zheng Z, Bari AA, Behnke E, Elias WJ, Desalles AA. Multi-institutional evaluation of deep brain stimulation targeting using probabilistic connectivity-based thalamic segmentation. J Neurosurg. 2011; 115(5):995–1004

[49] Rozanski VE, Vollmar C, Cunha JP, et al. Connectivity patterns of pallidal DBS electrodes in focal dystonia: a diffusion tensor tractography study. Neuroimage. 2014; 84:435–442

[50] Hana A, Hana A, Dooms G, Boecher-Schwarz H, Hertel F. Depiction of dentatorubrothalamic tract fibers in patients with Parkinson's disease and multiple sclerosis in deep brain stimulation. BMC Res Notes. 2016; 9:345

[51] Chazen JL, Sarva H, Stieg PE, et al. Clinical improvement associated with targeted interruption of the cerebellothalamic tract following MR-guided focused ultrasound for essential tremor. J Neurosurg. 2018; 129: 15–323

[52] Gutman DA, Holtzheimer PE, Behrens TE, Johansen-Berg H, Mayberg HS. A tractography analysis of two deep brain stimulation white matter targets for depression. Biol Psychiatry. 2009; 65(4):276–282

[53] Riva-Posse P, Choi KS, Holtzheimer PE, et al. A connectomic approach for subcallosal cingulate deep brain stimulation surgery: prospective targeting in treatment-resistant depression. Mol Psychiatry. 2018; 23(4):843–849

[54] Makris N, Rathi Y, Mouradian P, et al. Variability and anatomical specificity of the orbitofrontothalamic fibers of passage in the ventral capsule/ventral striatum (VC/VS): precision care for patient-specific tractography-guided targeting of deep brain stimulation (DBS) in obsessive compulsive disorder (OCD). Brain Imaging Behav. 2016; 10(4):1054–1067

[55] Schlaepfer TE, Bewernick BH, Kayser S, Mädler B, Coenen VA. Rapid effects of deep brain stimulation for treatment-resistant major depression. Biol Psychiatry. 2013; 73(12):1204–1212

[56] Dougherty DD, Rezai AR, Carpenter LL, et al. A randomized sham-controlled trial of deep brain stimulation of the ventral capsule/ventral striatum for chronic treatment-resistant depression. Biol Psychiatry. 2015; 78(4):240–248

[57] Holtzheimer PE, Husain MM, Lisanby SH, et al. Subcallosal cingulate deep brain stimulation for treatment-resistant depression: a multisite, randomised, sham-controlled trial. Lancet Psychiatry. 2017; 4(11):839–849

[58] Holtzheimer PE, Mayberg HS. Stuck in a rut: rethinking depression and its treatment. Trends Neurosci. 2011; 34(1):1–9

[59] Maier-Hein KH, Neher PF, Houde JC, et al. The challenge of mapping the human connectome based on diffusion tractography. Nat Commun. 2017; 8(1):1349

[60] Jbabdi S, Johansen-Berg H. Tractography: where do we go from here? Brain Connect. 2011; 1(3):169–183

[61] Thomas C, Ye FQ, Irfanoglu MO, et al. Anatomical accuracy of brain connections derived from diffusion MRI tractography is inherently limited. Proc Natl Acad Sci U S A. 2014; 111(46):16574–16579

[62] Slavin KV, Thulborn KR, Wess C, Nersesyan H. Direct visualization of the human subthalamic nucleus with 3 T MR imaging. AJNR Am J Neuroradiol. 2006; 27(1):80–84

[63] Lenglet C, Abosch A, Yacoub E, De Martino F, Sapiro G, Harel N. Comprehensive in vivo mapping of the human basal ganglia and thalamic connectome in individuals using 7 T MRI. PLoS One. 2012; 7(1):e29153

[64] Vaughan JT, Garwood M, Collins CM, et al. 7 T vs. 4T: RF power, homogeneity, and signal-to-noise comparison in head images. Magn Reson Med. 2001; 46 (1):24–30

[65] Haacke EM, Xu Y, Cheng YC, Reichenbach JR. Susceptibility weighted imaging (SWI). Magn Reson Med. 2004; 52(3):612–618

[66] Abosch A, Yacoub E, Ugurbil K, Harel N. An assessment of current brain targets for deep brain stimulation surgery with susceptibility-weighted imaging at 7 tesla. Neurosurgery. 2010; 67(6):1745–1756, discussion 1756

[67] Xiao Y, Zitella LM, Duchin Y, et al. Multimodal 7 T imaging of thalamic nuclei for preclinical deep brain stimulation applications. Front Neurosci. 2016; 10:264

[68] Noecker AM, Choi KS, Riva-Posse P, Gross RE, Mayberg HS, McIntyre CC. StimVision software: examples and applications in subcallosal cingulate deep brain stimulation for depression. Neuromodulation. 2018; 21(2):191–196

[69] Lipsman N, Woodside DB, Giacobbe P, et al. Subcallosal cingulate deep brain stimulation for treatment-refractory anorexia nervosa: a phase 1 pilot trial. Lancet. 2013; 381(9875):1361–1370

[70] Lozano AM, Fosdick L, Chakravarty MM, et al. A phase II study of Fornix deep brain stimulation in mild Alzheimer's disease. J Alzheimers Dis. 2016; 54 (2):777–787

[71] Fisher R, Salanova V, Witt T, et al. SANTE Study Group. Electrical stimulation of the anterior nucleus of thalamus for treatment of refractory epilepsy. Epilepsia. 2010; 51(5):899–908

[72] Boccard SG, Pereira EA, Aziz TZ. Deep brain stimulation for chronic pain. J Clin Neurosci. 2015; 22(10):1537–1543

7 Closed-Loop Stimulation Methods: Current Practice and Future Promise

Vivek P. Buch, Andrew I. Yang, Timothy H. Lucas, H. Isaac Chen

Abstract

Deep brain stimulation and other neuromodulatory therapies have traditionally been performed in the absence of real-time feedback and with constant stimulation parameters (open-loop stimulation). Although this approach has been quite successful, the clinical outcomes are now approaching a plateau. In the development of the next generation of neuromodulatory therapies, an emerging concept showing significant promise is closed-loop stimulation or adaptive neuromodulation in which a real-time feedback signal triggers or modifies stimulation. Theoretically, closed-loop strategies are superior to conventional open-loop stimulation for several reasons, including a wider therapeutic window, improved efficacy, and prolonged battery life. According to control theory, three parts comprise closed-loop stimulation systems: a feedback signal, a module that extracts features from the signal and interprets them, and a stimulation paradigm. Myriad options exist for each of these components, which lead to both the complexity and exciting possibilities of closed-loop strategies. The objective of this chapter is to provide an overview of these options, as well as the commercially available closed-loop systems and limited clinical data that has been accrued thus far. Then follows a discussion of the scientific and technological challenges that need to be overcome for broad clinical adoption of closed-loop neuromodulation. An understanding of these principles will be crucial for practitioners of neuromodulation to partake in the process of designing closed-loop systems and realizing their full potential.

Keywords: Activa PC + S, adaptive DBS, beta oscillation, closed-loop stimulation, feedback signal, NeuroPace, responsive neuromodulation

7.1 Introduction

Current deep brain stimulation (DBS) technologies are built upon simplistic circuits and control algorithms that deliver stimulation constitutively and require an iterative process of adjusting parameters to optimize clinical efficacy.[1,2] This "open-loop" stimulation paradigm lacks internal feedback. Recently, more intuitive "closed-loop" or "adaptive" paradigms have been developed which integrate real-time physiological feedback signals (▶ Fig. 7.1). These techniques promise to improve outcomes in patients with existing indications for neuromodulation, such as movement disorders,[3,4,5,6,7] and expand indications for additional disease states.[8]

There are several putative advantages of adaptive DBS (aDBS) over existing technologies. Closed-loop modulation of stimulation parameters could improve symptom control in conditions characterized by frequent symptom fluctuations, as in Parkinson's disease (PD)[9] or essential tremor (ET). In diseases characterized by episodic symptoms, such as seizure disorders, closed modulation would intervene at the point of seizure onset. In addition, aDBS would decrease the on-stimulation intervals by eliminating current delivery when symptoms are absent (e.g., during sleep), thereby extending battery life. Further, feedback control would modulate gain functions to reduce unwanted stimulation-induced side effects. Reducing unnecessary stimulation may reduce off-target effects that result from maladaptive plasticity.[10] Finally, closed-loop modulation would reduce the number of visits to physician office and parameter setting changes, which in turn could lower healthcare delivery costs.

With these advantages come some disadvantages. The engineering trade-off of closed-loop systems is that they must be designed for very specific applications. The optimal control strategy for PD will not likely be optimal for dystonia, epilepsy, or ET. Thus, the number of independent systems will grow. Also, as the control mechanisms become increasingly sophisticated, the internal mechanisms and functionality will be less apparent to the surgeon end-user. Similar design evolution has been observed in car engines. While the standard engines developed in the 1970s and 1980s employed common design features that permitted the neighborhood mechanic access for routine repairs, the highly computerized and customized engines manufactured nowadays require specialized technicians and complex diagnostic equipment for basic repairs. It is thus incumbent on functional neurosurgeons and other clinicians involved in neuromodulation to understand the fundamentals of aDBS. This chapter reviews these principles in the context of emerging systems and their intended disease indications, and reviews future direction on our immediate horizon.

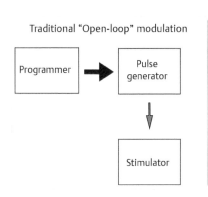

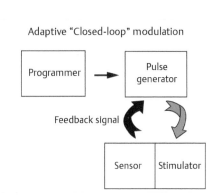

Fig. 7.1 Schematic representation of neuromodulation strategies. Color of arrows indicates signal type (*black* = input, *green* = activating signal, *red* = deactivating signal). Size of arrow indicates relative importance.

7.2 Approaches to Closed-Loop Neuromodulation

7.2.1 Considerations for Designing an Optimal System

The governing principles of closed-loop systems are derived from a field of engineering known as control theory that was first formally conceptualized in the mid 1800s by physicist James Clerk Maxwell[11] and was further developed over the next century.[12,13,14] Broadly speaking, feedback control theory dictates there should be three linked components: a controller, a system, and a sensor. The controller exerts an effect on the system known as the control action, which produces a measurable system output known as the process variable (PV). The PV, measured by the sensor, then informs the controller in the form of a feedback signal. The controller will then compare the PV to the programmed system set point (SP) and calculate an error measurement (PV − SP). Based on this error measurement, the controller will modulate its control action on the system (▶ Fig. 7.2). One of the most common examples of applied control theory is centralized heating. The controller is the heater unit, the system is the room temperature, and the sensor is the thermostat. The heater is turned on or off (control action) based on the thermostat reading (PV) compared to the desired temperature (SP).

Closed-loop neuromodulation applies control theory to translational devices. In control theory parlance, systems stimulate the nervous system (control action) in response to physiological signals (PV) relative to a desired physiological state (SP). Understanding control theory as it is applied to neuromodulation devices affords neurosurgeons and engineers a common language that facilitates communication and accelerates the pace of translation.

Several fundamental considerations influence the conversation (▶ Table 7.1). First, each disease condition requires a specific design solution. For example, intractable epilepsy requires a device with sensitive, customized algorithms for detecting seizure onsets within a narrow temporal window. Rapid seizure detection, in turn, must trigger recurrent stimulation to effectively suppress seizure propagation before seizure spread. By contrast, the disease state of ET is characterized by much slower time-scale oscillations and may consequently only require basic phase-amplitude algorithms averaged over long time sweeps to trigger suppressive stimulation. Thus, the device functionality must be specific to the disease state. Beyond disease specificity, the device must be tunable within a dynamic range to match patient-specific disease characteristics. This is because there is variability in physiological control signals within disease states. Returning to the epilepsy example, patients may have multiple seizure types and seizure onset detection may evolve over time. Accordingly, devices must have the capacity to be both disease- and patient-specific.

Second, there are engineering trade-offs between size, weight, power, and cost. Termed SWAP-C in aerospace engineering, the design trade-offs are equally applicable to medical device development. Increasingly, devices are designed for low-power architecture, compact form factor, and minimal weight.[15,16,17] When operationalized, these trade-offs mean that systems often sacrifice circuit complexity—and hence algorithm flexibility—for lower power consumption requirements and reduced device size. Reduced complexity leads to lower unit production costs and lower barriers to entry into the competitive device market. Of course, lower complexity means less programming flexibility. Neurosurgeons and engineers must work together to maximize idealized device features within design constraints.

Table 7.1 Criteria for designing closed-loop systems

Criteria	Design parameter considerations
Indication	Disease-specific physiology dictates ideal control algorithm and stimulation paradigm
Complexity	Increasingly complex parameters lead to increased sophistication but decreased feasibility
Clinical acceptability	Characteristics of electrodes, battery, and interface affect ergonomics of daily use and longevity
Stage of technology	Proven effectiveness of existing technology must be weighed against potential benefits of new technology

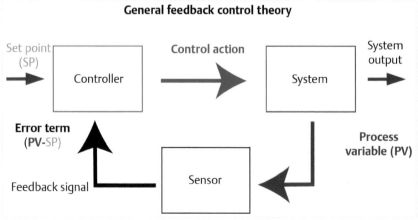

General feedback control theory

Fig. 7.2 Box diagram of general feedback control theory.

Third, system design elements must be acceptable to patients who have limited capacity to interface with the system directly. Electrodes, chassis, connector cables, and external peripherals must operate with little or no disruption in normal life activities of the patients. Increasing invasiveness of a device can become a barrier to patient adoption. For instance, in our experience, many patients refuse to undergo placement of Neuro-Pace® systems because of the requirement of a craniectomy and the limitation on future brain MRI. Devices which require battery replacement obligate patients to undergo multiple surgeries, a further barrier to wide adoption. Vagal nerve stimulators can produce painful cervical sensations or repeated urges to swallow that patients find dissatisfying. These and other factors diminish device adoption and must be considered in the early phase of development.

To provide further insight into possible approaches for closed-loop neuromodulation, the subsequent sections will summarize sources of feedback, stimulation strategies and control algorithms, and the small but growing literature on clinical outcomes with aDBS.

7.2.2 Sources of Feedback Signals

The main feature of aDBS is real-time modulation driven by physiological signals. Many signal sources have been considered (▶ Fig. 7.3). Current versions of aDBS rely upon a single feedback signal, but future devices will likely utilize multiple signals in parallel.

Single- and multi-unit activity

Extracellular action potentials are a robust source of discrete physiological data. Because individual neurons may be tuned to specific behavior features, such as the direction of extremity motion[18] and the orientation of visual stimuli,[19] devices may be highly precise in signal input. This type of information drives a variety of human brain–computer interfaces (BCIs), including systems for controlling neuroprosthetics,[20] graphical user interfaces,[21] and functional electrical stimulation.[22,23]

Extracellular action potential recordings require high electrical impedance. Therefore, multielectrode arrays, such as the

Utah array (Blackrock Microsystems, LLC, Salt Lake City, UT) that consists of a 10 × 10 array of electrodes, are used. Besides its use in BCIs, the Utah array has also been used to study the spread of the ictal wavefront in seizures.[24] Michigan probes and microwire constructions are other methods of chronically recording neurons. Future arrays, such as those being developed by MIT's Media Lab, promise thousands of contacts for chronic recording. As the number of input channels increases, so too must the complexity of the circuitry and computational processing to analyze this data.

Despite the advantage of highly discrete input signals afforded with single- or multi-unit activity, certain drawbacks limit their use as feedback signals. The technology available for recording this activity in patients allows only small areas of the brain to be sampled. Also, these arrays are designed for the cortical surface. There are few solutions for subcortical targets. Single-unit recording quality is also finite, owing to the inherent mismatch in material properties between the brain and electrodes.[25] Small shifts in electrode position, build-up of impedance over time, or loss of individual neurons due to damage results in unstable source signals. Thus, chronic applications require simplifying decoding algorithms[26] or frequent recalibration[21] to maintain performance over time. These challenges limit long-term durability of penetrating arrays and may prevent their widespread adoption for translational indications.

Local field potentials

Local field potentials (LFPs) represent the integrated analog synaptic inputs into cortical layers rather than the discrete spike activity of those neurons (i.e., postsynaptic activity).[27] This oscillatory activity is classified by dominant frequency ranges (▶ Table 7.2) and it plays a role in brain functions like memory formation[28] and temporal binding of neural activity.[29] Interactions exist between LFPs across frequency bands (e.g., theta-gamma coupling in the coding of multi-item messages[30]) and between LFPs and the firing of individual neurons that may contribute to disease states such as PD.

With existing technology, LFPs are thought to be a reliable source for signal detection.[31] LFP recordings benefit from the fact that they can be recorded with low-impedance electrodes

Currently implemented feedback signals

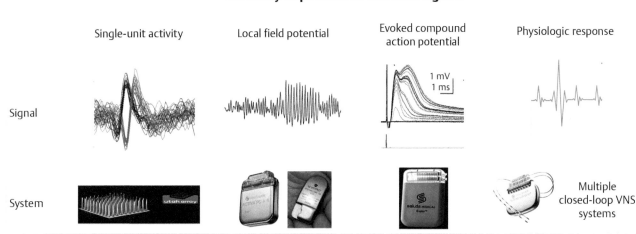

Fig. 7.3 Types of currently used feedback signals and corresponding systems.

Table 7.2 Types of local field potentials

Oscillation	Frequency (Hz)
Delta	1–4
Theta	4–10
Alpha	10–14
Beta	14–36
Low gamma	36–70
High gamma	>70

with larger contact surface areas. These electrodes cause less local tissue damage. Accordingly, LFPs are less sensitive to changes in electrode impedance caused by tissue destruction and gliosis. The relaxation of the electrode size constraint enables large sheets of electrode arrays to be deployed over the brain surface. Moreover, LFPs can be reliably recorded from concentric ring electrodes, as in the case of depth electrode contacts. Thus, LFPs can be recorded from deep structures safely for long durations. This relaxed electrode design feature makes it possible to record and stimulate from the same lead,[32] which is a major advantage for neuromodulatory devices. Highly flexible graphene arrays further improve tissue–electrode compliance matching and demonstrate superior performance over millions of duty cycles of stimulation and recording.[33] Penetrating, high-impedance electrodes use sharp tips that erode and breakdown in the presence of electrolytic charge buildup during stimulation, and consequently have limited utility in chronic stimulation paradigms.

The accessibility of LFP data in humans has elucidated a number of biomarkers for closed-loop neuromodulation. Beta oscillations in PD are a prominent example. Though the causal significance of beta oscillations in PD pathology remains unclear, their strong association with PD symptoms makes them a potentially useful feedback signal for closed-loops systems. While neural activity within the globus pallidus of healthy rhesus monkeys is not synchronized, treatment with 1-methyl-4-phenyl-1,2,3,6-tetrahydropyridine (MPTP) induces periodic oscillations in a significant fraction of neurons.[34] Similarly, oscillations in the 15 to 30 Hz band are a prominent feature of subthalamic nucleus (STN) recordings in PD patients.[35,36,37] The power of beta oscillations in the basal ganglia is related to symptom severity in PD, as it is increased when dopamine is depleted[38,39,40] and reduced during voluntary movement[39,41,42] and by DBS.[43,44,45] Moreover, low-frequency stimulation (20 Hz) of the STN in patients modestly slows motor activity.[46] The origin of these beta oscillations is not completely clear, although there is evidence to suggest roles of both the motor cortex[47,48,49] and the STN–globus pallidus pars externa circuit.[50,51]

Other LFP relationships are also being explored. Recently, it was demonstrated that DBS reduces coupling between the phase of beta oscillations and broadband amplitude in the motor cortex.[52] In addition to beta oscillations, dopamine influences the power of low-frequency bands[40,53] and non-beta frequencies may be better correlated with PD symptoms.[54]

LFP signals may be used in novel ways, such as in temporary applications for brain *rehabilitation* following injury. This concept is made possible by a number of electrode arrays which dissolve over time, as their use is no longer needed. Examples include resorbable silicon electrodes that dissolve after pre-programmed durations and do not require removal.[55]

Peripheral electromyography and inertial recordings

Clinical phenotypes are important manifestations of neurological disease. For movement disorders, real-time information concerning extremity function is a natural feedback source for closed-loop neuromodulation. Surface electromyography[56,57] and multi-axis accelerometers[58,59,60] can monitor tremor amplitude. Such functionality may even be built into smart watches.[59]

As these systems mature to clinical reality, wireless data fidelity and security will become driving factors in design. Environmental electromagnetic noise that is present in everyday life—will influence the utility of these devices and corresponding control algorithms. Cell phones, smart watches, activity monitors, and other sources of wireless signal may confound wireless medical device communication. In the modern era, engineers must design communication systems with the understanding that systems may be hacked (intentionally or unintentionally). Thus, secure, high-fidelity communication protocols must be developed.

Other signals

Although neural activity is most often measured electrically, there are other sources of physiological signals that may be tapped. In PD, symptoms arise due the loss of striatal dopamine from substantia nigra inputs. DBS may increase striatal dopamine release.[61] Thus, Dopamine metabolite concentration could serve as a biomarker of stimulation efficacy. Indeed, microdialysis has been used to assess extracellular neurotransmitter levels during the placement of DBS leads.[62] Similar to insulin pumps that use blood glucose measures to adjust insulin release, it is not difficult to imagine a system that monitors neurotransmitter levels to modulate stimulation. Such a system could be used in movement disorders or neuropsychiatric conditions, such as refractory depression. Alternatively, carbon fiber electrodes can be used to detect electroactive molecules, such as dopamine, adenosine, and oxygen, in real-time using fast-scanning cyclic voltammetry or amperometry techniques.[63] These methods are primarily being tested in animal models.[63,64] Feasibility in a human subject has been demonstrated,[65] though the long-term viability of this technology remains to be studied.

As reliable biomarkers are identified in other diseases or cognitive states, neuroengineering design principles may be applied. An emerging example is the use of prefrontal cortex signals of volition as control signals in psychiatric disorders.[66] In obsessive compulsive disorder (OCD), for instance, the volition to induce stimulation could enable a patient to intentionally "will" the system to trigger stimulations when obsessive thoughts are particularly intrusive.[67]

7.2.3 Control Systems and Stimulation Paradigms

Control systems depend on the disease- or state-specific biomarkers. In epilepsy, control systems are based on seizure detection algorithms.[68,69,70,71] In PD, beta oscillatory features are the candidate biomarkers. Specifically, amplitude and phase appear to be salient features. Amplitude-modulated approaches trigger stimulation when the amplitude of beta oscillations

Table 7.3 Stimulation paradigms in closed-loop systems

Paradigm	Closed-loop triggered stimulation
Binary	Predetermined stimulation parameters "on" or "off"
Graded	Changes in shape, intensity, frequency, pulse width, or location
Coordinated reset	Short bursts of high-frequency pulse trains
Hybrid	Coincident detection, phase-amplitude coupling, spike-phase coupling, central-peripheral biomarker pairing

Table 7.4 Current clinical indications for closed-loop neuromodulation

Indication	System	Feedback signal	Closed-loop target
Parkinson's disease	PC + S	Neural beta oscillations	Basal ganglia (STN, GPi)
Epilepsy	RNS VNS	Neural time-series Heart rate	Epileptogenic foci CN X
Chronic pain	SCS	Dorsal column ECAP	Pain fibers

Abbreviations: CN, cranial nerve; ECAP, evoked compound action potential; GPi, globus pallidus interna; RNS, responsive neurostimulator; SCS, spinal cord stimulation; STN, subthalamic nucleus; VNS, vagal nerve stimulator.

reaches a certain threshold. In contrast, phase-modulated approaches trigger stimulations at a particular phase of the oscillation that can either attenuate or potentiate the oscillation.[72]

Once a suitable feature has been identified, a number of stimulation paradigms are possible (▶ Table 7.3). The simplest strategy is binary modulation, in which preset stimulation parameters are triggered when feature criteria are satisfied. Cardiac sensitivity with Model 106 Aspire VNS (LivaNova PLC, London, United Kingdom previously Cyberonics, Inc., Houston, TX) is an example. When a rapid increase in heart rate is detected, the VNS runs a stimulation routine. Step-wise or graded responses are an alternative strategy. In this scenario, one or more stimulation parameters are modulated once feature criteria are met.[31] Paradigms can implement numerous steps to create near-continuous changes in stimulation intensity as driven by the feedback signal.[6] The specific method for defining the relationship between feedback and stimulation will likely rely upon different aspects of control theory.[5,6,7] Stimulation variables in this paradigm could include stimulation amplitude steps, pulse train, frequency, pulse width, electrode channel, and more complex combinations of parameters. Another paradigm is the coordinated reset. This method desynchronizes network activity and inhibits negative plasticity effects through short bursts of high-frequency pulse trains.[73,74,75] Finally, hybrid paradigms use complex feedback signals, such as coincident detectors, spike-phase, and central-peripheral detectors. These use input schemes that integrate information from multiple sources simultaneously. A hypothetical example of such a system could include one that detects beta oscillations in motor cortex and peripheral tremor oscillations from a wearable accelerometer to modulate PD tremor.

7.3 Existing Technology Platforms and Clinical Data (▶ Table 7.4)

7.3.1 Adaptive Deep Brain Stimulation

Activa PC + S device parameters

The Activa PC + S (Medtronic Inc., Minneapolis, MN) has been approved for investigational purposes in the United States. This system offers the same therapeutic stimulation variables as the clinically approved Activa PC (i.e., pulse widths, frequencies, amplitudes, and constant voltage versus constant current). In addition, the form factor is similar. The Activa PC + S uses the standard Medtronic leads and can accommodate up to two leads with four electrodes each for a total of eight channels of concurrent stimulation or sensing. Similar to prior Medtronic DBS platforms, the Activa PC + S is optimized for stimulation, and frequent recording may lead to rapid battery depletion.[76] A rechargeable system capable of sensing (Activa RC + S) is under development.

Up to two channels from each lead can be selected for recording of the voltage time series/LFP or spectral power in prespecified bandwidths (2.5–500 Hz, bandwidth ± 1.5/8/16 Hz).[77] Time series can be post-processed offline, whereas spectral power can be used for real-time calculations, allowing the use of internal triggers for data collection.[78] Data can be collected via two modes. The external trigger mode allows for recording that is started and stopped manually and has a sampling rate of 200 to 800 Hz. The auto-detect mode stores data continuously in a temporary buffer at a sampling rate of 200 to 422 Hz and saves segments of data when spectral power satisfies specified conditions. It can store up to 8 minutes of data with a sampling rate of 800 Hz.[79] The Sensing Programmer (Medtronic Inc., Minneapolis, MN) is used to control and manage these data using a wireless telemetry system.

Algorithms to analyze sensed information in real-time and control stimulation are not inbuilt and must be programmed on an external computer that can be connected to Activa PC + S via the Nexus-D system (Medtronic Inc., Minneapolis, MN), a bidirectional data port. Algorithms that have shown success with the in-the-loop computer can be incorporated into Activa PC + S using Nexus-D. One example is the use of spectral decomposition of LFPs from Tourette's disease patients implanted with the Activa PC + S. This data was used to train support vector machine (SVM) classifiers differentiating "tic" from "no-tic" data and fed back to control closed-loop stimulation.[80]

In PD, the Activa PC + S has been used in preclinical primate models for sensing data from sensorimotor cortex and proximal forelimb muscle,[78] as well as from the STN and globus pallidus.[81] Human recordings using the Activa PC + S have been obtained from the STN[82,83,84,85,86] and motor cortex.[85] This system has yielded stable recordings from the STN and motor cortex for over a year in PD patients.[79] The abovementioned studies recorded LFP signals in frequency ranges correlating with movement (i.e., beta and gamma ranges). None of these studies closed the loop by using control signals to alter stimulation.

Clinical data for aDBS

Initial evidence that closed-loop stimulation may be effective in treating movement disorders came from nonhuman primate (NHP) data. Rosen and colleagues found that a short burst of globus pallidus interna (GPi) stimulation (i.e., 7 pulses at 130 Hz) is more effective at alleviating parkinsonian akinesia than constant stimulation when the burst was triggered on spikes in GPi or motor cortex.[87] The delay in stimulation was selected to coincide with subsequent oscillatory bursts associated with tremors and pathological corticobasal ganglia synchronization.

Following this animal study, the concept of aDBS was applied to movement disorder patients using either custom platforms or the Activa PC + S system as acute studies at the time of lead implantation (i.e., during the period when electrode extension cables were externalized, prior to implantation of the pulse generator). In the first study of eight PD patients, unilateral stimulation was delivered when STN beta power crossed a threshold.[88] Motor symptoms, as measured by the Unified Parkinson's Disease Rating Scale (UPDRS), improved by 27% with aDBS as compared to constant stimulation. In addition, stimulation times were reduced by 55%. Importantly, random stimulation that was not triggered by beta activity was inferior to aDBS. In a follow-up study in four PD patients, bilateral aDBS triggered on beta amplitude showed that gait and extremity symptoms improved with aDBS (decrease in UPDRS scores by 43%).[89] Another study of 10 PD patients, again using beta modulation bilaterally, found that aDBS was superior to constant stimulation and had fewer speech side effects.[90] These studies highlight how bioinspired hypothesis testing can be conducted in patients undergoing clinical procedures.

Beta-modulated aDBS has been applied in a number of other case studies and pilot studies. A single PD patient demonstrated a trend toward superior outcomes compared to constant stimulation when triggering on beta activity during a battery change procedure.[91] Adaptive voltage triggered on beta power was noted to improve bradykinesia and rest dyskinesia.[31] The principle of coordinated resets was noted to improve motor symptoms in six patients.[92] Lastly, both phase-[93] and amplitude-responsive[59,94] stimulation has been applied to the treatment of essential and dystonic tremors using external devices to measure tremor activity. The latter two studies combined the Activa PC + S with a wearable smart watch to measure tremor activity. Both of these studies used a scalar approach to amplitude-responsive stimulation, in which stimulation voltage was varied based on the amplitude of the control signal.

In Tourette's syndrome, the Activa PC + S was used to record from the thalamic centromedian–parafascicular (CM–PF) complex and motor cortex, and spectral power in 1 to 100 Hz range was utilized to classify behavioral states as tic versus volitional movement.[80] Although the features that were most discriminating varied throughout the study time period, an SVM classifier retrained over time was able to accurately predict these behavioral states. A study currently underway by the same group integrates tic features from CM–PF complex in the 1 to 10 Hz

range and motion features in hand motor cortex in the beta range to adaptively deliver stimulation.[95] Other studies using the Activa PC + S for OCD targeting ventral capsule/ventral striatum (VC/VS) and major depressive disorder targeting subgenual cingulate gyrus (Cg25) are currently underway (ClinicalTrials. gov Identifiers: NCT03457675 & NCT01984710, respectively).

7.3.2 Closed-Loop Stimulation for Epilepsy

RNS device parameters

The Responsive Neurostimulation System (RNS, NeuroPace, Inc., Mountain View, CA) can accommodate one or two recording and stimulating leads with four electrodes each.[96] The leads are either depth or cortical strip electrodes that are targeted to seizure foci. Stimulation parameters include current amplitude, frequency, pulse width, burst duration, and a daily limit on the number of stimulation therapies delivered. Stimulation can be delivered between any combination of electrodes, including monopolar stimulation with respect to the stimulator chassis, analogous to DBS. Unlike DBS, however, the chassis is implanted in the head.

In comparison to the Activa PC + S, RNS is configured, by default, for closed-loop stimulation. There are three built-in algorithms that detect electrographic changes that may progress to electrographic and/or clinical seizures. The half-wave algorithm is used to detect spikes and rhythmic activity in specific frequency ranges using the amplitude of, and distance between, local minima/maxima pairs.[97] The line-length algorithm identifies changes in frequency and amplitude by averaging the absolute sample-to-sample amplitude differences within a short-term sliding window and compares it to the same metric over a long-term sliding window.[98] Lastly, the area algorithm measures overall signal energy by calculating the average absolute area under the curve over a short-term window and likewise compares it to the value measured from a longer-term window.[99] The specific parameters can be customized by the physician to optimize the accuracy and latency of seizure detection. Also, in contrast to Activa PC + S, RNS is optimized for continuous recording and short, intermittent stimulation, and frequent stimulation will lead to rapid battery depletion.[76]

Clinical effectiveness of the RNS system

The RNS system has been implanted in patients with refractory epilepsy (partial motor, complex, and/or secondarily generalized seizures) with up to two seizure foci. In a prospective, randomized controlled trial, seizure reduction was significantly greater with therapeutic stimulation (40% reduction) compared to the sham stimulation control group (17% reduction) over the course of a 12-week blinded evaluation period.[96] There was no difference in efficacy in patients with mesial temporal lobe epilepsy versus neocortical epilepsy, in those with one versus two seizure foci, or in those who had undergone previous vagal nerve stimulator (VNS) or epilepsy surgery. The responder rate (percentage of patients in which seizures were reduced by ≥ 50%) increased from 29% at the end of blinded evaluation period to 43% at 1 year and 46% at 2 years.[100] Subsequent follow-up studies of this patient cohort demonstrated a further increase in the responder rate to 64.6% with a median reduction of 70% in seizure frequency using the last observation carried forward methodology.[101] While these improvements in response over time may reflect improvements in device programming, there is also the possibility that chronic stimulation results in beneficial modulation of the epileptic network itself.

7.3.3 Closed-Loop Vagal Nerve Stimulation

As an open-loop stimulation device for seizures, VNSs deliver pulses at preset intervals (e.g., 30 seconds on, 5 minutes off), and can deliver additional stimulation by on-demand external application of a magnet over the pulse generator.[102] This on-demand stimulation is often not fully utilized due to various reasons, including cognitive impairment, ictal immobilization, nocturnal seizures, or lack of seizure auras. Evidence show that a large proportion of seizures are associated with a significant rise in heart rate,[103] and the framework for the Aspire SR™ device (LivaNova PLC, London, United Kingdom) utilizes this fact. This closed-loop VNS device incorporates an additional stimulation mode in which an EKG sensor monitors heart rate and delivers stimulation when it detects a rapid rise in heart rate.

The Aspire SR algorithm detects near-term (foreground) heart rate and compares it to a baseline (background) heart rate over a 5-minute period and delivers stimulation in response to a 20 to 70% increase in ictal heart rate, sustained for 1 second. The threshold can be adjusted in 10% increments to tailor treatment for individual variations in ictal tachycardia and baseline level of physical activity. Stimulation parameters include current amplitude, frequency, pulse width, and "on" time that can be different between the two modes (normal mode, magnet mode). Additionally, in normal mode, the "off" time is also specified.

The first prospective trial of Aspire SR (E-36) evaluated 30 implanted patients during short-term monitoring in an epilepsy-monitoring unit (EMU). Successful seizure detection, defined as therapeutic stimulation triggered within 2 minutes of seizure onset, was achieved in 41% patients.[104] Stimulation delivered during seizure activity resulted in event termination in 59% patients. Another prospective trial (US E-37) in 20 implanted patients, also performed in the EMU setting, showed seizure detection in 35% of ictal events (likewise defined as treatment delivered within 2 minutes of seizure onset) and seizure termination in 61% of those events.[105] In this study, the ictal heart rate threshold was customized for each patient based on historical trends of ictal elevations in heart rate. Defining the ideal heart rate threshold for triggering stimulation remains a challenge, especially given the variability in ictal heart rate not only across patients but also across seizures in an individual patient. There have not yet been any trials comparing the efficacy of Aspire SR to its open-loop predecessor.

7.3.4 Closed-Loop Spinal Cord Stimulation

Spinal cord stimulation (SCS) has been demonstrated to be an effective therapy for neuropathic pain after its introduction into clinical use in the 1960s.[106,107] It was recognized early that posture influences the effective stimulation amplitude, likely because changes in body position affect the distance between the stimulating electrodes and the spinal cord.[108,109] Moreover, the threshold voltage required to induce paresthesias for different positions varied across patients, that is, the threshold was lowest when supine in some patients while it was lowest when sitting in others.[108]

The RestoreSensor system (Medtronic Inc., Minneapolis, MN) was designed with a three-axis accelerometer that senses the body's position and activity, and accordingly adjusts stimulation amplitude. The system requires training where accelerometer data are correlated with multiple positions, for example, upright, prone, supine, left lateral decubitus, and right lateral decubitus. Stimulation settings for all or a subset of the positions are programmed to meet specific patient requirements. Stimulation settings include cycling versus continuous stimulation modes, pulse width, frequency, amplitude, and number of active electrodes. The two leads of eight electrodes each are typically targeted to spinal cord levels such that the induced paresthesias cover most of the area of perceived pain.[110]

A prospective, randomized controlled trial on RestoreSensor (Medtronic Inc., Minneapolis, MN) comparing automatic position-adaptive stimulation (AdaptiveStim) to the traditional manual adjustment showed that 87% of patients in the treatment arm met the primary objective of improved pain control without loss of convenience or improved convenience without loss in pain relief.[111] Pain scores in the treatment arm were decreased compared to the manual adjustment arm, but this difference was not statistically significant.

7.4 Outstanding Questions and New Horizons

7.4.1 Effects of Closed-Loop Stimulation on the Underlying Mechanism of DBS

Initial theories on the mechanism of open-loop DBS were based on the clinical similarity of DBS, particularly with high-frequency stimulation (HFS; ≥ 100 Hz), and lesioning. DBS was thought of as "functional lesioning" or "jamming the circuit."[112] The contemporary understanding of the DBS mechanisms of action is far more complex. The therapeutic benefit of DBS occurs over a time course of seconds, as in case of tremor in PD and ET, to months, such as dystonia and OCD symptoms. This implies that there are multiple mechanisms at work.[113] These mechanisms include: (1) modulation of neural networks, including the disruption of pathological information flow/communication[114,115] (2) synaptic plasticity-mediated changes in network activity or connectivity, akin to neuronal changes seen in natural behaviors, e.g., learning; and (3) anatomic changes mediated by neuroprotection or neurogenesis.[113]

For most current clinical applications, DBS utilizes HFS. Closed-loop stimulation using specific biomarkers is a different stimulation paradigm altogether, characterized by temporally irregular pulse trains and much lower average stimulation frequencies. It may be the case that different mechanisms of action are engaged. As an example, amplitude-responsive DBS in PD was found to selectively suppress long-duration beta bursts while conventional constant stimulation decreased global beta activity.[116] Closed-loop neuromodulation could also have more directed effects on altering the activity of neuronal networks as evidenced by the gradual increase in responder rate over time with the RNS system.[101] A better understanding of how closed-loop stimulation affects neural circuitry in the brain will enable further improvements in the efficacy and specificity of aDBS.

7.4.2 Accelerating Improvements in Control Algorithms Using Machine Learning

Although guidelines exist to guide the decision-making process,[2] programming of DBS parameters has traditionally been a process of trial and error that is highly subjective and time-consuming. Because of the many combinations of stimulation settings, programming is highly dependent on the skills and experience of the clinician. For closed-loop stimulation, programming is likely to be even more complex and laborious as not only stimulation but sensing parameters also need to be optimized for each patient. During the RNS pivotal trial, initial optimization of sensing and stimulation parameters occurred over a 4-week period prior to the evaluation of clinical efficacy.[96] However, programming changes to further optimize outcomes were made continuously at a median rate of three changes per year per subject (range of one to seven).[101]

Another factor complicating the programming process is the so-called moving target. Patient disease states as well as therapeutic efficacy with open-loop DBS change over time;[117] this usually requires recalibration of stimulation parameters. This phenomenon reflects changes in patients' needs and may result from disease progression or the development of tolerance to stimulation. Several studies suggest the prevalence of tolerance to be in the 10% range.[117,118,119,120,121] Changes in the phenotype of many neurologic diseases are more complex than worsening in the severity of symptoms. In eight PD patients with Vim DBS for tremor followed for a mean of 49 months, tremor ceased to be a major source of disability in two patients as levodopa-induced dyskinesia, motor fluctuations, and bradykinesia worsened.[119] Furthermore, in three patients tremor severity declined, obviating the need for thalamic DBS.[119] With closed-loop neuromodulatory strategies, additional complexity could be introduced by the disappearance of certain biomarkers over time.

Due to these considerations, it may be the case that humans soon will not be able to provide adequate adaptability and flexibility to optimize the programming of closed-loop systems. One potential solution is the application of machine-learning algorithms to closed-loop neuromodulation. Under supervised frameworks, algorithms are manually trained on a data set to identify patterns of neuronal activity that correlate with a particular behavioral or pathological state.[122] In contrast, unsupervised machine-learning frameworks enable algorithms to be applied naively to neuronal data with minimal a priori assumptions about what features, i.e. biomarkers, may be most relevant or what stimulation parameters are most effective. Patterns are recognized and segregated based on the data themselves. Generally, machine-learning algorithms are composed of three components: feature extraction, dimensionality reduction, and pattern classification. The algorithm must not only have high accuracy but also computational efficiency to allow for online, real-time detection.[123] Preclinical work in an ovine model has employed the SVM method to classify seizures during concurrent stimulation.[32]

7.4.3 Using Multiple Feedback Signals

Many neurological diseases affect multiple behavioral conditions and underlying neural networks. For example, in PD, the motor symptoms of tremor, bradykinesia, rigidity, and postural instability are often accompanied by cognitive, autonomic, and psychiatric deficits. One biomarker may be insufficient to properly address the optimized treatment of multiple symptoms. Combinations of multiple feedback signals could be considered. Determining the optimal combinations will require an improved comprehension of the underlying circuitry, careful empiric testing, and perhaps the use of machine-learning algorithms, as described above. Issues such as redundancy of information from multiple biomarkers and the need for additional hardware will need to be addressed to design the most efficient closed-loop systems.

In PD, different aspects of beta oscillatory activity could potentially provide feedback information for bradykinesia and rigidity. These factors include the amplitude of the oscillation,[124] low beta (13–20 Hz) versus high beta (21–35 Hz) spectral power,[48] cross-frequency coupling between beta and other frequency bands,[52] and high-gamma oscillations.[125] Although some features of beta correlate specifically with rigidity/akinesia, the exact relation between different beta features and the numerous motor symptoms of PD remains to be fully understood. In contrast, alpha activity within the pedunculopontine nucleus correlates with gait instability and could provide useful feedback information for this symptom.[126] Combining different frequency bands and analytical paradigms may be required to create multiple feedback signals to target various symptoms.

Recording signals from various brain regions could also have potential benefits. These include improved accuracy of the detection algorithm, higher signal-to-noise ratios, and minimization of stimulation and external artifacts, thereby providing more robust control signal. Although some LFPs may be generated locally, many studies of PD have demonstrated coherent activity throughout the motor basal ganglia–thalamocortical circuit.[127] Recording activity from multiple nodes of this network could provide confirmation that pathological beta oscillations are being suppressed throughout the network. Ongoing studies with the Activa PC + S in Tourette's syndrome combine recordings from motor cortex and the CM–PF complex with the former acting as a general motion detector and the latter yielding tic-specific data.[95]

Finally, several different types of signals (e.g., LFP, EMG, biochemical signals, etc.) from multiple regions could be combined to provide potentially synergistic feedback.[7] This approach may be best suited for controlling disparate symptoms with different physical manifestations.

7.5 Conclusion

Closed-loop stimulation techniques are slowly filtering into clinical practice and are sure to become more prevalent in the near future. This strategy promises to improve outcomes, broaden the application of neuromodulation, cause fewer side effects, and utilize resources more efficiently. To achieve these objectives, an enormous array of recording sources, stimulation paradigms, and control systems is available for consideration and testing. It is likely that these options will further expand with new technological developments and advances in neuroscience and engineering, generating even greater numbers of possible systems. The opportunity currently exists to define how searches within this parameter space are conducted, endeavors that will be driven, in large part, by scientists, engineers, and industry. Clinicians can and should participate in this discourse, but they will need to be familiar with the relevant principles and knowledge bases in order to do so. Active collaboration among neurosurgeons, neurologists, and other members of DBS community will be crucial for realizing the possibilities of closed-loop neuromodulation.

References

[1] Bronstein JM, Tagliati M, Alterman RL, et al. Deep brain stimulation for Parkinson disease: an expert consensus and review of key issues. Arch Neurol. 2011; 68(2):165

[2] Volkmann J, Moro E, Pahwa R. Basic algorithms for the programming of deep brain stimulation in Parkinson's disease. Mov Disord. 2006; 21 Suppl 14: S284–S289

[3] Arlotti M, Rosa M, Marceglia S, Barbieri S, Priori A. The adaptive deep brain stimulation challenge. Parkinsonism Relat Disord. 2016; 28:12–17

[4] Beudel M, Brown P. Adaptive deep brain stimulation in Parkinson's disease. Parkinsonism Relat Disord. 2016; 22 Suppl 1:S123–S126

[5] Carron R, Chaillet A, Filipchuk A, Pasillas-Lépine W, Hammond C. Closing the loop of deep brain stimulation. Front Syst Neurosci. 2013; 7:112

[6] Meidahl AC, Tinkhauser G, Herz DM, Cagnan H, Debarros J, Brown P. Adaptive deep brain stimulation for movement disorders: the long road to clinical therapy. Mov Disord. 2017; 32(6):810–819

[7] Parastarfeizabadi M, Kouzani AZ. Advances in closed-loop deep brain stimulation devices. J Neuroeng Rehabil. 2017; 14(1):79

[8] Lo MC, Widge AS. Closed-loop neuromodulation systems: next-generation treatments for psychiatric illness. Int Rev Psychiatry. 2017; 29(2): 191–204

[9] Ahlskog JE, Muenter MD. Frequency of levodopa-related dyskinesias and motor fluctuations as estimated from the cumulative literature. Mov Disord. 2001; 16(3):448–458

[10] Chen HI, Attiah M, Baltuch G, Smith DH, Hamilton RH, Lucas TH. Harnessing plasticity for the treatment of neurosurgical disorders: an overview. World Neurosurg. 2014; 82(5):648–659

[11] Maxwell JC. (1868). On Governors. Proceedings of the Royal Society of London. 16: 270–283. doi:10.1098/rspl.1867.0055. JSTOR 112510

[12] Flugge-Lotz, Irmgard; Titus, Harold A. (October 1962). "Optimum and Quasi-Optimum Control of Third and Fourth-Order Systems" (PDF). Stanford University Technical Report (134): 8–12

[13] Steffano JD, Stubberud AR, Williams IJ. Feedback and control systems. Schaums outline series, McGraw-Hill; 1967

[14] Weiner N. Cybernetics: or control and communication in the animal and the machine. Paris, (Hermann & Cie) & Camb. Mass. (MIT Press) ISBN 978-0-262-73009-9; 1948, 2nd revised ed. 1961

[15] Kakkar V. An ultra low power system architecture for implantable medical devices. IEEE Access. 2018:1

[16] Liu X, Zhang M, Subei B, Richardson AG, Lucas TH, Van der Spiegel J. The PennBMBI: design of a general purpose Wireless Brain-Machine-Brain Interface System. IEEE Trans Biomed Circuits Syst. 2015; 9(2):248–258

[17] Liu X, Zhang M, Xiong T, et al. A fully integrated wireless compressed sensing neural signal acquisition system for chronic recording and brain machine interface. IEEE Trans Biomed Circuits Syst. 2016; 10(4):874–883

[18] Georgopoulos AP, Schwartz AB, Kettner RE. Neuronal population coding of movement direction. Science. 1986; 233(4771):1416–1419

[19] Hubel DH, Wiesel TN. Receptive fields, binocular interaction and functional architecture in the cat's visual cortex. J Physiol. 1962; 160:106–154

[20] Hochberg LR, Bacher D, Jarosiewicz B, et al. Reach and grasp by people with tetraplegia using a neurally controlled robotic arm. Nature. 2012; 485 (7398):372–375

[21] Jarosiewicz B, Sarma AA, Bacher D, et al. Virtual typing by people with tetraplegia using a self-calibrating intracortical brain-computer interface. Sci Transl Med. 2015; 7(313):313ra179

[22] Ajiboye AB, Willett FR, Young DR, et al. Restoration of reaching and grasping movements through brain-controlled muscle stimulation in a person with tetraplegia: a proof-of-concept demonstration. Lancet. 2017; 389(10081): 1821–1830

[23] Bouton CE, Shaikhouni A, Annetta NV, et al. Restoring cortical control of functional movement in a human with quadriplegia. Nature. 2016; 533 (7602):247–250

[24] Smith EH, Liou JY, Davis TS, et al. The ictal wavefront is the spatiotemporal source of discharges during spontaneous human seizures. Nat Commun. 2016; 7:11098

[25] Judy JW. Neural interfaces for upper-limb prosthesis control: opportunities to improve long-term reliability. IEEE Pulse. 2012; 3(2):57–60

[26] Chestek CA, Gilja V, Nuyujukian P, et al. Long-term stability of neural prosthetic control signals from silicon cortical arrays in rhesus macaque motor cortex. J Neural Eng. 2011; 8(4):045005

[27] Buzsáki G, Anastassiou CA, Koch C. The origin of extracellular fields and currents—EEG, ECoG, LFP and spikes. Nat Rev Neurosci. 2012; 13(6):407–420

[28] Buzsáki G, Moser EI. Memory, navigation and theta rhythm in the hippocampal-entorhinal system. Nat Neurosci. 2013; 16(2):130–138

[29] Singer W, Gray CM. Visual feature integration and the temporal correlation hypothesis. Annu Rev Neurosci. 1995; 18:555–586

[30] Lisman JE, Jensen O. The θ-γ neural code. Neuron. 2013; 77(6):1002–1016

[31] Rosa M, Arlotti M, Ardolino G, et al. Adaptive deep brain stimulation in a freely moving Parkinsonian patient. Mov Disord. 2015; 30(7):1003–1005

[32] Stanslaski S, Afshar P, Cong P, et al. Design and validation of a fully implantable, chronic, closed-loop neuromodulation device with concurrent sensing and stimulation. IEEE Trans Neural Syst Rehabil Eng. 2012; 20(4):410–421

[33] Lu Y, Lyu H, Richardson AG, Lucas TH, Kuzum D. Flexible neural electrode array based-on porous graphene for cortical microstimulation and sensing. Sci Rep. 2016; 6:33526

[34] Nini A, Feingold A, Slovin H, Bergman H. Neurons in the globus pallidus do not show correlated activity in the normal monkey, but phase-locked oscillations appear in the MPTP model of parkinsonism. J Neurophysiol. 1995; 74 (4):1800–1805

[35] Levy R, Hutchison WD, Lozano AM, Dostrovsky JO. High-frequency synchronization of neuronal activity in the subthalamic nucleus of parkinsonian patients with limb tremor. J Neurosci. 2000; 20(20):7766–7775

[36] Levy R, Hutchison WD, Lozano AM, Dostrovsky JO. Synchronized neuronal discharge in the basal ganglia of parkinsonian patients is limited to oscillatory activity. J Neurosci. 2002b; 22(7):2855–2861

[37] Weinberger M, Mahant N, Hutchison WD, et al. Beta oscillatory activity in the subthalamic nucleus and its relation to dopaminergic response in Parkinson's disease. J Neurophysiol. 2006; 96(6):3248–3256

[38] Brown P, Oliviero A, Mazzone P, Insola A, Tonali P, Di Lazzaro V. Dopamine dependency of oscillations between subthalamic nucleus and pallidum in Parkinson's disease. J Neurosci. 2001; 21(3):1033–1038

[39] Levy R, Ashby P, Hutchison WD, Lang AE, Lozano AM, Dostrovsky JO. Dependence of subthalamic nucleus oscillations on movement and dopamine in Parkinson's disease. Brain. 2002a; 125(Pt 6):1196–1209

[40] Priori A, Foffani G, Pesenti A, et al. Rhythm-specific pharmacological modulation of subthalamic activity in Parkinson's disease. Exp Neurol. 2004; 189 (2):369–379

[41] Cassidy M, Mazzone P, Oliviero A, et al. Movement-related changes in synchronization in the human basal ganglia. Brain. 2002; 125(Pt 6):1235–1246

[42] Foffani G, Bianchi AM, Baselli G, Priori A. Movement-related frequency modulation of beta oscillatory activity in the human subthalamic nucleus. J Physiol. 2005; 568(Pt 2):699–711

[43] Eusebio A, Thevathasan W, Doyle Gaynor L, et al. Deep brain stimulation can suppress pathological synchronisation in parkinsonian patients. J Neurol Neurosurg Psychiatry. 2011; 82(5):569–573

[44] Giannicola G, Marceglia S, Rossi L, et al. The effects of levodopa and ongoing deep brain stimulation on subthalamic beta oscillations in Parkinson's disease. Exp Neurol. 2010; 226(1):120–127

[45] Rosa M, Giannicola G, Servello D, et al. Subthalamic local field beta oscillations during ongoing deep brain stimulation in Parkinson's disease in hyperacute and chronic phases. Neurosignals. 2011; 19(3):151–162

[46] Chen CC, Litvak V, Gilbertson T, et al. Excessive synchronization of basal ganglia neurons at 20 Hz slows movement in Parkinson's disease. Exp Neurol. 2007; 205(1):214–221

[47] Brown P. Abnormal oscillatory synchronisation in the motor system leads to impaired movement. Curr Opin Neurobiol. 2007; 17(6):656–664

[48] Fogelson N, Williams D, Tijssen M, van Bruggen G, Speelman H, Brown P. Different functional loops between cerebral cortex and the subthalamic area in Parkinson's disease. Cereb Cortex. 2006; 16(1):64–75

[49] Pavlides A, Hogan SJ, Bogacz R. Computational models describing possible mechanisms for generation of excessive beta oscillations in Parkinson's disease. PLOS Comput Biol. 2015; 11(12):e1004609

[50] Holgado AJ, Terry JR, Bogacz R. Conditions for the generation of beta oscillations in the subthalamic nucleus-globus pallidus network. J Neurosci. 2010; 30(37):12340–12352

[51] Tachibana Y, Iwamuro H, Kita H, Takada M, Nambu A. Subthalamo-pallidal interactions underlying parkinsonian neuronal oscillations in the primate basal ganglia. Eur J Neurosci. 2011; 34(9):1470–1484

[52] de Hemptinne C, Swann NC, Ostrem JL, et al. Therapeutic deep brain stimulation reduces cortical phase-amplitude coupling in Parkinson's disease. Nat Neurosci. 2015; 18(5):779–786

[53] Alonso-Frech F, Zamarbide I, Alegre M, et al. Slow oscillatory activity and levodopa-induced dyskinesias in Parkinson's disease. Brain. 2006; 129(Pt 7): 1748–1757

[54] Thevathasan W, Pogosyan A, Hyam JA, et al. Alpha oscillations in the pedunculopontine nucleus correlate with gait performance in parkinsonism. Brain. 2012; 135(Pt 1):148–160

[55] Yu KJ, Kuzum D, Hwang SW, et al. Bioresorbable silicon electronics for transient spatiotemporal mapping of electrical activity from the cerebral cortex. Nat Mater. 2016; 15(7):782–791

[56] Basu I, Tuninetti D, Graupe D, Slavin KV. Adaptive control of deep brain stimulator for essential tremor: entropy-based tremor prediction using surface-EMG. Conf Proc IEEE Eng Med Biol Soc. 2011; 2011:7711–7714

[57] Yamamoto T, Katayama Y, Ushiba J, et al. On-demand control system for deep brain stimulation for treatment of intention tremor. Neuromodulation. 2013; 16(3):230–235, discussion 235

[58] Basu I, Graupe D, Tuninetti D, et al. Pathological tremor prediction using surface electromyogram and acceleration: potential use in 'ON-OFF' demand driven deep brain stimulator design. J Neural Eng. 2013; 10(3):036019

[59] Malekmohammadi M, Herron J, Velisar A, et al. Kinematic adaptive deep brain stimulation for resting tremor in Parkinson's disease. Mov Disord. 2016; 31(3):426–428

[60] Shukla P, Basu I, Graupe D, Tuninetti D, Slavin KV. A neural network-based design of an on-off adaptive control for deep brain stimulation in movement disorders. Conf Proc IEEE Eng Med Biol Soc. 2012; 2012:4140–4143

[61] Lee KH, Blaha CD, Garris PA, et al. Evolution of deep brain stimulation: human electrometer and smart devices supporting the next generation of therapy. Neuromodulation. 2009; 12(2):85–103

[62] Kilpatrick M, Church E, Danish S, et al. Intracerebral microdialysis during deep brain stimulation surgery. J Neurosci Methods. 2010; 190(1):106–111

[63] Grahn PJ, Mallory GW, Khurram OU, et al. A neurochemical closed-loop controller for deep brain stimulation: toward individualized smart neuromodulation therapies. Front Neurosci. 2014; 8:169

[64] Chang SY, Kimble CJ, Kim I, et al. Development of the Mayo Investigational Neuromodulation Control System: toward a closed-loop electrochemical feedback system for deep brain stimulation. J Neurosurg. 2013; 119(6): 1556–1565

[65] Kishida KT, Sandberg SG, Lohrenz T, et al. Sub-second dopamine detection in human striatum. PLoS One. 2011; 6(8):e23291

[66] Widge AS, Moritz CT. Pre-frontal control of closed-loop limbic neurostimulation by rodents using a brain-computer interface. J Neural Eng. 2014; 11 (2):024001

[67] Widge AS, Dougherty DD, Moritz CT. Affective brain-computer interfaces as enabling technology for responsive psychiatric stimulation. Brain Comput Interfaces (Abingdon). 2014; 1(2):126–136

[68] Baldassano S, Wulsin D, Ung H, et al. A novel seizure detection algorithm informed by hidden Markov model event states. J Neural Eng. 2016; 13(3): 036011

[69] Baldassano SN, Brinkmann BH, Ung H, et al. Crowdsourcing seizure detection: algorithm development and validation on human implanted device recordings. Brain. 2017; 140(6):1680–1691

[70] Echauz J, Esteller R, Tcheng T, et al. Long-term validation of detection algorithms suitable for an implantable device. Epilepsia. 2001; 42 Suppl 7:35–36

[71] Kossoff EH, Ritzl EK, Politsky JM, et al. Effect of an external responsive neurostimulator on seizures and electrographic discharges during subdural electrode monitoring. Epilepsia. 2004; 45(12):1560–1567

[72] Azodi-Avval R, Gharabaghi A. Phase-dependent modulation as a novel approach for therapeutic brain stimulation. Front Comput Neurosci. 2015; 9:26

[73] Lourens MA, Schwab BC, Nirody JA, Meijer HG, van Gils SA. Exploiting pallidal plasticity for stimulation in Parkinson's disease. J Neural Eng. 2015; 12(2): 026005

[74] Popovych OV, Lysyansky B, Rosenblum M, Pikovsky A, Tass PA. Pulsatile desynchronizing delayed feedback for closed-loop deep brain stimulation. PLoS One. 2017; 12(3):e0173363

[75] Tass PA. A model of desynchronizing deep brain stimulation with a demand-controlled coordinated reset of neural subpopulations. Biol Cybern. 2003; 89 (2):81–88

[76] Neuropace. (2014). RNS System Clinical Summary. (https://www.neuropace.com/manuals/ClinicalSummary.pdf. Accessed April 27, 2018

[77] Stanslaski S, Cong P, Carlson D, et al. An implantable bi-directional brain-machine interface system for chronic neuroprosthesis research. Conf Proc IEEE Eng Med Biol Soc. 2009; 2009:5494–5497

[78] Ryapolova-Webb E, Afshar P, Stanslaski S, et al. Chronic cortical and electromyographic recordings from a fully implantable device: preclinical experience in a nonhuman primate. J Neural Eng. 2014; 11(1):016009

[79] Swann NC, de Hemptinne C, Miocinovic S, et al. Chronic multisite brain recordings from a totally implantable bidirectional neural interface: experience in 5 patients with Parkinson's disease. J Neurosurg. 2018; 128:605–616

[80] Shute JB, Okun MS, Opri E, et al. Thalamocortical network activity enables chronic tic detection in humans with Tourette syndrome. Neuroimage Clin. 2016; 12:165–172

[81] Connolly AT, Muralidharan A, Hendrix C, et al. Local field potential recordings in a non-human primate model of Parkinson's disease using the Activa PC + S neurostimulator. J Neural Eng. 2015; 12(6):066012

[82] Houston B, Blumenfeld Z, Quinn E, Bronte-Stewart H, Chizeck H. Long-term detection of Parkinsonian tremor activity from subthalamic nucleus local field potentials. Conf Proc IEEE Eng Med Biol Soc. 2015; 2015:3427–3431

[83] Neumann WJ, Staub F, Horn A, et al. deep brain recordings using an implanted pulse generator in Parkinson's disease. Neuromodulation. 2016; 19 (1):20–24

[84] Quinn EJ, Blumenfeld Z, Velisar A, et al. Beta oscillations in freely moving Parkinson's subjects are attenuated during deep brain stimulation. Mov Disord. 2015; 30(13):1750–1758

[85] Swann NC, de Hemptinne C, Miocinovic S, et al. Gamma oscillations in the hyperkinetic state detected with chronic human brain recordings in Parkinson's disease. J Neurosci. 2016; 36(24):6445–6458

[86] Trager MH, Koop MM, Velisar A, et al. Subthalamic beta oscillations are attenuated after withdrawal of chronic high frequency neurostimulation in Parkinson's disease. Neurobiol Dis. 2016; 96:22–30

[87] Rosin B, Slovik M, Mitelman R, et al. Closed-loop deep brain stimulation is superior in ameliorating parkinsonism. Neuron. 2011; 72(2):370–384

[88] Little S, Pogosyan A, Neal S, et al. Adaptive deep brain stimulation in advanced Parkinson's disease. Ann Neurol. 2013; 74(3):449–457

[89] Little S, Beudel M, Zrinzo L, et al. Bilateral adaptive deep brain stimulation is effective in Parkinson's disease. J Neurol Neurosurg Psychiatry. 2016a; 87 (7):717–721

[90] Little S, Tripoliti E, Beudel M, et al. Adaptive deep brain stimulation for Parkinson's disease demonstrates reduced speech side effects compared to conventional stimulation in the acute setting. J Neurol Neurosurg Psychiatry. 2016b; 87(12):1388–1389

[91] Piña-Fuentes D, Little S, Oterdoom M, et al. Adaptive DBS in a Parkinson's patient with chronically implanted DBS: a proof of principle. Mov Disord. 2017; 32(8):1253–1254

[92] Adamchic I, Hauptmann C, Barnikol UB, et al. Coordinated reset neuromodulation for Parkinson's disease: proof-of-concept study. Mov Disord. 2014; 29 (13):1679–1684

[93] Cagnan H, Pedrosa D, Little S, et al. Stimulating at the right time: phase-specific deep brain stimulation. Brain. 2017; 140(1):132–145

[94] Herron JA, Thompson MC, Brown T, Chizeck HJ, Ojemann JG, Ko AL. Chronic electrocorticography for sensing movement intention and closed-loop deep brain stimulation with wearable sensors in an essential tremor patient. J Neurosurg. 2017; 127(3):580–587

[95] Deeb W, Giordano JJ, Rossi PJ, et al. Proceedings of the Fourth Annual Deep Brain Stimulation Think Tank: a review of emerging issues and technologies. Front Integr Neurosci. 2016; 10:38

[96] Morrell MJ, RNS System in Epilepsy Study Group. Responsive cortical stimulation for the treatment of medically intractable partial epilepsy. Neurology. 2011; 77(13):1295–1304

[97] Gotman J. Automatic recognition of epileptic seizures in the EEG. Electroencephalogr Clin Neurophysiol. 1982; 54(5):530–540

[98] Esteller R, Echauz J, Tcheng T, Litt B, Pless B. Line length: an efficient feature for seizure onset detection. In Engineering in Medicine and Biology Society, 2001. Proceedings of the 23rd Annual International Conference of the IEEE (Vol. 2, pp. 1707–1710). IEEE

[99] Litt B, Esteller R, Echauz J, et al. Epileptic seizures may begin hours in advance of clinical onset: a report of five patients. Neuron. 2001; 30(1):51–64

[100] Heck CN, King-Stephens D, Massey AD, et al. Two-year seizure reduction in adults with medically intractable partial onset epilepsy treated with responsive neurostimulation: final results of the RNS System Pivotal trial. Epilepsia. 2014; 55(3):432–441

[101] Geller EB, Skarpaas TL, Gross RE, et al. Brain-responsive neurostimulation in patients with medically intractable mesial temporal lobe epilepsy. Epilepsia. 2017; 58(6):994–1004

[102] Morris GL, III. A retrospective analysis of the effects of magnet-activated stimulation in conjunction with vagus nerve stimulation therapy. Epilepsy Behav. 2003; 4(6):740–745

[103] Eggleston KS, Olin BD, Fisher RS. Ictal tachycardia: the head-heart connection. Seizure. 2014; 23(7):496–505

[104] Boon P, Vonck K, van Rijckevorsel K, et al. A prospective, multicenter study of cardiac-based seizure detection to activate vagus nerve stimulation. Seizure. 2015; 32:52–61

[105] Fisher RS, Afra P, Macken M, et al. Automatic vagus nerve stimulation triggered by ictal tachycardia: clinical outcomes and device performance—The U.S. E-37 Trial. Neuromodulation. 2016; 19(2):188–195

[106] Cameron T. Safety and efficacy of spinal cord stimulation for the treatment of chronic pain: a 20-year literature review. J Neurosurg. 2004; 100(3) Suppl Spine:254–267

[107] Shealy CN, Mortimer JT, Reswick JB. Electrical inhibition of pain by stimulation of the dorsal columns: preliminary clinical report. Anesth Analg. 1967; 46(4):489–491

[108] Cameron T, Alo KM. Effects of posture on stimulation parameters in spinal cord stimulation. Neuromodulation. 1998; 1(4):177–183

[109] Olin JC, Kidd DH, North RB. Postural changes in spinal cord stimulation perceptual thresholds. Neuromodulation. 1998; 1(4):171–175

[110] Kumar K, Buchser E, Linderoth B, Meglio M, Van Buyten JP. Avoiding complications from spinal cord stimulation: practical recommendations from an international panel of experts. Neuromodulation. 2007; 10(1):24–33

[111] Schultz DM, Webster L, Kosek P, Dar U, Tan Y, Sun M. Sensor-driven position-adaptive spinal cord stimulation for chronic pain. Pain Physician. 2012; 15(1):1–12

[112] Benabid AL, Benazzouz A, Hoffmann D, Limousin P, Krack P, Pollak P. Long-term electrical inhibition of deep brain targets in movement disorders. Mov Disord. 1998; 13 Suppl 3:119–125

[113] Herrington TM, Cheng JJ, Eskandar EN. Mechanisms of deep brain stimulation. J Neurophysiol. 2016; 115(1):19–38

[114] Chiken S, Nambu A. Mechanism of deep brain stimulation: inhibition, excitation, or disruption? Neuroscientist. 2016; 22(3):313–322

[115] Gradinaru V, Mogri M, Thompson KR, Henderson JM, Deisseroth K. Optical deconstruction of parkinsonian neural circuitry. Science. 2009; 324(5925): 354–359

[116] Tinkhauser G, Pogosyan A, Little S, et al. The modulatory effect of adaptive deep brain stimulation on beta bursts in Parkinson's disease. Brain. 2017; 140(4):1053–1067

[117] Shih LC, LaFaver K, Lim C, Papavassiliou E, Tarsy D. Loss of benefit in VIM thalamic deep brain stimulation (DBS) for essential tremor (ET): how prevalent is it? Parkinsonism Relat Disord. 2013; 19(7):676–679

[118] Koller WC, Lyons KE, Wilkinson SB, Troster AI, Pahwa R. Long-term safety and efficacy of unilateral deep brain stimulation of the thalamus in essential tremor. Mov Disord. 2001; 16(3):464–468

[119] Kumar R, Lozano AM, Sime E, Lang AE. Long-term follow-up of thalamic deep brain stimulation for essential and parkinsonian tremor. Neurology. 2003; 61(11):1601–1604

[120] Lyons KE, Koller WC, Wilkinson SB, Pahwa R. Long term safety and efficacy of unilateral deep brain stimulation of the thalamus for parkinsonian tremor. J Neurol Neurosurg Psychiatry. 2001; 71(5):682–684

[121] Papavassiliou E, Rau G, Heath S, et al. Thalamic deep brain stimulation for essential tremor: relation of lead location to outcome. Neurosurgery. 2008; 62 Suppl 2:884–894

[122] Deo RC. Machine learning in medicine. Circulation. 2015; 132(20):1920–1930

[123] Mohammed A, Zamani M, Bayford R, Demosthenous A. Toward on-demand deep brain stimulation using online Parkinson's disease prediction driven by dynamic detection. IEEE Trans Neural Syst Rehabil Eng. 2017; 25(12): 2441–2452

[124] Hammond C, Bergman H, Brown P. Pathological synchronization in Parkinson's disease: networks, models and treatments. Trends Neurosci. 2007; 30 (7):357–364

[125] Yang AI, Vanegas N, Lungu C, Zaghloul KA. Beta-coupled high-frequency activity and beta-locked neuronal spiking in the subthalamic nucleus of Parkinson's disease. J Neurosci. 2014; 34(38):12816–12827

[126] Fraix V, Bastin J, David O, et al. Pedunculopontine nucleus area oscillations during stance, stepping and freezing in Parkinson's disease. PLoS One. 2013; 8(12):e83919

[127] Brown P, Williams D. Basal ganglia local field potential activity: character and functional significance in the human. Clin Neurophysiol. 2005; 116(11): 2510–2519

8 Parkinson's Disease Application

Charles B. Mikell, Bradley Ashcroft

Abstract

Deep brain stimulation (DBS) can be used to alleviate the motor and cognitive symptoms of Parkinson's disease (PD). The therapeutic benefit of DBS is equivalent to both the maximal "on-time" and symptom reduction conferred by classic dopamine drugs, and it allows a reduction in the use of medication to manage symptoms. Several structures have been studied and used as targets, chief among them being the subthalamic nucleus and the globus pallidus pars interna. Mutliple techniques can be utilized to target these structures. Frame-based and frameless approaches can be used to guide the implant, while different magnatic resonance imaging modalities can be combined with microelectrode recording to identify and confirm the correct target and electrode placement. DBS offers a therapeautic benefit and should be considered for PD patients whose symptoms are no longer well controlled by medication.

Keywords: Parkinson's disease, deep brain stimulation, subthalamic nucleus, globus pallidus interna, frame-based, frameless, targeting

> "The thing about Parkinson's disease is, it gets worse."
> – Guy Schwartz, MD

8.1 Introduction

Parkinson's disease (PD) is a devastating degenerative illness that affects movement, gait, and thinking of a patient. As of 2010, more than 630,000 Americans suffered from PD; the number is projected to double by 2040.[1] Neurologists usually treat PD patients with drugs that augment dopamine transmission; levodopa-based agents are generally first-line treament for most patients.[2] Although these agents are effective in a majority of patients with PD, the response to these agents starts declining with time or the benefit is tempered due to intolerable side effects associated with increased dosing requirements. The major motor symptoms of PD include rigidity, tremors, bradykinesia, and gait and posture abnormalities. In addition, many nonmotor symptoms can manifest, such as depression/anxiety, fatigue, worsening sense of smell, and cognitive changes. Patients whose symptoms are responsive to dopamine drugs yet are not well controlled or patients experiencing worsening on/off periods and/or receiving ineffective doses should be considered as surgical candidates.

Although originally considered for patients with severe PD, recent evidence suggests that movement disorder surgery should be considered relatively early in the course of the disease. The Medtronic Deep Brain Stimulation (DBS) system is now Food and Drug Administration (FDA) labeled for patients who have had 4 years of symptoms with motor fluctuations that are not controlled, in addition to patients with longer-duration disease. This labeling was updated in response to data from the EARLYSTIM trial in which patients with 4 years of disease were randomized to surgery or best medical therapy.[3] Patients who underwent surgery had gains in quality of life, as assessed by the Parkinson's Disease Questionnaire (PDQ-39),[3,4] whereas patients in the medical therapy arm remained the same or their disease progressed. Because of this improvement in quality of life, DBS should be considered as soon as movement symptoms are not fully controlled with medication; it is only going to get worse.

8.2 Patient Selection

PD patients are generally older and may suffer from multiple comorbidities. Some younger patients are also surgical candidates, but these are the exceptions, given the increasing incidence of PD with age.[5] In general, DBS is not a highly morbid surgery, and some very elderly patients are candidates for surgery. There is no age cutoff in our opinion, though treatment decisions have to be individualized based on discussions between the patient, his or her family, and a multidisciplinary team including the neurologist, surgeon, and other caregivers (i.e., neuropsychologist, physical therapist). Treatment decisions should be informed by Dr. Schwartz's truism: the disease is only going to get worse.

The most important consideration in determining candidacy for DBS is whether the patient's symptoms respond to dopaminergic medication. Symptoms that respond to carbidopa/levodopa, or dopamine agonists can generally be expected to improve with surgery. Cardinal symptoms of PD, including rigidity, tremor, and bradykinesia, almost always respond to dopamine equivalents and can, therefore, be counted upon to respond to surgery.[6] Tremor can be a relative exception to this general rule as tremor is often quite responsive to DBS even when resistant to medical therapy. However, gait symptoms are more complicated. According to early reports, stride length and velocity improve with DBS without benefit for freezing.[7,8] More recent evidence suggest that high-frequency DBS may worsen freezing, while low-frequency (60 Hz) DBS improves it.[9,10] We have found that patients whose gait symptoms respond to medication will generally improve with stimulation, though we inform the patient of the uncertainty during the informed consent discussion. We relate our experience, while acknowledging that literature on the topic does not show a consistent benefit for gait with surgery. Finally, voice symptoms are a special case; we have seen both amelioration and aggravation of hypophonia. The response to DBS in this case is not clearly linked to prior response to medication. One report used cluster analysis to identify subtypes of voice dysfunction after DBS; while some patients have dysarthria related to corticobulbar stimulation, patients with low volume actually *benefit* from subthalamic nucleus (STN) DBS.[11] One group has hypothesized that this variability has to do with variations in the location of the dentatorubrothalamic tracts in DBS patients.[12] As a general rule, symptoms that get better with medication also get better with surgery.

Due to the high efficacy of DBS in the treatment of PD, DBS should be considered in dopamine-responsive PD patients as soon as motor symptoms are not fully controlled with medication or side effects become bothersome, because the disease is only going to get worse. To determine responsiveness to dopaminergic medication, most centers score the patient with the United Parkinson's Disease Rating Scale (UPDRS) when the patient is both on and off medication; a decrease of 30% in the UPDRS-III is considered to be appropriate for consideration of surgery.[13] Of note, tremor symptoms are often well controlled by stimulation, but may respond to levodopa only at very high or poorly tolerated doses, and thus some tremor-predominant PD patients may be excellent candidates for DBS, without a 30% decrease in the UPDRS.[14]

According to the FDA-approved labeling of both of the commercially available devices, patients should have experienced 4 years of symptoms prior to surgery. However, at present it is more common that a patient is referred for surgery after living with the disease for many years. Though it would be unusual to consider surgery prior to 4 years of symptoms, we would consider offering surgery after explaining to the patient that this operation would constitute off-label therapy. We would also mention the caveat that Parkinson's-plus syndromes, distinguished by motor symptoms similar to PD that are unresponsive to dopamine drugs, as well as prominent autonomic or cognitive dysfunction are often only obvious after a few years of disease, and these syndromes do not respond well to DBS therapy. In addition, we do not think there is current evidence that DBS modifies the course of PD or is neuroprotective in human subjects, despite promising animal data.[15,16] Nonetheless, most patients with motor symptoms that were previously well controlled with medications but are not fully controlled with medicine now or those who are experiencing on/off fluctuations would benefit from surgery.

Despite the general success of DBS in PD, a number of absolute and relative contraindications exist. The only truly absolute contraindication is the presence of symptoms that do not respond to dopamine equivalents. This is a hallmark of Parkinson's-plus syndromes such as multiple system atrophy (MSA) and progressive supranuclear palsy. To establish whether and to what extent carbidopa/levodopa is helpful for the patient being considered for surgery, the treating physicians should judge whether the patient has been followed by a neurologist long enough to establish the diagnosis. Prominent dementia and autonomic symptoms (characteristic of MSA) may take several years to declare themselves. However, fainting and orthostatic hypotension, which may be present in MSA, are also common in PD, and may represent a side effect of carbidopa/levodopa more than a true symptom. In these cases, we do not hesitate to implant, though we may allow the disease to "play out" a bit longer to see if other symptoms of Parkinson's-plus syndromes appear. Nonetheless, for a first approximation, a weak or no response to dopamine should be considered an absolute contraindication to DBS.

Relative contraindications to DBS include cognitive impairment, medical comorbidities, and frailty. Cognitive impairment may be exacerbated by DBS. Some prior reports suggested globus pallidus pars interna (GPi) DBS is preferred in patients with cognitive problems; however, a recent meta-analysis suggested that although declines occur across a broader spectrum of cognitive functions with STN DBS, the treatments are largely similar in their cognitive effects.[17] Many centers obtain preoperative neuropsychological assessments to identify patients at serious risk for cognitive decline. Serious medical comorbidities

may make the surgery itself dangerous. Finally, general frailty, which can be defined as general poor health, vulnerability to poor wound healing and infection, and limited physiological reserve aside from a disease process,[18,19] may limit the patient's ability to tolerate a lengthy procedure. Frail patients tend to have a more challenging and prolonged postoperative course, and they may require discharge to inpatient rehabilitation. Notably, independent of frailty, we do not consider age a contraindication as both young and old PD patients can be frail; thus, it is more useful to consider frailty than age. Frailty predicts surgical morbidity, mortality, and discharge institutionalization.[20,21,22] These are relative and not absolute contraindications, and should be discussed with the patient and his or her caregivers as part of the informed consent discussion. An important consideration in this discussion should also be the lack of other effective treatment modalities.

8.3 Goals of Treatment

After it has been determined that a patient is a suitable candidate for DBS, clinicians should communicate clearly the goals of surgery. We explain that the most important goal is prolonging the "on time," in which the patient can do the things he or she needs to do. In large, randomized trials, DBS improves "on time" by 4 hours a day.[23,24] With STN surgery, medication doses can usually be decreased by 30 to 50% on average, while GPi surgery allows for a lesser decrease;[24,25] however, there is still a marked increase in "on time" and an equivalent UPDRS benefit. With all surgical targets, patients should expect improvements in all of the symptom domains that are treated by medication, including rigidity, bradykinesia, and tremor. An important caveat for patient expectations is that the patients are typically as good after surgery as their "best on." Surgery does not cure PD, and it is important to emphasize that the patient may still expect significant disability. In addition, the nonmotor symptoms of PD are typically not well treated with DBS. In sum, we try to underpromise and overdeliver.

A common question is how long the treatment effect is expected to last. In long-term follow-up studies, patients continue to benefit from DBS for many years, and are generally doing better at 5 or even 10 years of follow-up than patients treated with medical therapy.[26,27] However, the disease does continue to progress ("it gets worse") and the severity of motor symptoms will inevitably increase. Non-dopamine-responsive symptoms, such as cognitive and autonomic problems, may contribute to disability more significantly in the later course of the disease. In general, the goal of treatment is to treat dopamine-responsive symptoms for a prolonged period, even though the disease progresses. However, each patient will have his or her own goals and these must be taken into consideration in the surgical plan.

8.4 Target Selection

Selection of a surgical target depends on the surgeon's and the patient's personal goals for treatment. The best-characterized targets for DBS in PD are STN and GPi. Though randomized trials have not demonstrated superiority of one target over the other, many neurologists favor STN implantation simply because

Table 8.1 Relative advantages and disadvantages of the STN and GPi as implantation targets for DBS treatment of PD[30]

Target	Advantages	Disadvantages
Subthalamic nucleus	Surgically safe with proper targeting	Surrounded by more critical structures
	Robust visualization via 3 Tesla MRI and microelectrode recording	More difficult to program
	Greater reduction of dosing of concurrent medication	Smaller size compared to GPi
	More commonly targeted due to slightly greater improvement in motor output	Generally requires bilateral implantation to achieve therapeutic advantage
	Surgeons are typically more familiar with the STN	Risk of adverse neurocognitive effects
	Very clear intraoperative effects	Risk of voice impairment
Globus pallidus pars interna	Equivalent of on-time benefit compared to STN	Significant motor improvement, though slightly better in STN vs. GPi
	Surrounded by fewer critical structures	Less familiar to some surgeons
	Larger size and easier to target for programming as compared to STN	Lesser reduction in dosing of medication
	Unilateral GPi implantation may offer greater therapeutic outcome compared to unilateral STN implantation	Evidence for superior cognitive outcome relative to STN implantation may be questionable and limited
	May be more appropriate for the elderly and frail patients	

Abbreviations: DBS, deep brain stimulation; GPi, globus pallidus pars interna; MRI, magnetic resonance imaging; PD, Parkinson's disease; STN, subthalamic nucleus.

many patients prefer to take less medication. GPi implantation, however, does have several advantages. Some trials have suggested that GPi implantation has less cognitive morbidity than STN implantation,[24,28] though this evidence has been called into question.[17] In addition, GPi is surrounded by fewer critical structures than STN, thus making implantation and programming more forgiving. Also, unilateral GPi implants are more beneficial than unilateral STN implants, so frail patients who may not very well tolerate bilateral surgery may benefit from staged (or unilateral) GPi implantation.[29] Other relative advantages and disadvantages of STN and GPi are summarized in ▶ Table 8.1.

8.4.1 Less Frequently Used Targets

VIM thalamus

Tremor control is the chief benefit of stimulation of the ventral intermediate (VIM) nucleus of thalamus.[31,32] However, STN and GPi surgery also control tremor in addition to rigidity and bradykinesia, so VIM surgery for Parkinson's is second line.

Zona incerta/posterior subthalamic area

This area lies between the posterior STN and the red nucleus, and stimulating it has excellent benefit for control of tremor;[33] at least one randomized trial comparing zona incerta stimulation with VIM stimulation is ongoing.[34] However, several groups have reported benefit in bradykinesia and rigidity from stimulation of this area.[35,36,37] A larger randomized trial is required to confirm efficacy.

Centromedian/parafascicular nucleus

In early studies, lesions of the central nuclei of the thalamus lead to improvements in rigidity and tremor.[38] DBS of the centromedian nucleus improves freezing of gait[39] and may also treat dyskinesia.[40] Experience is limited to very small series, however.

Pedunculopontine nucleus

The pedunculopontine nucleus is a cholinergic brainstem nucleus that has been proposed as a DBS target in PD for reducing gait-related symptoms, especially freezing.[41] Early reports of unilateral and/or bilateral stimulation of this region, some using ostensibly stimulatory low-frequency settings, describe improvement in freezing.[42,43,44] However, a recent systematic review described wide variation in implantation techniques and settings, as well as variability of response, and ultimately expressed skepticism about proposed benefit.[45,46] Further studies and/or registries of implanted patients may be useful in understanding the role of this target.

Nucleus basalis of Meynert

Recently, a small clinical trial explored stimulation of the nucleus basalis of Meynert for the alleviation of dementia symptoms in PD.[47] Despite a slight improvement in the patients' Neuropsychiatric Inventory, the study found no significant difference in cognitive improvement. Nonetheless, implantation surgery and stimulation were both well tolerated in all patients in this and other trials. Cognitive decline is otherwise untreatable, so further studies on this target will probably be conducted in PD and other dementing illnesses.[47,48]

8.5 Benefits of DBS

As mentioned above, the benefit of DBS mostly consists of improvements in "on time." Patients should be counseled that DBS will only make them as good as their "best on," and that they should still expect significant disability from PD. There are also benefits for other dopamine-responsive symptoms of the disease, such as tremor, rigidity, and bradykinesia. Medication-induced dyskinesias, as well as other medication side effects (such as orthostatic hypotension and constipation), can also improve after DBS as medication doses go down. Some general benefits of DBS are listed in ▶ Table 8.2.

Table 8.2 General benefits for the use of DBS in the treatment of PD

Benefits of DBS treatment for PD	
Provides significant improvement to combined motor scores	Allows a reduction in concurrent medications: reduction of side effects, reduction of variable drug efficacy
Increases mobility	Less drug-induced dyskinesia
Rapidly and reliably achieves the threshold of maximum benefit conferred by dopamine drugs	Electrical stimulation works synergistically with chemical stimulation from drugs to enhance therapeutic effect
Improves the length of maximum functional benefit (on-time) compared to dopamine drugs	Direct electrical stimulation may be neuroprotective, though data is limited

Abbreviations: DBS, deep brain stimulation; PD, Parkinson's disease.

8.6 Risks of DBS

The risks associated with DBS can be grouped into immediate surgical risks and long-term issues. Immediate risks of DBS include bleeding with the electrode pass that may result in permanent neurological deficits (0.7–7%),[49] infection (2.2–8%),[50,51] perioperative seizure, and a confusional state characterized by low arousal, poor cognitive function, and balance problems for the perioperative period (2–20%).[24,52] We counsel patients that the first three risks are on the order of low, single-digit percentages in the literature. There is some evidence that number of microelectrode passes correlates with hemorrhage, but the data are equivocal.[53] Frail patients and patients with significant cortical atrophy should be counseled that surgery may require a longer recovery period relative to other patients, and they may require discharge to acute rehabilitation. In the long term, these patients generally do well.

Long-term risks of DBS include hardware complications, such as infection and erosions, and side effects from stimulation. The leads and lead extensions do occasionally fracture and require revision.[54,55] Reported risks include: lead fracture (1.4–3%), lead erosion/infection (1.7–10%), and lead migration (3–12%).[55,56,57] Implanted pulse generator (IPG) malfunctions are distinctly rare. More commonly, prominent scars can develop around the leads and cause a restriction of head movement termed as "bowstringing."[58] This condition is often managed conservatively but can also require revision. Finally, stimulation can cause untoward side effects, such as face pulling (if the electrode is near the internal capsule or other critical structures), and these can be dose limiting. As the disease progresses, patients' stimulation needs may increase and dose-limiting capsular effects can become a problem, even if they were not present in the starting. In rare instances, the electrode may require revision to a more medial or posterior position. Tantalizingly, the availability of directional stimulation may prevent the need for such revisions, but no data are available on this yet.[59]

8.7 Techniques

DBS implantation techniques may be frame-based or frameless, and may or may not use microelectrode recording (MER). At our institution, we combine a frameless technique (STarFix) with MER, and we do simultaneous bilateral recording and implantation. However, surgeon preferences vary widely, and there are advantages and disadvantages of each technique. We have described all techniques in the subsequent text.

8.7.1 Frame-based Implantation

Most neurosurgeons use a frame-based implantation technique, utilizing either the Cosman-Robert-Wells (CRW) or Leksell frames. Both frames must be applied preoperatively, and then a localizer scan must be obtained. There is some discomfort with both head frames which varies widely between patients. Additionally, some patients want that the frame be applied under general anesthesia, which may prolong the OR time. Nonetheless, head frames are simple to use, accurate, and reliable.

8.7.2 Frameless Implantation

Several frameless implantation techniques are available. The Medtronic Nexframe™ system is a bone-fiducial based system in which a plastic tower attaches to bone anchors which are also used for stereotactic registration. Nexframe can be combined with MER,[60] intraoperative MRI,[61] or CT[62] to optimize lead location. While the Nexframe was used for the original intraoperative MRI-based implantations, the newer system ClearPoint™ (MRI Interventions, Irvine, CA) has taken over the bulk of MRI-guided DBS placements. ClearPoint is also a skull-mounted device that is designed for intraoperative imaging inside the MRI environment. It can be used in both "intraoperative" MRIs, as well as regular, closed-bore MRIs.[61] Finally, the STarFix™ platform (FHC Inc., Bowdoin, ME) is another bone-fiducial based system which uses 3D-printed single-use frames for targeting.[63] We use STarFix, for several reasons: low upfront capital investment, ease of use, and capacity to perform simultaneous bilateral implantation.

8.7.3 Stereotactic Targeting: Subthalamic nucleus

The STN is the most common DBS target in PD. Surgery depends on precise placement of the electrode in the dorsolateral portion of the STN, which is usually accomplished with a combination of image-based targeting and MER. Several methods are available for targeting.

Direct (image-guided) targeting

Modern, 3-Tesla MRI scanners are usually able to visualize the STN as an almond-shaped, T2-hypointense structure, just lateral to the red nucleus (▶ Fig. 8.1).[64] Reports of targeting STN with magnetic susceptibility-weighted imaging are also available as it is high in iron content.[65,66] In both of these reports, as well as another description of direct targeting,[67] the authors also used MER. This suggested that the targeting was reasonably robust since the correct location could be confirmed through two reliable methods.

AC-PC coordinate-based targeting

Many neurosurgeons use coordinate-based targeting from a line drawn between the anterior and posterior commissures.

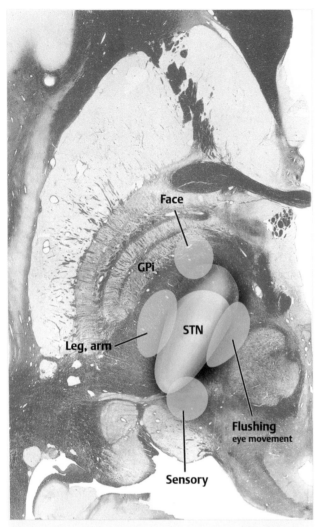

Fig. 8.1 The subthalamic nucleus is a small, almond-shaped structure just lateral to the red nucleus. Off-target stimulation effects can provide a clue about which direction the electrode should be moved in.

Generally, the STN is targeted 11 to 12 mm lateral to the mid-commissural point, 3 mm posterior, and 4 mm inferior.[68] This approach is time-honored but dates back to the time before advanced neuroimaging was available. This approach is generally combined with MER,[68] though it may also be combined with impedance measurement and macrostimulation to confirm targeting.[69,70]

Red nucleus targeting

Another imaging-guided technique utilizes the red nucleus (RN) as an internal reference to identify the STN.[71] The STN is consistently about 3 mm lateral to the RN. Taking care to identify the thickest slice of the RN in the mediolateral dimension, we choose a target 3 mm lateral to this slice in line with the anterior border of the RN and 2 mm inferior to the superior border of the RN. According to a report, RN-based targeting was found to be superior to coordinate-based and direct targeting,[71] though this paper predates wide availability of 3 T MRI. At present, there are data supporting the use of several imaging-based techniques (when MRI is available).

Refining the target: microelectrode recording in STN

After a stereotactic target has been identified, most surgeons use an entry site at the coronal suture, just lateral to the ventricles. From there, surgeons frequently confirm the target using MER. In addition to confirming the target, many surgeons will designate between one and four additional trajectories surrounding the center trajectory to the target, corresponding to the five holes in the Ben Gun apparatus (see Chapter 3, Microelectrode Recording Methods). MER has the advantage of confirming the location of STN, its borders, and surrounding structures. MER is used to identify kinesthetic neurons, which encode the movement of joints within limbs affected by the disease as well as tremor cells.

Most surgeons start 10 or 15 mm above the STN with their recording. Typical structures encountered are described in ► Table 8.3.

Table 8.3 Neurophysiological characteristics of structures encountered while mapping STN[72,73,74]

STN structure and divisions/cell types		MER neurophysiology
Thalamus	Reticular nucleus Lateropolaris nucleus VOA nuclei	6–10 mm prior to target there is a bimodal population of: • Bursting cells (15 ± 19 Hz) • Nonbursting cells (28 ± 19 Hz)
Zona incerta	Homogenous population	Minimal cell activity
Subthalamic nucleus	Mostly tonic/high-frequency cells that have kinesthetic responses Some irregular/long pause cells that have kinesthetic responses Some oscillatory/slow activity cells 32–40% cells are kinesthetically sensitive • All kinesthetically sensitive neurons are in the dorsal two-third of the nucleus • 78% are in the dorsal one-third of the nucleus	Increased background activity Mean frequency 37 ± 17 Hz • 25–45 Hz spiking between 3–8 mm in length Relatively low number of bursting cells • 8 versus 50% in thalamus • May be synchronized to tremor Tremor cells frequently found with tremor patients (4–6 Hz) Movement-stimulated in 26%, inhibited in 4%
Substantia nigra	Mostly tonic/high frequency	Relatively regular firing pattern 71 ± 23 Hz

Abbreviations: MER, microelectrode recording; STN, subthalamic nucleus; VOA, ventralis oralis anterior.

8.7.4 Stereotactic Targeting: Globus Pallidus Pars Interna

The GPi is the next most common DBS target in PD. Similar to the STN targeting, a combination of image-based targeting and MER can be used to properly target the structure.

Direct targeting

GPi is more easily visualized on MRI than the STN. Most surgeons select an area in the posteroventral GPi (where motor-encoding neurons are located), just above the optic tract[75] and medial to the internal medullary lamina and globus pallidus externa. These structures are reasonably well seen on proton density or T2-weighted MRI.[76] However, when image-based targeting was combined with MER, the central target was only used 64% of the time, suggesting that direct targeting of GPi is comparable in efficacy to direct (image-guided) targeting of STN.

Coordinate-based targeting

Given the high visibility of GPi, it is unusual to rely purely on coordinates, except when MRI is unavailable. The traditional GPi target is 20 to 22 mm lateral to the midcommisural point, 2 to 3 mm anterior, and 3 to 6 mm inferior. This corresponds to an area where so-called tremor cells (cells whose firing is entrained to the patient's tremor) and cells that respond to limb movement are located.[77]

8.7.5 Target Confirmation

MER in STN

MER is commonly used to (1) confirm the boundaries of the STN, and (2) identify kinesthestic cells corresponding to hand, arm, and leg areas affected by PD (tremor cells are a related phenomenon). In general, a cannula is advanced to a depth of 10 to 20 mm above the target and a tungsten microelectrode is advanced from there by fractions of a millimeter until cells that have characteristics associated with STN are detected. In the ideal MER pass, we identify thalamic cells, followed by a brief interlude in the silent zona incerta, and subsequently identify 5 mm of the highly cellular STN, as well as a clear border with substantia nigra. Each of these areas has characteristic firing rates and patterns (▶ Table 8.3). In particular, kinesthetic cells are a giveaway that the neurons in question are in STN.

In practice, detection is intrinsically challenging, and we often detect a smaller piece of STN than we had hoped. We use two MER cannulas, as a compromise between the passing of multiple tracts through the frontal lobe and the amount of useful information gathered. In general, the depth at which we encounter the STN in each tract informs our next pass. The STN is shaped like an almond, with the pointy tip facing medial and inferior; thus, if the STN is encountered later than expected, the target is usually more lateral or posterior. If the STN is encountered early, we are usually quite dorsal or lateral. Another helpful landmark is the thalamus; if only a modest amount of thalamus is obtained, you are usually lateral.

In general, we use MER as a tool for confirmation of the imaging-based targeting. MER generally enjoys a popularity that outstrips it usefulness; in the era when STN and RN were difficult to visualize on MRI, it was indispensable, but at present, excellent imaging-based targeting is available that is comparable in accuracy than MER alone.[57] While there is some intuitive appeal to the idea of confirming the somatotopy of the STN, evidence suggest that stimulation in the somatotopically relevant portion of the STN is indirect and limited to imaging studies showing that active contacts are in the same anterodorsal region as the hand- and leg-responsive cells of the STN.[78] Finally, the availability of directional DBS may allow more direct, specific targeting of sections within the STN in order to achieve maximum benefit from stimulation. In summary, MER is useful in DBS, but it is not critical.

MER in GPi

In general, GPi is a more forgiving target than STN because of its larger size and fewer nearby eloquent structures (▶ Fig. 8.1 and ▶ Fig. 8.2). Motor-encoding and tremor cells are prevalent,

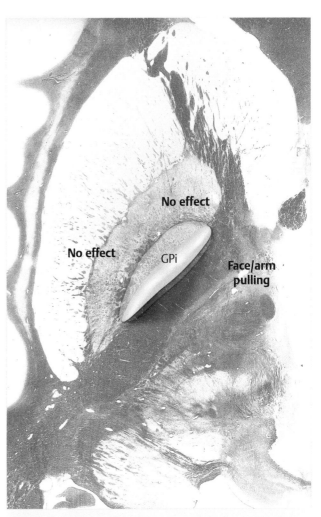

Fig. 8.2 The globus pallidus is the most medial component of the lentiform nucleus. As a target, it is much more forgiving than the subthalamic nucleus; off-target stimulation generally causes no ill effects, unless the electrode is extremely far from the target.

Table 8.4 Neurophysiological characteristics of structures encountered while mapping GPi[77,79,80]

GPi structure and divisions/cell types		MER neurophysiology
GPe	20% regular cells 71.1% irregular cells 8.9% bursting cells	Regular tonic high activity Lower activity but more bursting approaching medial lamina • Mean FR 52 ± 18 Hz • Range 45–60 Hz
Medial pallidal lamina	1–2 mm thick	Decreased electrical activity relative to GPe • Regular tonic 5–30 Hz
GPi	External segment Incomplete pallidal lamina Internal segment 29.3% regular cells 65.9% irregular cells 4.8% bursting and pausing cells Kinesthetic responses detectable to both active and passive movement Tremor cells may be present	More intense, high-amplitude electrical activity relative to GPe • Mean FR 96 ± 23 Hz • Frequency spread 20–200 Hz bursting and pausing in outer GPi More regular and lower amplitude approaching the optic tract
Optic tract	Regular, nonbursting, very low amplitude cells	Sharp decrease in electrical activity at the inferior edge of GPi Clear spikes when shining light in eyes

Abbreviations: GPe, globus pallidus pars externa; GPi, globus pallidus pars interna; MER, microelectrode recording.

similar to STN, and the neurons sound subjectively similar. Most neurosurgeons will first encounter GPe, then listen for a period of silence corresponding to the internal medullary lamina, and then identify GPi neurons. GPi neurons encode movement and tremor, similar to STN neurons. The key difference is the presence of the optic tract just below the posteroventral GPi. A bright light shone in the eyes will cause increased firing of neurons in the optic tract, which is usually easy to hear. If this is not identified, the targeting should be changed, as the electrophysiology is described in ▶ Table 8.4.

Macrostimulation in STN

STN is surrounded by several eloquent structures, and useful information can be gained by stimulating them (▶ Fig. 8.1). Cranial nerve nuclei and associated white matter tracts are found medially; if the electrode is too medial, there will be gaze deviation. The internal capsule is anterior and lateral; if the electrode is too lateral or anterior, there may be face or arm pulling. The medial lemniscus is posterior; paresthesias are elicited by posterior stimulation. The substantia nigra is inferior to the STN, and anxiety and autonomic effects can be elicited if the electrode is too deep. If side effects are noted during test stimulation, the surgeon should consider whether the eliciting voltage (as in constant-voltage systems like Medtronic) or amplitude (as in constant-current systems like Abbott Infinity) is acceptable. If not, the electrode should be repositioned. It is also possible to perform mapping with the FHC microelectrode cannula in a manner similar to electrode stimulation; we find this has no benefit over macrostimulation with the permanent electrode.

Macrostimulation in GPi

As stated previously, GPi is a generally more forgiving target due to its relatively larger size and the fact that current spread into GPe is not associated with symptoms (▶ Fig. 8.2). However, the internal capsule is medial and posterior to GPi and stimulation there can result in face or leg pulling, analogous to STN. The optic tract is deep to GPi its and stimulation can result in

scotomata or flashes of light (phosphenes). However, these are not uniformly seen in the same area as the evoked spikes from light stimulation, for reasons that are unclear.[80]

When the electrode is optimally positioned in either GPi or STN, there may be immediate improvements in tremor and rigidity from a "microlesion" effect. With stimulation, the patient should experience further improvements in the cardinal symptoms of PD, that is, tremor, rigidity, and bradykinesia, with minimal side effects. Dyskinesias are often seen as well, which are interpreted as meaning that the electrode is recapitulating the effects of the medication.

8.8 After Surgery

Electrodes are secured and tunneled under the skin, and the IPG is placed in a second surgery 1 to 2 weeks later. The patient may go to a floor- or stepdown-level bed if he or she is young, but elderly and/or frail patients are observed overnight in the ICU. In especially frail patients, we either stage the electrodes and the IPG, or occasionally try to do the entire procedure in a single day (both electrodes and the IPG) to minimize surgeries. In these cases, the patients generally benefit from discharge to a rehabilitation facility, rather than to home. However, most patients are able to be discharged home without complication.

We (and others) wait a period of 2 to 4 weeks before initial programming to let microlesion effects dissipate. A detailed discussion of programming is outside the scope of this chapter, but we will summarize the approach. After wound checks by the surgeon, the patient visits the neurologist off-medication for a monopolar survey of the electrodes. In the monopolar survey, the neurologist systematically documents the setting (either current amplitude or voltage, depending on the system) at which there is therapeutic benefit, and then the setting at which there are side effects. The "therapeutic window" is the range of settings between the therapeutic and the side-effect-producing amplitudes. Over a period of several months, we adjust the stimulation settings and decrease medication doses correspondingly. The overall goal is to make the patient to be more "stimulation dependent" and less "medication dependent."

Because of the constant nature of the stimulation, this change is associated with increased "on time" and decreased side effects.

8.9 Summary and Conclusion

DBS robustly improves clinical outcomes and quality of life for patients with PD. Surgical intervention should be considered relatively early in the course of the disease, before non-medication-responsive symptoms predominate. The goal of treatment is to prolong the length of time during the day in which the patient has satisfactory symptomatic relief, without dyskinesias; several studies suggest this benefit lasts around 4 to 6 hours per day. However, DBS is not a cure; it is important to counsel the patient to expect significant disability from PD, whether he or she has undergone surgery or not. It is also important to explain the risks of surgery, such as stroke or lack of benefit. With expectations appropriately adjusted, DBS is an excellent option and generally straightforward to perform. We suggest that MER be used as an adjunct to imaging-based targeting, but macrostimulation alone is also reasonable. After surgery, the patient should expect a 6-month period before the full benefit is obtained. Given the excellent results of DBS in most patients, we feel justified in recommending it to all patients with early motor complications of PD, because it only gets worse.

References

[1] Kowal SL, Dall TM, Chakrabarti R, Storm MV, Jain A. The current and projected economic burden of Parkinson's disease in the United States. Mov Disord. 2013; 28(3):311–318

[2] Holloway RG, Shoulson I, Fahn S, et al. Parkinson Study Group. Pramipexole vs levodopa as initial treatment for Parkinson disease: a 4-year randomized controlled trial. Arch Neurol. 2004; 61(7):1044–1053

[3] Schuepbach WM, Rau J, Knudsen K, et al. EARLYSTIM Study Group. Neurostimulation for Parkinson's disease with early motor complications. N Engl J Med. 2013; 368(7):610–622

[4] Martinez-Martin P, Jeukens-Visser M, Lyons KE, et al. Health-related quality-of-life scales in Parkinson's disease: critique and recommendations. Mov Disord. 2011; 26(13):2371–2380

[5] Van Den Eeden SK, Tanner CM, Bernstein AL, et al. Incidence of Parkinson's disease: variation by age, gender, and race/ethnicity. Am J Epidemiol. 2003; 157(11):1015–1022

[6] Fahn S, Oakes D, Shoulson I, et al. Parkinson Study Group. Levodopa and the progression of Parkinson's disease. N Engl J Med. 2004; 351(24):2498–2508

[7] Allert N, Volkmann J, Dotse S, Hefter H, Sturm V, Freund HJ. Effects of bilateral pallidal or subthalamic stimulation on gait in advanced Parkinson's disease. Mov Disord. 2001; 16(6):1076–1085

[8] Stolze H, Klebe S, Poepping M, et al. Effects of bilateral subthalamic nucleus stimulation on parkinsonian gait. Neurology. 2001; 57(1):144–146

[9] Moreau C, Defebvre L, Destée A, et al. STN-DBS frequency effects on freezing of gait in advanced Parkinson disease. Neurology. 2008; 71(2):80–84

[10] Xie T, Kang UJ, Warnke P. Effect of stimulation frequency on immediate freezing of gait in newly activated STN DBS in Parkinson's disease. J Neurol Neurosurg Psychiatry. 2012; 83(10):1015–1017

[11] Tsuboi T, Watanabe H, Tanaka Y, et al. Distinct phenotypes of speech and voice disorders in Parkinson's disease after subthalamic nucleus deep brain stimulation. J Neurol Neurosurg Psychiatry. 2015; 86(8):856–864

[12] Fenoy AJ, McHenry MA, Schiess MC. Speech changes induced by deep brain stimulation of the subthalamic nucleus in Parkinson disease: involvement of the dentatorubrothalamic tract. J Neurosurg. 2017; 126(6):2017–2027

[13] Bronstein JM, Tagliati M, Alterman RL, et al. Deep brain stimulation for Parkinson disease: an expert consensus and review of key issues. Arch Neurol. 2011; 68(2):165

[14] Morishita T, Rahman M, Foote KD, et al. DBS candidates that fall short on a levodopa challenge test: alternative and important indications. Neurologist. 2011; 17(5):263–268

[15] Musacchio T, Rebenstorff M, Fluri F, et al. Subthalamic nucleus deep brain stimulation is neuroprotective in the A53T α-synuclein Parkinson's disease rat model. Ann Neurol. 2017; 81(6):825–836

[16] Wallace BA, Ashkan K, Heise CE, et al. Survival of midbrain dopaminergic cells after lesion or deep brain stimulation of the subthalamic nucleus in MPTP-treated monkeys. Brain. 2007; 130(Pt 8):2129–2145

[17] Combs HL, Folley BS, Berry DT, et al. Cognition and depression following deep brain stimulation of the subthalamic nucleus and globus pallidus pars internus in Parkinson's disease: a meta-analysis. Neuropsychol Rev. 2015; 25(4):439–454

[18] Partridge JS, Harari D, Dhesi JK. Frailty in the older surgical patient: a review. Age Ageing. 2012; 41(2):142–147

[19] Xue QL. The frailty syndrome: definition and natural history. Clin Geriatr Med. 2011; 27(1):1–15

[20] Farhat JS, Velanovich V, Falvo AJ, et al. Are the frail destined to fail? Frailty index as predictor of surgical morbidity and mortality in the elderly. J Trauma Acute Care Surg. 2012; 72(6):1526–1530, discussion 1530–1531

[21] Robinson TN, Wu DS, Stiegmann GV, Moss M. Frailty predicts increased hospital and six-month healthcare cost following colorectal surgery in older adults. Am J Surg. 2011; 202(5):511–514

[22] Sündermann S, Dademasch A, Praetorius J, et al. Comprehensive assessment of frailty for elderly high-risk patients undergoing cardiac surgery. Eur J Cardiothorac Surg. 2011; 39(1):33–37

[23] Deuschl G, Schade-Brittinger C, Krack P, et al. German Parkinson Study Group, Neurostimulation Section. A randomized trial of deep-brain stimulation for Parkinson's disease. N Engl J Med. 2006; 355(9):896–908

[24] Follett KA, Weaver FM, Stern M, et al. CSP 468 Study Group. Pallidal versus subthalamic deep-brain stimulation for Parkinson's disease. N Engl J Med. 2010; 362(22):2077–2091

[25] Vitek JL. Deep brain stimulation for Parkinson's disease. A critical re-evaluation of STN versus GPi DBS. Stereotact Funct Neurosurg. 2002; 78(3–4):119–131

[26] Aviles-Olmos I, Kefalopoulou Z, Tripoliti E, et al. Long-term outcome of subthalamic nucleus deep brain stimulation for Parkinson's disease using an MRI-guided and MRI-verified approach. J Neurol Neurosurg Psychiatry. 2014; 85(12):1419–1425

[27] Moro E, Lozano AM, Pollak P, et al. Long-term results of a multicenter study on subthalamic and pallidal stimulation in Parkinson's disease. Mov Disord. 2010; 25(5):578–586

[28] Okun MS, Fernandez HH, Wu SS, et al. Cognition and mood in Parkinson's disease in subthalamic nucleus versus globus pallidus interna deep brain stimulation: the COMPARE trial. Ann Neurol. 2009; 65(5):586–595

[29] Zahodne LB, Okun MS, Foote KD, et al. Greater improvement in quality of life following unilateral deep brain stimulation surgery in the globus pallidus as compared to the subthalamic nucleus. J Neurol. 2009; 256(8):1321–1329

[30] Obeso JA, Olanow CW, Rodriguez-Oroz MC, Krack P, Kumar R, Lang AE, Deep-Brain Stimulation for Parkinson's Disease Study Group. Deep-brain stimulation of the subthalamic nucleus or the pars interna of the globus pallidus in Parkinson's disease. N Engl J Med. 2001; 345(13):956–963

[31] Benabid AL, Pollak P, Gervason C, et al. Long-term suppression of tremor by chronic stimulation of the ventral intermediate thalamic nucleus. Lancet. 1991; 337(8738):403–406

[32] Benabid AL, Pollak P, Louveau A, Henry S, de Rougemont J. Combined (thalamotomy and stimulation) stereotactic surgery of the VIM thalamic nucleus for bilateral Parkinson disease. Appl Neurophysiol. 1987; 50(1–6):344–346

[33] Plaha P, Khan S, Gill SS. Bilateral stimulation of the caudal zona incerta nucleus for tremor control. J Neurol Neurosurg Psychiatry. 2008; 79(5):504–513

[34] Skogseid IM. (2017, May 31, 2017). A Controlled Comparison of Two DBS Targets for Upper Extremity Action Tremor (Tremorstim). Retrieved from https://clinicaltrials.gov/ct2/show/NCT03156517

[35] Plaha P, Ben-Shlomo Y, Patel NK, Gill SS. Stimulation of the caudal zona incerta is superior to stimulation of the subthalamic nucleus in improving contralateral parkinsonism. Brain. 2006; 129(Pt 7):1732–1747

[36] Velasco F, Carrillo-Ruiz JD, Salcido V, Castro G, Soto J, Velasco AL. Unilateral stimulation of prelemniscal radiations for the treatment of acral symptoms of Parkinson's disease: long-term results. Neuromodulation. 2016; 19(4):357–364

[37] Velasco F, Jiménez F, Pérez ML, et al. Electrical stimulation of the prelemniscal radiation in the treatment of Parkinson's disease: an old target revised with new techniques. Neurosurgery. 2001; 49(2):293–306, discussion 306–308

[38] Adams JE, Rutkin BB. Lesions of the centrum medianum in the treatment of movement disorders. Confin Neurol. 1965; 26(3):231–245

[39] Mazzone P, Stocchi F, Galati S, et al. Bilateral implantation of centromedian-parafascicularis complex and GPi: a new combination of unconventional targets for deep brain stimulation in severe Parkinson's disease. Neuromodulation. 2006; 9(3):221–228

[40] Stefani A, Peppe A, Pierantozzi M, et al. Multi-target strategy for parkinsonian patients: the role of deep brain stimulation in the centromedian-parafascicularis complex. Brain Res Bull. 2009; 78(2–3):113–118

[41] Pahapill PA, Lozano AM. The pedunculopontine nucleus and Parkinson's disease. Brain. 2000; 123(Pt 9):1767–1783

[42] Moro E, Hamani C, Poon YY, et al. Unilateral pedunculopontine stimulation improves falls in Parkinson's disease. Brain. 2010; 133(Pt 1):215–224

[43] Plaha P, Gill SS. Bilateral deep brain stimulation of the pedunculopontine nucleus for Parkinson's disease. Neuroreport. 2005; 16(17):1883–1887

[44] Stefani A, Lozano AM, Peppe A, et al. Bilateral deep brain stimulation of the pedunculopontine and subthalamic nuclei in severe Parkinson's disease. Brain. 2007; 130(Pt 6):1596–1607

[45] Thevathasan W, Debu B, Aziz T, et al. Movement Disorders Society PPN DBS Working Groupin collaboration with the World Society for Stereotactic and Functional Neurosurgery. Pedunculopontine nucleus deep brain stimulation in Parkinson's disease: A clinical review. Mov Disord. 2018; 33(1):10–20

[46] Wang JW, Zhang YQ, Zhang XH, Wang YP, Li JP, Li YJ. Deep brain stimulation of pedunculopontine nucleus for postural instability and gait disorder after parkinson disease: a meta-analysis of individual patient data. World Neurosurg. 2017; 102:72–78

[47] Gratwicke J, Zrinzo L, Kahan J, et al. Bilateral deep brain stimulation of the nucleus basalis of meynert for parkinson disease dementia: a randomized clinical trial. JAMA Neurol. 2018; 75(2):169–178

[48] Kuhn J, Hardenacke K, Lenartz D, et al. Deep brain stimulation of the nucleus basalis of Meynert in Alzheimer's dementia. Mol Psychiatry. 2015; 20(3):353–360

[49] Binder DK, Rau G, Starr PA. Hemorrhagic complications of microelectrode-guided deep brain stimulation. Stereotact Funct Neurosurg. 2003; 80(1–4):28–31

[50] Blomstedt P, Hariz MI. Hardware-related complications of deep brain stimulation: a ten year experience. Acta Neurochir (Wien). 2005; 147(10):1061–1064, discussion 1064

[51] Umemura A, Jaggi JL, Hurtig HI, et al. Deep brain stimulation for movement disorders: morbidity and mortality in 109 patients. J Neurosurg. 2003; 98(4):779–784

[52] Appleby BS, Duggan PS, Regenberg A, Rabins PV. Psychiatric and neuropsychiatric adverse events associated with deep brain stimulation: a meta-analysis of ten years' experience. Mov Disord. 2007; 22(12):1722–1728

[53] Ben-Haim S, Asaad WF, Gale JT, Eskandar EN. Risk factors for hemorrhage during microelectrode-guided deep brain stimulation and the introduction of an improved microelectrode design. Neurosurgery. 2009; 64(4):754–762, discussion 762–763

[54] Lyons KE, Wilkinson SB, Overman J, Pahwa R. Surgical and hardware complications of subthalamic stimulation: a series of 160 procedures. Neurology. 2004; 63(4):612–616

[55] Oh MY, Abosch A, Kim SH, Lang AE, Lozano AM. Long-term hardware-related complications of deep brain stimulation. Neurosurgery. 2002; 50(6):1268–1274, discussion 1274–1276

[56] Fenoy AJ, Simpson RK, Jr. Risks of common complications in deep brain stimulation surgery: management and avoidance. J Neurosurg. 2014; 120(1):132–139

[57] Morishita T, Hilliard JD, Okun MS, et al. Postoperative lead migration in deep brain stimulation surgery: incidence, risk factors, and clinical impact. PLoS One. 2017; 12(9):e0183711

[58] Miller PM, Gross RE. Wire tethering or 'bowstringing' as a long-term hardware-related complication of deep brain stimulation. Stereotact Funct Neurosurg. 2009; 87(6):353–359

[59] Rebelo P, Green AL, Aziz TZ, et al. Thalamic directional deep brain stimulation for tremor: spend less, get more. Brain Stimul. 2018; 11(3):600–606

[60] Kelman C, Ramakrishnan V, Davies A, Holloway K. Analysis of stereotactic accuracy of the Cosman-Robert-Wells frame and Nexframe frameless systems in deep brain stimulation surgery. Stereotact Funct Neurosurg. 2010; 88(5):288–295

[61] Starr PA, Martin AJ, Ostrem JL, Talke P, Levesque N, Larson PS. Subthalamic nucleus deep brain stimulator placement using high-field interventional magnetic resonance imaging and a skull-mounted aiming device: technique and application accuracy. J Neurosurg. 2010; 112(3):479–490

[62] Burchiel KJ, McCartney S, Lee A, Raslan AM. Accuracy of deep brain stimulation electrode placement using intraoperative computed tomography without microelectrode recording. J Neurosurg. 2013; 119(2):301–306

[63] Konrad PE, Neimat JS, Yu H, et al. Customized, miniature rapid-prototype stereotactic frames for use in deep brain stimulator surgery: initial clinical methodology and experience from 263 patients from 2002 to 2008. Stereotact Funct Neurosurg. 2011; 89(1):34–41

[64] Slavin KV, Thulborn KR, Wess C, Nersesyan H. Direct visualization of the human subthalamic nucleus with 3 T MR imaging. AJNR Am J Neuroradiol. 2006; 27(1):80–84

[65] Lefranc M, Derrey S, Merle P, et al. High-resolution 3-dimensional T2*-weighted angiography (HR 3-D SWAN): an optimized 3-T magnetic resonance imaging sequence for targeting the subthalamic nucleus. Neurosurgery. 2014; 74(6):615–626, discussion 627

[66] Rasouli J, Ramdhani R, Panov FE, et al. Utilization of quantitative susceptibility mapping for direct targeting of the subthalamic nucleus during deep brain stimulation surgery. Oper Neurosurg (Hagerstown). 2018; 14(4):412–419

[67] Tonge M, Kocabicak E, Ackermans L, Kuijf M, Temel Y. Final electrode position in subthalamic nucleus deep brain stimulation surgery: a comparison of indirect and direct targeting methods. Turk Neurosurg. 2016; 26(6):900–903

[68] Bakay RA. Movement Disorder Surgery: The Essentials. 1st ed. Thieme; 2008

[69] Foltynie T, Zrinzo L, Martinez-Torres I, et al. MRI-guided STN DBS in Parkinson's disease without microelectrode recording: efficacy and safety. J Neurol Neurosurg Psychiatry. 2011; 82(4):358–363

[70] Yoshida F, Martinez-Torres I, Pogosyan A, et al. Value of subthalamic nucleus local field potentials recordings in predicting stimulation parameters for deep brain stimulation in Parkinson's disease. J Neurol Neurosurg Psychiatry. 2010; 81(8):885–889

[71] Andrade-Souza YM, Schwalb JM, Hamani C, et al. Comparison of three methods of targeting the subthalamic nucleus for chronic stimulation in Parkinson's disease. Neurosurgery. 2005; 56(2) Suppl:360–368, discussion 360–368

[72] Benazzouz A, Breit S, Koudsie A, Pollak P, Krack P, Benabid AL. Intraoperative microrecordings of the subthalamic nucleus in Parkinson's disease. Mov Disord. 2002; 17 Suppl 3:S145–S149

[73] Hutchison WD, Allan RJ, Opitz H, et al. Neurophysiological identification of the subthalamic nucleus in surgery for Parkinson's disease. Ann Neurol. 1998; 44(4):622–628

[74] Rodriguez-Oroz MC, Rodriguez M, Guridi J, et al. The subthalamic nucleus in Parkinson's disease: somatotopic organization and physiological characteristics. Brain. 2001; 124(Pt 9):1777–1790

[75] Vayssiere N, Hemm S, Cif L, et al. Comparison of atlas- and magnetic resonance imaging-based stereotactic targeting of the globus pallidus internus in the performance of deep brain stimulation for treatment of dystonia. J Neurosurg. 2002; 96(4):673–679

[76] O'Gorman RL, Shmueli K, Ashkan K, et al. Optimal MRI methods for direct stereotactic targeting of the subthalamic nucleus and globus pallidus. Eur Radiol. 2011; 21(1):130–136

[77] Lozano AM, Hutchison WD. Microelectrode recordings in the pallidum. Mov Disord. 2002; 17 Suppl 3:S150–S154

[78] Saint-Cyr JA, Hoque T, Pereira LC, et al. Localization of clinically effective stimulating electrodes in the human subthalamic nucleus on magnetic resonance imaging. J Neurosurg. 2002; 97(5):1152–1166

[79] Bour LJ, Contarino MF, Foncke EM, et al. Long-term experience with intraoperative microrecording during DBS neurosurgery in STN and GPi. Acta Neurochir (Wien). 2010; 152(12):2069–2077

[80] Lozano A, Hutchison W, Kiss Z, Tasker R, Davis K, Dostrovsky J. Methods for microelectrode-guided posteroventral pallidotomy. J Neurosurg. 1996; 84(2):194–202

9 Essential Tremor Application

June Y. Guillet, Abhijeet Gummadavelli, Dwaine Cooke, Jason Gerrard

Abstract

Tremor is the most common movement disorder and essential tremor (ET) affects a significant portion of the population that increases with age. Although ET can be identified with a handful of clinical tests, the Movement Disorder Society has recently published The Essential Tremor Rating Assessment Scale (TET-RAS) to provide a consistent and more accurate measure of ET severity and disability. The medical treatment of ET has a 50 to 60% response rate with beta blockers (propranolol) and primidone having level A recommendations as initial therapy. In addition to the initial failure rate, 10 to 15% of responders will develop tolerance within 1 year of treatment, and the failure rate increases over time. Surgical treatment of patients with ET has been proven to be safe and highly efficacious. Deep brain stimulation (DBS) to the ventral intermediate (Vim) or ventrolateral (VL) thalamus is the gold standard for surgical treatment of ET with a reported average of 80 to 85% improvement in tremor. Unilateral or bilateral DBS to the Vim nucleus of the thalamus is the most commonly utilized target. The Vim is not well visualized on magnetic resonance imaging for direct image-guided targeting, and therefore, traditional awake surgery remains the most common technique utilized in cases of ET. Well-established potential surgical and stimulation side effects, including dysphagia, dysarthria, and disequilibrium, are more likely to occur with bilateral Vim DBS. Patients who are unable or unwilling to undergo undergo DBS surgery may have clinically significant improvement in tremor with less invasive thalamotomy techniques such as gamma knife thalamotomy and high-frequency focused ultrasound.

Keywords: deep brain stimulation, essential tremor, ventrolateral thalamus/Vim, thalamotomy, surgical technique

9.1 Presentation

Essential tremor (ET) is one of the most common neurological movement disorders, estimated to affect 0.4 to 1% of the world's population with an increasing prevalence (4–7%) in people over 65 years of age.[1] The diagnostic hallmark of ET on physical examination is a regular 8 to 12-Hz recurrent and progressive kinetic tremor usually affecting both upper extremities. The tremor may also be postural in nature or increased in severity with certain postures. ET may also affect the head, face, voice, and/or lower extremities. ET is usually bilateral and symmetric, in contrast to the resting tremor of Parkinson's disease (PD) that is often unilateral or asymmetric. Unilateral tremor or progression is less common in ET and may predict worse prognosis.[2] Recent studies have also suggested nonmotor symptoms of ET may also affect or exacerbate cognitive, psychiatric, and sensory disabilities.[3] A careful clinical exam is critical as it is reported that 37% of ET patients are misdiagnosed.[4] The differential diagnosis of an observed tremor on exam includes PD, hyperthyroidism, dystonic tremor, Wilson's disease, drug effects, and physiological tremor. ET may be distinguished from other entities on the basis of history and physical exam. Lab tests and nuclear imaging are less commonly needed or utilized. ET may be distinguished from a Parkinsonian tremor, which classically presents as a predominant resting tremor in the setting of associated bradykinesia. Dystonic tremor is often associated with limb posturing. Physiological tremor is heightened by emotional states and does not include head tremor. Recent neurophysiological studies propose a Tremor Stability Index to help determine the kinematic characteristics of tremor in order to distinguish the most likely pathologic classification of the tremor with 92% accuracy.[5]

9.1.1 Classification of Essential Tremor

A consensus for tremor classification was proposed by the Movement Disorder Society in 1998 that provided a useful syndromic and clinical classification to identify the ET syndrome.[5] The International Parkinson and Movement Disorder Society Task Force on tremor classification is undergoing reclassification by updates in genetic, pathophysiologic, and pathologic evidence of ET pathogenesis.[6] The utility of classification in ET is to attempt to uncover pathophysiologically homogenous groups in order to help assess prognosis and customize the treatment options. The ET syndrome can be subclassified by genetic predisposition (hereditary and sporadic subgroups), age of onset (early and late onset; cutoff at 65 years of age), and anatomic distribution of tremor (isolated arm, arm and head, other focal tremors). Hereditary ET is clinically significant and fully penetrant by 60 years of age.[1] An older age of onset of ET is less likely hereditary and has been associated with more rapid progression of the disease.[1] Faster rate of progression has also been reported in patients with involvement of head tremor as opposed to an isolated arm tremor.[7] Earlier age of onset of ET is associated with a familial form.[1]

9.1.2 Tremor Severity

The severity of ET may be described by the severity of the observed tremor, impairment of activities of daily living (Bain and Findley Tremor activities of daily living [ADL] questionnaire), and impact on quality of life (Quality of Life in Essential Tremor [QUEST] questionnaire).[5]

The impairment related to ET may be visualized with simple writing (writing name and sentence), or drawing (Archimedes spiral) tasks. The Fahn–Tolosa–Marin (FTM) tremor rating scale is widely used to quantify ET severity based on tremor location (Part A: arms, head, face, etc., rated from 1–4, at rest, with posture, and with action), specific motor tasks (Part B: handwriting, spiral drawing, pouring), and functional disabilities (Part C: speaking, eating, drinking, etc.).[6] The widespread use of the FTM tremor rating scale often lead it to be referred to as the Clinical Tremor Rating Scale (CRST). Due to limitations of the FTM scale in severe ET, the Tremor Research Group has published a comprehensive ET rating scale known as The Essential Tremor Rating Assessment Scale (TETRAS) that has high reliability especially for head and upper extremity tremor.[7] Tremor rating scales in ET are further discussed later in this chapter.

9.2 Genetics

More than 50% of patients with ET have a positive family history, suggesting the importance of genetic influence.[8] ET is thought to be conferred in an autosomal-dominant fashion.[9] Analysis in mono- and dizygotic twins have shown that monozygotic twins have a significantly higher concordance rate.[10] However, problems in genetic studies including phenotypically heterogeneous samples, small sample sizes, and difficulties in reproducibility limit these studies' impacts.[11] A number of genes have been linked to ET through genome-wide association studies (GWAS), mapping studies, linkage analysis, and exome sequencing. Linkage studies found three loci of interest ETM1–3 related to ET: ETM1, a polymorphism in the *DRD3* gene (chromosome 13q13.31) that encodes a dopamine-receptor subtypes found in numerous areas of the brain including regions of the cerebellum[12]; ETM2 locus mapped to *HS1BP3* gene (hematopoetic lineage cell-specific protein binding protein 3, Ch 2p25-p22)[13]; ETM3 locus (6p23) with unclear related gene expression.[14] A recent linkage analysis showed relation of Ch 5q35 to ET.[15] Whole exome sequencing in a French-Canadian ET family discovered a nonsense-mediated mRNA decay of the *FUS* gene product (fused in sarcoma, Ch 16p11).[16] Polymorphisms indicated by GWAS studies have suggested other genes of interest including *LINGO1* (Leucine rich repeat and Ig domain containing 1, involved in intracellular signaling in response of myelin-associated inhibitors) (chromosome 15q24)[17]; *SLC1A2* (Ch 11p13) whose gene product EAAT2 glutamate reuptake transporter is highly expressed in the inferior olive[18]; STK32B (a serine/threonine kinase), PPARGC1A (a transcriptional activator), and CTNNA3 (a cell adhesion molecule) were linked with ET.[19] The genetic landscape of ET is complex, and although numerous candidate genes of interest have been found, no clear causative genes have been studied, in part due to the phenotypic and diagnostic variability inherent in the populations.[20] Interestingly, a number of these genes may be localized to cerebellar and olivary circuitry, implicating their role in the cerebellum and inferior olive in effecting the network oscillation thought to underlie ET.[21]

9.3 Pathophysiology and Tremor Circuitry

The olivocerebellar hypothesis of tremor pathophysiology is the predominant theory of disturbance underlying the rhythmic network oscillation of ET.[22] Initial data from harmaline-induced tremor animal models and human neurophysiological studies in ET patients pointed toward electrophysiologic dysfunction of the inferior olivary nucleus (ION) as the origin of ET

dysfunction. The bursting oscillatory nature of pathologic ION cells was spread to the extremities via the reticulo- and vestibulospinal pathways.[23,24] However, more recent data questioned the involvement of ION as the postmortem neuropathological examination of ET patients showed no structural difference in the ION and neuroimaging studies showed no ION activation.[25,26]

Latest data are suggestive of a cerebellar hypothesis.[27] Neuroimaging data from resting state functional magnetic resonance imaging (fMRI) in ET patients (matched with controls) showed intrinsic variations in network properties compared to control patients specifically in the cerebellum, pre- and postcentral gyri, supplementary motor area (SMA), and paracentral lobule.[28] Postmortem pathophysiological evidence from ET patients show changes that include structural (Purkinje cell morphology) and functional (Purkinje-basket cell and Purkinje-climbing fiber interface dysfunction) components[29] as well as pathological findings ('torpedoes' and Bergmann glia).[30] At the cellular level, this process may be driven by Purkinje neuron loss, as evidenced by studies of decreased cell counts and increased intercell distance in ET patients compared to controls.[31] In this sense, ET shares the feature of specific cell loss as seen in cases of other neurodegenerative diseases. Neuroimaging, pathological, and electrophysiological studies suggest that the tremor circuitry involves olivo-cerebello-thalamo-cortical connections. The ION is the primary input of climbing fibers to the cerebellar Purkinje inhibitory cells; the output of the cerebellar Purkinje cells is to the deep cerebellar nuclei, which then target the VL thalamus. The output of VL thalamus include motor and premotor cortices. Interestingly, the pathological and electrophysiological characteristics of the tremor may be determined by the specific nature of dysfunction within the circuit; tremors may be generated by mechanical oscillations, reflex-driven oscillations, centrally driven oscillations, or oscillations driven by feedforward or feedback loops.[22] ET is thought to be a centrally driven tremor; the structural and functional changes in the olivocerebellar network generate rhythmic disinhibition of the thalamus. The tremor oscillation is effected by gamma-aminobutyric acid (GABA)ergic dysfunction of the cerebellar dentate nuclei as they project to the thalamus. Neurochemical studies have supported this GABAergic dysfunction in the cerebellum.[32] Noninvasive transient manipulation of the cerebellar circuit with transcranial alternating current stimulation allowed for entraining the neural oscillation in ET patients.[33]

9.4 Diagnostic Testing

There are no tests to diagnose ET; the diagnosis is made typically on clinical evaluation with the presence of the typical kinetic/postural tremor. Standard neuroimaging with computed tomography (CT) and MRI scans of the head is usually normal and demonstrate no specific findings for ET.[34] However, specialized imaging with single-photon emission CT (SPECT) and ioflupain 123 I (DaTSCAN) may be used to rule out other causes of tremor such as PD.[35,36,37] The exact mechanism of ET has not been completely understood, but diffusion tensor imaging (DTI) performed on patients with ET demonstrated increased apparent diffusion coefficient in the red nucleus suggestive of cell loss as a result of a neurodegenerative disorder.[38] Several structural and functional imaging studies have identified pathology involving the cerebellum (dentate nucleus, vermis, and superior and inferior cerebellar peduncles), the ION, the red nucleus, the thalamus, the cortex, and the interconnecting pathways.[34] The clinical significance and the application of such findings is still not clear.

9.4.1 Testing and Grading Scales for Essential Tremor

The simple bedside tests for essential tremor include:
- Arm extension test.
- Finger-to-nose test.
- Heel shin test.
- Drawing a spiral.
- Drawing a straight line.
- Archimedes spiral.
- Signing of name.
- Pouring water from one cup to the next back and forth.
- Having the patient utter a single sound such as "aaahhh" or "eeehhh" and hold it for as long as possible.

The presence of a tremor and its characteristics in terms of its frequency and amplitude are noted while certain functions are tested. The finger-to-nose test is the most useful screening test in a general population and is usually abnormal in approximately 50% of patients with ET.[29] To exclude normal subjects, tests such as a sustained arm extension, drawing a spiral, and pouring of water have been very effective.[29,39]

There are several grading scales and screening instruments for ET. Tremor grading scales that were recommended by the task force of the Movement Disorder Society include[40]:

- The Essential Tremor Rating Assessment Scale (TETRAS).
- The Fahn–Tolosa–Marin Tremor Rating Scale (FTM).
- Quality of Life in Essential Tremor Questionnaire.
- Bain and Findley Clinical Tremor Rating Scale.
- Bain and Findley Spirography Scale.
- Bain and Findley Tremor activities of daily living scale.
- Washington Heights-Inwood Genetic Study of Essential Tremor (WHIGET) Tremor Rating Scale, Version 2.

The Movement Disorder Society task force further recommended the WHIGET Tremor Rating Scale, version 1 as a screening tool for ET.[40] In this system, patients were categorized as having possible, probable, or definite ET. The tremor (postural and kinetic) was rated as 0 to 3 grade based on motor task performance. The presence of grade 2 or more makes the diagnosis of ET definite.[40] TETRAS is a short, valid, and easy-to-use scale that was designed for clinical assessment of severity of ET.[7] It rates the presence of tremors in a range of 0 to 4 for 10 test items (▶ Table 9.1).

The Fahn–Tolosa–Marin Tremor Rating Scale

This scale is divided into three main parts A, B, and C, where part A (items 1–9) looks at the amplitude of rest, postural, and kinetic tremors in specific anatomic sites (face, tongue, voice, head, bilateral upper and lower extremities, and the trunk; part B (items 10–14) evaluates the degree of tremor in handwriting, drawing, and pouring; and part C (items 15–21) assesses activities of daily living (speaking, eating, drinking, hygiene, dressing, writing, and working).[6,40] This scale utilizes a 5-point grading scheme with a maximum total of 144 points (▶ Table 9.2). The total score is calculated as a percentage of 144. In addition, a global assessment percentage score for the examiner (▶ Table 9.3) and for the patient (▶ Table 9.4) can be obtained based on their subjective assessment of the patient's ability to perform the activities of daily living.[6]

Table 9.1 The Essential Tremor Rating Assessment Scale (TETRAS)[40]

Test	1	2	3	4
Head (tremor amplitude)	<0.5 cm	0.5 –<2.5 cm	2.5–5 cm	>5 cm
Face	Minimal	Noticeable	Present in most facial muscle contractions	Disfiguring
Tongue				
Voice	Minimal, mainly during "aaah" or "eee"	Noticeable during "aaah" or "eee" but minimal during speech	Obvious during speech	Some words incomprehensible
Upper limb	Minimal	1 –<3 cm	5 –<10 cm	20 cm or greater
Lower limb	Minimal	Mild	<5 cm	>5 cm
Spirals	Minimal	Obvious	Portions not discernible	Figure not discernible
Handwriting	Minimal	Obvious but legible	Some words illegible	Completely illegible
Dot approximation	Minimal	1 –<3 cm	5 –<10 cm	>20 cm
Standing	Minimal	Obvious	Moderate	Severe

Table 9.2 The Fahn–Tolosa–Marin Tremor Rating Full Scale and Worksheet[6]

	Task	0 Normal	1 Mildly abnormal	2 Moderately abnormal	3 Markedly abnormal	4 Severely abnormal
A	**(1–9) Tremor** 1 – At rest 2 – While holding posture 3 – While performing action	None	Amplitude < 0.5 cm	Amplitude 0.5–1 cm	Amplitude 1–2 cm	Amplitude > 2 cm
B	**(10) Handwriting** The patient signs his or her name, writes the date, and writes the standard sentence: "This is a sample of my best handwriting."	None	Slightly untidy, tremulous	Legible but with considerable tremor	Illegible	Inability to keep pencil/pen on the paper, or has to stabilize with contralateral limb
	(11–13) Drawing (A, B, C) Patient is instructed to connect points on a drawing without crossing lines. Each hand is tested individually. Example: Items A and B – Archimedes spirals and C – a straight line within a narrow rectangular box	Normal	Slightly tremulous	Moderately tremulous or frequent crossing of lines	Accomplishes the task with great difficulty usually with several errors	Inability to complete the drawing
	(14) Pouring Individually assessing the patient's ability to pour water from firm plastic cups (8-cm tall) filled upto within 1 cm of the top	Normal	No water is spilled, but more caution exercised than seen in patient without tremor	Spills up to 10% of water	Spills between 10–50% of water	Spills most of the water
C	**(15) Speaking** Includes spastic dysphonia	Normal	Mild tremulousness (only when patient is nervous)	Mild voice tremor	Moderate voice tremor	Severe voice tremor
	(16) Feeding Other than liquids	Normal	Can bring all solids to the mouth, rarely spilling	Frequently spilling, has to bring head halfway toward the food	Has to hold cup or glass with two hands in order to have a drink	Needs help to feed
	(17) Drinking	Normal	Can still use a spoon, but not if completely full	Unable to use spoon, uses cup or glass	Can drink from cup or glass, but needs two hands	Must use straw
	(18) Hygiene	Normal	More cautious than the average person when performing tasks	Able to do everything but with errors	Unable to do fine tasks like shaving or putting on lipstick	Inability to do any fine movement activity
	(19) Dressing	Normal	Able to do everything	Able to do everything but with errors	Unable to do most of the fine tasks	Requires assistance even for gross motor activities
	(20) Writing	Normal	Legible, writes letters	Legible, but no longer writes letters	Illegible	Unable to sign checks or other documents
	(21) Working	Tremor does not interfere with job	Able to work, but needs to be more careful than the average person	Able to do everything, but with errors	Unable to do regular job. May have change to a different job because of the tremor. There is usually limitation in performance of household activities such as ironing	Unable to do any outside job, housework also very limited

Score Sheet
Part A

Tremor location	Rest	Posture	Action/intention
1. Face			
2. Tongue			
3. Voice			
4. Head			
5. Right upper extremity			
6. Left upper extremity			
7. Trunk			
8. Right lower extremity			
9. Left lower extremity			
			TOTAL

Part B

	Right	Left
10. Handwriting (dominant only)		
11. Drawing A		
12. Drawing B		
13. Drawing C		
14. Pouring		
	TOTAL	

Part C

15. Speaking		
16. Eating		
17. Drinking		
18. Hygiene		
19. Dressing		
20. Writing		
21. Working		
	TOTAL	

Table 9.3 Global assessment percentage score by the examiner

Score	Impairment (%)
0	No functional disability
1	Mild disability (1–24% impaired)
2	Moderate disability (25–49% impaired)
3	Marked disability (50–74% impaired)
4	Severe disability (75–100% impaired)

Table 9.4 Follow-up assesment table

Score	Improvement/decline (%)
+ 3	Marked improvement (50–100% improved)
+ 2	Moderate improvement (25–49% improved)
+ 1	Mild improvement (10–24% improved)
0	Unchanged
−1	Mild worsening (10–24% worse)
−2	Moderate to marked worsening (25–49%)
−3	Marked worsening (50–100%)

The scoring below (▶ Table 9.4) can be used to subjectively follow the patient during visits.

The TETRAS and FTM, used in the context of kinetic tremors, have been shown to correlate very closely; however, the TETRAS scale has an advantage due to its simplicity and its lack of the ceiling effect seen with the FTM when assessing severe tremor.[41]

9.5 The Medical Management of Essential Tremor

The medical management of ET is largely dependent on the use of beta-adrenergic antagonists (propranolol), anticonvulsants (primidone), second-generation antipsychotics (clozapine), antidepressants (mirtazapine), and alcohol and botulinum toxin A (Botox injections).[42,43]

Both propranolol and primidone are first line in the pharmacological management of ET.[42,43] Propranolol causes blockade of the peripheral beta-2 adrenoceptor and results in a 50 to 70% response in individuals with ET, particularly causing a reduction in the tremor amplitude affecting the upper and lower extremities.[42] However, it should be avoided in patients with asthma and diabetes mellitus. The starting dose of propranolol is 40 mg every 12 hours and it is usually titrated to a daily maintenance dose of 120 to 320 mg given every 8 to 12 hours.[42] Like propranolol, primidone offers a 50 to 70% response, by reducing the tremor frequency.[42] Due to its sedative effects, this anticonvulsant medication is less tolerable in the young patients. Other drugs, such as topiramate, are usually considered in cases of failure of the first-line therapy. Clozapine has been shown to demonstrate good effect on tremors of the upper extremity. Botulinum toxin is a good option for head and neck tremors. However, its effectiveness is limited to 3-month intervals and for head and neck tremors only as it causes undesirable weakness in the extremities.[43] Botulinum toxin can be effective in upper extremity tremors, but the patient must be willing to deal with the resulting weakness.

9.6 Surgical Management of Essential Tremor

9.6.1 Surgical Patient Selection

One of the most challenging obstacles in deep brain stimulation (DBS) surgery is picking the right candidate. Many centers, such as ours, utilize a collaborative, multidisciplinary preoperative assessment of patients consisting of movement disorder neurologists, a functional neurosurgeon, neuropsychologists, a patient coordinator, and physical, speech and occupational therapists. Each potential candidate for surgery is systematically evaluated and then presented, reviewed and discussed, typically in a movement disorders or DBS conference. The group reviews the risks and benefits of surgery and a consensus is reached by the team. This individualized, committee evaluation process helps to ensure that the surgical management of a patient's disease achieves successful results.[44,45] The evaluation assesses each patient's tremor characteristics, its impact on that patient's quality of life, the number of failed medications and duration of therapy, patient's medical and psychological comorbidities, and the strength of patient's support system for the postoperative management of the implanted devices. In addition, the ability of the patient to cope with known potential side effects such as imbalance or dysarthria is also analyzed.

9.6.2 Tremor Evaluation

For ET patients, tremor in the arms and hands are most common, but head tremor (40% of patients), voice tremor (20% of patients), and leg or trunk tremors (20% of patients) are also seen.[46,47] The surgery is most benifical for the patients with ET who typically have an intention tremor located in the distal upper extremities, rather than proximally, such as the shoulder or the head. Voice tremor has also been more difficult to manage with DBS, but bilateral procedures have shown significant responses.[45,48]

Characteristically, most patients referred for surgery have a medication-refractory ET.[46,49] While there has not been a standardized guideline, the American Academy of Neurology recommends level A evidence that primidone and propranolol should be offered to patients who desire treatment for limb tremor.[47] As mentioned in the section above, most patients would have been treated with a medical therapy but have less than optimal symptomatic control. Careful evaluation by a movement disorder specialist helps categorize the features of the tremor and also helps determine the etiology, distinguishing how likely surgery will be beneficial for each patient.[50]

9.6.3 Quality of Life

Tremors seen in ET patients can be very debilitating and disruptive to a patient's ability to perform activities of daily living as well as to their function in society through employment and social interactions. In severe cases, performing activities of daily living, such as feeding, drinking, writing, or communicating can be quite challenging.[47] Patients should have realistic expectations about the improvement that should be expected with DBS or thalamotomy. The ability to change stimulation with DBS can be quite an advantage since one can modulate the effects to improve efficacy of tremor control and to control side effects. In addition, modern DBS generators are capable of holding multiple stimulation programs and patients can select between stimulation programs depending on whether they require precise tremor control or they can tolerate some tremor for a reduction in side effects such, as those effecting speech. Reports have shown that both head tremor and voice tremor responses to DBS can be variable and uncertain.[45] Therefore, patients with severe head, neck, or voice tremors must be counseled on the lower likelihood of optimal treatment for these types of tremors relative to tremors of the upper extremities.

9.6.4 Comorbidities

As with any elective surgery, the patient's risks for safely undergoing the surgery must be evaluated. Preoperative medical evaluation and clearance is commonly obtained with attention to the relevant specifics of the patient's medical or anesthesia history (i.e., hypertension, diabetes, anesthesia complications). Particular attention should be payed to the patients with pulmonary or cardiovascular issues that may increase the risk of airway compromise during a frame-based surgery that utilizes conscious sedation. It is typical for patients to undergo laboratory evaluation, including coagulation panel, and patients over the age of 65 years often undergo screening with electro-cardiography (EKG) and chest X-ray. Further preoperative evaluation is done as per the patient's medical history. In addition, the neuropsychiatric evaluation provides important information regarding the patient's cognitive function and psychiatric or mood disorders. Recent longitudinal studies have shown an association between ET and cognitive impairment or dementia. Careful consideration should be given to patients with significant cognitive impairment or psychiatric condition. Cognitive, psychotic, and mood disorders, severe brain atrophy, and alcoholism preclude an individual from getting DBS.[46,48] Furthermore, patient participation is needed for optimal intraoperative testing during microelectrode recording (MER), and stimulation mapping and testing.[50] Age of the patient and life expectancy must also be taken into account. Specific to DBS for ET, patients with preexisting dysarthria and dysphagia are cautioned as thalamic stimulation can possibly worsen these issues.[47,51]

9.6.5 Strength of Support System

Patients, who undergo DBS implantation, and their families must understand that the therapy is a lifelong commitment with numerous postoperative visits for reprogramming, and end-of-life generator replacements.[45] Recent introduction of rechargeable batteries within the pulse generators can reduce the repeated surgeries for end-of-life generator replacements, but would require recharging of the device at home. Having a strong support system helps unburden patients with logistical issues, such as remembering the different appointments, traveling to the different facilities, emotional support during recovery or in the event of complications, side effects or unexpected outcomes, and vigilance for recharging, hardware failures or infections.

9.7 Surgical Interventions

9.7.1 Deep Brain Stimulation—Stereotactic Frame

The operative day begins with placing the stereotactic frame on the patient. The patient is instructed not take his/her tremor medications that morning in order to facilitate intraoperative testing. The time-out procedure is performed, and the patient receives intravenous lines for the administration of sedatives, antibiotics, and antihypertensives if necessary. A mild and/or short-acting sedative can be utilized to assist with placement of the stereotactic frame. It is important to understand the potential impact of any medications on the MERs. The scalp is cleansed and prepared. The stereotactic frame is then applied after local anesthesia. We prefer a mixture of short-acting and long-lasting local anesthetics (e.g., Lidocaine and bupivicaine) mixed in the ratio 9:1 with sodium bicarbonate injected into the pin sites for the stereotactic frame placement. The frame is carefully aligned to be parallel to the anterior commissure (AC)-posterior commissure (PC) and as symmetric as possible. Ear bars are used to minimize lateral movement or rotation during placement. Once the frame is satisfactorily secured, high-fidelity, high-resolution imaging is obtained with the fiducial box applied to the frame for localization. Both CT and MRI may be utilized for frame imaging. We prefer the use of CT imaging with the stereotactic frame in place. MRI with the stereotactic frame may

also be used, but is limited to 1.5 T MRI with head only send-receive coil. There are small but known distortions in MRI from the titanium frame and trials with the Leksell frame in 3 T MRI have suggested distortions that are too large for stereotactic procedures. If the patient traveled for the in-frame imaging, they are returned to the operating room and transferred to the operative table in the supine position. If they are utilized, the arterial line and foley are placed at this time during stereotactic planning. Close monitoring of the blood pressure is essential and although this may be done with repeat blood pressure cuff measures, we prefer intensive monitoring and control with an arterial line for continuous monitoring, especially in patients with preoperative hypertension. It is recommended that systolic blood pressure should be maintained below 140 mm Hg throughout the operation and especially during placement of electrodes.

9.7.2 Target and Trajectory Planning (▶ Fig. 9.1)

During this time, the stereotactic planning is performed on a computer planning station. At our institution, after localization of the stereotactic frame on CT imaging, this CT scan is fused with a high-quality preop MRI. There are a variety of sequences that can be utilized for stereotactic planning. We utilize a high-resolution anatomical T1 sequence magnetization-prepared rapid gradient echo (MPRAGE) with contrast and volumetric fluid-attenuated inversion recovery (FLAIR) or inversion recovery sequences for every case. MPRAGE sequences are utilized for accurate fusion, localization of the AC and PC, and trajectory planning. The second sequence is utilized for direct imaging-based confirmation of the target when feasible. Many institutions use the short tau inversion recovery (STIR) sequence for the grey-white differentiation for direct target verification. At our institution, this is best accomplished with a volumetric FLAIR sequence. We recommend collaborating with neuroradiology to develop a high-quality sequence for grey-white differentiation as this can vary depending on the particular MRI scanner(s) utilized. The ventral intermediate (Vim) target of the ventrolateral (VL) thalamus, however, is not well visualized on MRI and is, therefore, targeted via standard indirect coordinates. After the AC-PC line is established, the coordinates for the Vim target are mapped using typical stereotactic coordinates based on the PC point.

X: 11.5 mm lateral + ½ width of third ventricle
Y: Anterior to PC by 20% of AC-PC line length
Z: In the plane of the AC-PC line

Once the target is established, the trajectory is chosen with standard angles including anterior 60 to 75 degrees and lateral as parallel to the midsagittal plane as possible while avoiding the lateral ventricle. We strongly prefer to avoid the lateral ventricles for the Vim trajectory and only transverse the lateral ventricle when the target requires and provides an orthogonal pass through the ventricle. The trajectory is then adjusted as necessary to avoid blood vessels and sulci. The typical entry point is near the coronal suture, at 2.5 to 4.5 cm off the midline. Once the stereotactic planning is completed, the coordinates for the stereotactic frame system, including the X, Y, Z, ring, and arc settings are recorded. In bilateral cases, the average Y and Z are determined as necessary.

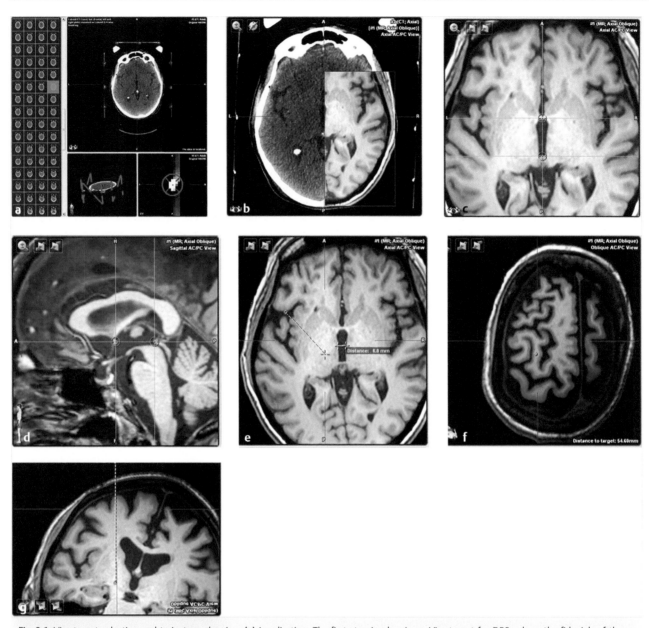

Fig. 9.1 Vim target selection and trajectory planning. **(a)** Localization: The first step in planning a Vim target for DBS, where the fiducials of the stereotactic frame on each axial CT image slice are chosen automatically by the BRAINLAB software program. The bottom left panel shows the axial CT image with three blue "N"s which represent the fiducials. The bottom right panel shows a blue circle around the chosen fiducial point in line with the chosen axial plane. **(b)** Fusion: The other imaging sequence, such as T1 MRI, are fused to the CT image. The fidelity of the fusion is inspected here showing satisfactory alignment of the CT and MRI images. **(c)** AC-PC localization: The anterior (AC) and posterior (PC) commissures are chosen on the MRI so that the AC point is the midpoint of the back edge of the anterior commissure and the PC point is the midpoint of the anterior edge of the posterior commissure (*green circles*). **(d)** The software then aligns the images parallel to the AC-PC line (*green line*). **(e)** Target selection: The consensus coordinates for the VIM target are: X coordinate is usually 11.5 mm lateral + ½ width of third ventricle, Y coordinate is anterior to PC by 20% of AC-PC line length, and the Z coordinate is in the Plane of the AC-PC line. (Crosshair indicates the R VIM target with dashed line indicating the trajectory). **(f)** The entry point is shown (*green dot*), which is near the coronal suture, usually about 2.5–4.5 cm off the midline. **(g)** The trajectory chosen is shown in the coronal plane (*dashed line*). Typical angles are anterior 60–75 degrees and lateral as parallel to the mid-sagittal plane, ensuring to avoid blood vessels and sulci.

The patient is then positioned in the semi-Fowler position with the neck in a comfortable position that does not compromise breathing, and the frame is fixed to the table. The approximate entry sites can be marked based on the coronal suture and midline, and the hair in this region is clipped. Alternatively, all hair can be clipped prior to frame placement but it is not required.

The proposed incision(s) is drawn on the appropriate side(s); we prefer a linear semicoronal incision, but other alternatives such as the semicircular incision(s) are also utilized. The scalp is then prepped in the typical fashion. The drapes and stereotactic system are then placed and assembled; this process varies somewhat depending on the system used and draping preference.

Many centers position a fluoroscopy system or intraoperative CT system into the field during draping. Local anesthetic is used to create an entire regional block around the operative site. The arc of the stereotactic system and electrode carrying system is now assembled and verified. The coordinates are double checked for the target and then a cannula is used to mark the entry site on the scalp and adjust the incision as needed.

The incision is made in the scalp and the site of the bur hole is marked using the cannula that is placed at target on the skull. The location of the entry site relative to the coronal suture and midline can be verified based on target planning. A high-speed perforator drill is used to make the 14.5-mm bur hole which is waxed immediately. The bur hole is then cleared of bone fragments and modified if needed. If a bur hole based DBS electrode locking device is utilized, this is placed and secured. The dura is then cauterized and opened in a cruciate fashion. A small corticectomy is made. The recording system X-Y stage, cannulae, and microdrive are then assembled. There are a variety of electrodes and platforms utilized and it is important to be intimately familiar with the design and functions of the particular platform that are being utilized. The cannulae are lowered into position. There are a variety of cannula types and lengths, designed to end either at the target or more commonly at a known distance above the target (i.e., 15 or 25 mm above target). Once the cannulae are in position, Gelfoam is placed in the bur hole and then a sealant is applied to seal off the bur hole and reduce the amount of cerebrospinal fluid leak leakage and potential brain shift. Microelectrode(s) are then placed into the cannula(s) and connected to the recording system. For the Vim target, we utilize two microelectrodes, one placed at the target and one in the position 2 mm posterior to the target for identification of the ventral caudal (Vc) nucleus.

Next, the MER is performed (see Chapter 9.7.3, Intraoperative Recordings and Mapping (p. 71)). Once the trajectory is chosen, fluoroscopy is aligned and the microelectrodes are removed and preparation is made for placement of the DBS electrode. Then, DBS electrode is placed through the final target cannula at the expected position with fluoroscopy or CT for verification. Macrostimulation is performed once the electrode is connected to the temporary stimulation device. The electrode is tested for efficacy and side effects, noting the voltages and which combination of contacts produced the effects. If any untoward side effects are observed at low or normal DBS currents, then the electrode should be removed and repositioned based on mapping results (see Chapter 9.7.3, Intraoperative Recordings and Mapping).

Once testing is finished, the electrode is secured in place and the cannula is removed from the brain. There are a variety of techniques used to secure the electrode into position, such as the Medtronic silicone burr hole fastening device and cap, methylmetacrylate with a straight titanium miniplate and screws, or the Medtronic Stimloc, St. Jude Guardian™, Boston Scientific SureTek™ burrhole covers. An additional imaging or scan is done to ensure stable location of the electrode. Finally, the electrode is removed from the recording platform and the cap is secured to the distal end of the electrode. A subgaleal pocket is made and the distal end of the electrode is tunneled there with excess wire loops fed into the pocket. The wound is copiously irrigated with 2 L of antibiotic irrigation, inspected for hemostasis, and closed in two layers.

9.7.3 Intraoperative Recordings and Mapping

Thalamic mapping via MERs and stimulation is critical for the correct placement of the DBS electrode. Electrodes positioned too posterior (sensory parasthesias – Vc) or too lateral (muscle contractions—internal capsule) can be difficult to utilize due to intolerable side effects. Once the microelectrode(s) are in position and connected to the recording system, they are advanced slightly and the impedance is checked. There are a variety of electrode types but the impedance is typically between 400 kΩ to 1 MΩ at 1000 kHz in order to record individual neurons. Electrodes with lower impedance will record more multi-unit or field potentials and may differentiate fewer single units during MERs. The characteristic neuronal firing patterns identified during MER are reviewed in later sections and ▶ Fig. 9.2 and ▶ Fig. 9.3. In addition, microstimulation through the recording electrode can be utilized for test stimulation mapping in addition to the recordings. For Vim targeting, we use two microelectrode tracts, the central target and the posterior tract in order to map the two nuclei of interest, i.e., the Vim nucleus that receives kinesthetic, vestibular, and cerebellar inputs for somatomotor control, and the Vc nucleus which is the sensory nucleus that receives input from both the medial lemniscus and the spinothalamic tracts.

Neuronal Responses During MER (▶ Fig. 9.3)

The final physiological target of the DBS electrode for ET has the distal tip of the electrode at the base of Vim nucleus, 2 to 4 mm anterior to the border of the Vc with the shaft of the electrode placed in the upper limb representation of Vim which lies ~ 13 to 16 mm from midline. During MER and mapping, the microdriver slowly advances the microelectrodes down through the tissue, and different cell types are encountered. The following neurons are frequently recorded along the trajectory path of the microelectrode:

- Kinesthetic neurons: These fire with passive movement of a joint of the contralateral hemibody. Usually, with movement of the joint, modulation or increased firing is heard. These neurons are located in the dorsal Vim as well as other thalamic and subthalamic nuclei.
- Tremor neurons: These tremors have discharges that correlate with the patient's tremor and are most commonly located in the Vim, sometimes in the Vc or ventral oralis posterior (Vop).
- Tactile neurons: These respond to sensory input, such as light touch or pressure. These neurons are located in the Vc nucleus as part of the sensory system. The recognition of tactile neurons prior to reaching target suggests that the tract is too posterior.
- Voluntary cells: These cells fire when the patient volitionally moves a part of his/her body. They are located in Vop, anterior to Vim typically.

Anatomy and Neurophysiology of Vim

Typically, a trajectory path toward Vim will pass through the dorsal thalamus. Thalamic neurons of the dorsal thalamus will often display the hallmark burst or tonic firing properties. The transition from dorsal to ventral thalamus is often marked by an increase in overall or background cellular activity and then kinesthetic and/or voluntary cells should be noted. It is typical

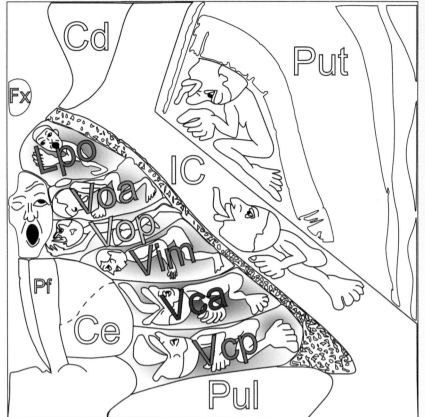

Fig. 9.2 Schematic diagram of thalamic somatotopy. Tremor reduction is best targeting Vim, specifically the aspect including the "arm" and "hand" regions. Primary foot kinesthetics are suggestive of lateral position while primarily, the face and jaw kinesthetic neurons are suggestive of medial electrode positioning. Electrodes placed too posteriorly will generate sustained paresthesias with stimulation due to the proximity to Vca (see Table 9.5). Thalamic structures are labeled using Hassler's classification of human thalamic anatomy: Ce, centromedian nucleus; Lpo, lateral posterior; Pf, parafasicular nucleus; Vca, ventral caudalis anterior; Vcp, ventral caudalis posterior; Vim, ventral intermediate nucleus; Voa, ventral oralis anterior. Extra-thalamic anatomy: Cd, caudate; Fx, fornix; Pul, pulvinar; Put, putamen.

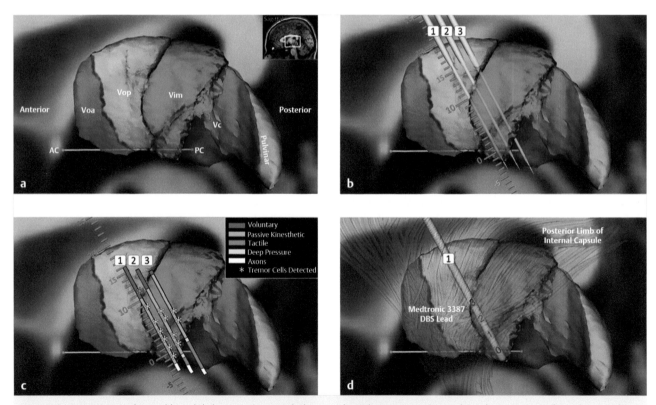

Fig. 9.3 **(a)** Sagittal view of ventral lateral thalamus is shown with the ventralis oralis anterior and ventralis oralis posterior (*yellow*), the ventralis intermedius (*green*) and the ventralis caudalis (*red*). The AC-PC line is shown as a *yellow line*. **(b)** Three parallel recording trajectories are shown in the parasagittal plane, which reveals the passes of these microelectrodes through Vop, Vim and in the posterior tracts Vc is encountered. A trajectory depth ruler (*red*) with target at zero is superimposed along track 1. **(c)** The three MER trajectories are color coded by the typical primary neuronal responses encountered, with tremor cells shown as asterisks (*). **(d)** Placement of DBS electrode in trajectory 1. This trajectory includes voluntary and kinesthetic neuronal responses, includes some tremor cells and does not enter VC shown by the lack of tactile or pressure responses. This tract minimizes the risk of significant parasthesias with stimulation. (Reprinted with the permission of Medtronic, Inc. ©2019).

to encounter some kinesthetic cells starting at 8 to 10 mm above target (▶ Fig. 9.3). In the ideal Vim trajectory, no tactile/sensory neurons are encountered prior to target. We utilize two recordings electrodes with the center and posterior tracts in the Bengun, which ideally matches trajectories 1 and 2 in ▶ Fig. 9.3. In this configuration, the posterior electrode transitions from Vim to Vc nuclei just prior to target (1–2 mm above target). The Vc nuclei can be identified by a transition in firing rates as well as the presence of tactile or pressure responsive neurons. Identification of the Vim/Vc transition provides confidence in the localization of the DBS electrode within the Vim nucleus. Electromyography (EMG) or modern accelerometer recordings can be utilized in conjunction with MERs to better identify tremor cells and monitor movement/tremor during DBS surgery (▶ Fig. 9.4).

Stimulation Mapping (▶ Fig. 9.4)

Once a good tract through the Vim nucleus is identified with MERs, the location of the tract can be verified with stimulation through the microelectrode. There are a variety of microelectrodes, some with contacts designed specifically for stimulation so as to avoid stimulating through the recording tip of the electrodes. These contacts have a known distance from the tip of the electrode. It is important to understand the contact that is stimulated and the current source density that results from the contact and stimulation utilized, as this will impact the effects of the stimulation. Microstimulation can then be performed to test for therapy and side effects. We mainly utilize microstimulation for side

effect testing, but in a good tract there is most often some clear modification of the patient's tremor with stimulation. The presence of side effects localizes the electrode too close to a critical structure (i.e., Vc nucleus or internal capsule) mandating repositioning of the electrode.

Once the appropriate placement for the DBS electrode has been achieved, the microelectrode(s) are removed and the permanent DBS electrode is lowered into position. There are multiple electrode spacings available but we typically use the 1.5 mm spacing between contacts (Medtronic model 3387). The DBS electrode is then connected to temporary stimulation device and macrostimulation is performed using bipolar settings. Several groups of contacts are used for macrostimulation testing and the therapy and side effects of each pair and current/voltage are recorded (▶ Table 9.5). Repositioning of the electrode is required if any untoward side effects, such as permanent parasthesias (Vc) or muscle contractions (internal capsule) at low current are observed. Side effects at high current and/or broad stimulation fields are commonly anticipated and do not necessarily mandate repositioning of the electrode.

9.7.4 Postoperative Management and Complications

For patients undergoing this technique, monitored anesthesia care or conscious sedation anesthesia is used. Patients typically wake up quickly, and are able to converse and follow commands, once the procedure is over. Postoperatively, patients are

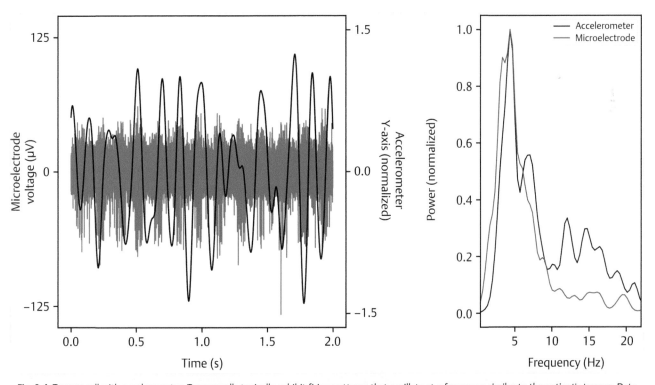

Fig. 9.4 Tremor cell with accelerometer. Tremor cells typically exhibit firing patterns that oscillate at a frequency similar to the patient's tremor. Data from an accelerometer attached to the patient's hand are time locked with the MER data recorded during intraoperative testing. The left panel shows two seconds of high pass filtered (300-900 Hz) microelectrode recordings (*red*). Overlaid is normalized, time-locked accelerometer data (*black*) showing phase locking. The oscillatory pattern of neuronal activity is similar to the frequency of the tremor movements recorded by the accelerometer. The right panel shows peak normalized power spectra of the broadband microelectrode (*red*) and accelerometer data. Both datasets show a similar peak near 5Hz. (Figure data produced by Shane Lee and Wael F. Asaad based on techniques reported in Schaeffer et al.[52])

Table 9.5 Recording and stimulation effects by location

Location[a]	MER observations (anatomical correlate)	Stimulation effects (anatomical correlate)
Posterior	• Cells responsive to deep pressure (anterior Vc, or "proprioceptive shell") • Cells responsive to tactile stimulation of the patient • Exit thalamus lower than expected	• Paresthesias that increase in severity with increasing stimulation (Vc nucleus)
Anterior	• Entry point into thalamus lower than expected • Cells responsive to voluntary patient movements (Vop) • Nontremor synchronous bursting cells present (Vop) • Tremor cells (Vop and Vim) • Exit thalamus higher than expected	• No effect (Voa) • Some improvement in tremor at higher stimulation thresholds (Vop)
Lateral	• Quiet stretch preceding late or no entry into Vim • Kinesthetic activity correlating with lower limb movements • Sensory responsive cells correlating with lower limb tactile stimuli (Vc)	• Dysarthria, muscle contractions (contracting muscles correspond to the region of the capsular homunculus) (internal capsule)
Medial	• Kinesthetic activity correlating with jaw movements (Vim) • If within Vc, sensory responsive cells correlating with oral/facial tactile stimuli	• Possible dysarthria in addition to tremor control (medial Vim) • No effect (CM/Pf, medial to Vim nucleus)
Superior[b]	• Low amplitude, sporadically firing cells (dorsal thalamus)	• No effect (dorsal thalamus) • Possible impact on tremor (dorsal Vim/Vop) • Lateral and dorsal: dysarthria, muscle contractions (internal capsule)
Inferior	• Low amplitude, sporadically firing cells (ZI, prelemniscal radiation)	• Possible impact on dyskinesias and/or tremor (ZI, prelemniscal radiation) • Ventral and medial: ataxia (brachium conjunctivum) • Ventral and posterior: paresthesias (medial lemniscus) • Ventral and lateral: dysarthria, muscle contractions (internal capsule)

Abbreviations: MER, microelectrode recording; Vc, ventral caudal; Vim, ventral intermediate; Voa, ventral oral anterior; Vop, ventral oral posterior; ZI, zona incerta.
[a] Relative to posteroventral Vim.
[b] Along the trajectory path.
Source: Reprinted with the permission of Medtronic, Inc. ©2019.

observed closely in the anesthesia recovery room, step down unit, or even intensive care unit. Frequent neurological checks are conducted in the first 2 to 4 hours postop; pain control and strict blood pressure parameters (systolic blood pressure less than 140 mm Hg) are instituted, ensuring that any change in neurological exam is caught immediately and that the patient does not have increased risk for raised intracranial pressure or venous bleeding. The patient's diet is advanced progressively as tolerated and all of their preop medications are resumed. If a Foley catheter was utilized during the surgery, it is removed postop and patients must pass a voiding trial prior to discharge.

The night after surgery, a postoperative CT or MRI scan is typically obtained to screen for any signs of complications, specifically hemorrhage or venous infarct, and for confirmation of lead placement. The majority of patients are discharged from the hospital the day after surgery, provided that they tolerate their usual diet, have adequate pain control on oral medications, pass the voiding trial, and are able to ambulate. Patients are sent home with wound care instructions, pain medication, and we prescribe a short course of oral antibiotics. Patients return after 1 to 4 weeks for the placement of the lead extension and implanted pulse generator within the chest wall (the Stage 2 procedure). This is, most often, an outpatient procedure. The generator is implanted in a subcutaneous chest pocket and the DBS lead is connected to the lead extension which is tunneled under the skin from the parietal scalp to the chest. The lead extension and IPG are typically placed on the

same side of the body as the electrode. At our institution, if two electrodes are implanted in a single surgery, the generator is preferentially placed on the right side of the chest, allowing the left side to be available for cardiac pacemakers or other devices.

9.7.5 Complications

The complications associated with DBS surgery occur during the procedure itself or during the long-term follow-up with the hardware or stimulation parameters. While steps and precautions are taken to minimize the risks for these complications, sometimes they are unavoidable.

Procedural complications

The most potentially devastating complication is hemorrhage with 2 to 4% risk for stereotactic procedures.[51,53] Placement of the microelectrodes or the DBS electrode lead through the parenchyma can cause rupture of small vessels or injury to a draining vein can lead to a venous infarct that subsequently hemorrhages, or it can cause a subdural hematoma. Although some hemorrhages are asymptomatic, small, and intraparenchymal; significant symptomatic, even devastating, or sometimes deadly, hemorrhages have also been reported.[45] Other immediate complications include postoperative nausea, headache, seizures, and perioperative confusion.[51,53]

Stimulation risks

Some are specific to instrumentation of the Vim are most commonly due to the close proximity to either the Vc nucleus or the medial lemniscus, causing parasthesias in 21% of patients that are ameliorated with decreased stimulation.[51] Other noted side effects are headache, ataxia, weakness or paresis (from activating corticospinal fibers), or dysarthria.[53]

Hardware complications

As with any implant, the hardware may present with complications. Infection, a troublesome complication, occurs at a rate of roughly 2 to 3% per lead.[53] To combat the infection, a dose of preoperative antibiotics is administered roughly 30 minutes prior to the incision and dose of perioperative intravenous antibiotics is repeated every 4 to 6 hours. The surgical wounds are vigorously irrigated with 1 L of antibiotic irrigation. Patients receive oral antibiotics for 3 days postoperatively.

In rare cases, incorrect placement of electrodes may also occur that may cause a variety of symptoms depending on the anatomical structure being stimulated. Patients may experience parasthesias, ataxia, dysarthria or dysphagia, paresis, hemiballism, or cognitive problems.[48] In these cases, if there is no hemorrhage, the effects should be reversed once the stimulation is discontinued. The electrode should be replaced in the appropriate location. In rare cases, when electrode location is satisfactory and stimulation side effects are not tolerated or therapy is unsatisfactory, the placement of rescue electrodes at another target can be considered. Furthermore, especially in patients with thin subcutaneous tissues, erosion of hardware through the skin may be an issue. Pain or a sensation of pulling in the neck, or pain in the chest pocket from scar contracture around the wire or generator can also occur. Also, lead migration may result in a delayed loss of tremor reduction efficacy, and wire fractures may result in the same reduction in efficacy or produce a shock-like sensation.

9.7.6 Deep Brain Stimulation—Frameless Techniques

There are several frameless stereotactic techniques that can be utilized for DBS surgery. Among these are the StarFix microTargeting Platform® (FHC Inc., Bowdoin, ME, USA), Nexframe® (Medtronic, Minneapolis, MN, USA), and robotic stereotactic platforms such as ROSA® (MedTech/Zimmer Biomet). The StarFix platform utilizes preop imaging obtained after the placement of bone fiducials in the skull. This volumetric imaging is then used to create the target and trajectory for DBS electrode placement. After surgical planning is completed, a customized platform is created that affixes to the patient's skull and provides the predetermined trajectory to target. The Nexframe® system utilizes a frameless neuronavigation system for targeting and trajectory planning. The robotic systems also use a frameless neuronavigation system coregistered with the patient's head combined with a robotic arm that produces the trajectory to target. For further details on these techniques, see Chapter 2, Customized Platform-based Stereotactic DBS Lead Placement Technique. Once these platforms are registered and attached, cerebral access obtained and cannula lowered into

the brain, the intraoperative recordings and mapping are conducted as described above.

9.8 Minimally Invasive Techniques

9.8.1 Gamma Knife Thalamotomy

Although stereotactic surgery with DBS or less frequent radio-frequency thermocoagulation are effective therapies for patients with medication-refractory ET, some patients may not be acceptable surgical candidates or unwilling to tolerate the risks associated with open surgery or unwilling to deal with long-term implanted hardware. For these patients, Gamma knife thalamotomy is a less invasive neurosurgical procedure that provides an alternative treatment for tremor that is refractory to medical therapy. There is no craniotomy or hardware involved and thus no risk of intracranial hemorrhage, infection, or hardware complications related to surgery. Patients having significant cardiac or respiratory diseases, immunosuppression, borderline or poor cognition, advanced age, anticoagulant use, and difficulty with compliance are examples of potential candidates for gamma knife thalamotomy.[54,55] In most cases, gamma knife thalamotomy can be performed in anticoagulated patients. There are no data to suggest any cognitive or memory risks associated with gamma knife thalamotomy. At our institution, the preprocedure evaluation for gamma knife thalamotomy is identical to that of DBS and the treatment method is determined by the DBS/Movement Disorder Council.

The gamma knife thalamotomy is performed with the application of the stereotactic frame in the same fashion as done in DBS surgery. This procedure does not require anesthesia other than local anesthetic at the pin site locations but often some mild sedation (i.e., midazolam) is used for patient comfort. Once the frame is placed, the patient undergoes imaging with a 1.5 T MRI scanner with both contrast-enhanced volumetric T1 (i.e., MPRAGE) and with sequences designed to identify the internal capsule and differentiate gray and white matter structures, for example, fast inversion recovery (STIR) or FLAIR sequences. The acquisition of preprocedure high-resolution MRI sequences allows the utilization of additional sequences such as DTI, STIR, etc., obtained on higher magnetic field scanners to be fused with the in-frame imaging and assist with final targeting. The initial targeting of the Vim is similar to DBS; however, there are some important differences. First, the target for gamma knife thalamotomy is the center of the thalamic region to be lesioned, whereas DBS target is typically the most ventral aspect of the nucleus of interest. Second, the final position of the gamma knife thalamotomy is determined by the MRI. The MPRAGE sequence is utilized for identification of the AC-PC line. Then the anterior-posterior location is determined, usually 5 to 6 mm posterior to the midcommissural point or 25% of the AC-PC distance + 1-mm anterior from the PC. Then, coronal reformats are used for placement of the target in the lateral and dorsoventral planes. Some groups have advocated for using the same lateral coordinate as DBS for initial targeting. A single 4-mm collimator is then targeted with isocenter at this location with maximum dose range of 130 to 140 Gy. A gamma angle of 110 degrees is utilized for gamma knife thalamotomy to create an isocenter volume that more closely matches the shape of the Vim nucleus. Then, the target is adjusted in the lateral and dorsoventral planes, according to the MRI sequences best differentiating gray and white matter structures, to place the target at the inferior-lateral border of the thalamus. There are various reports on this technique, with suggestions to place the 50% isodose line at the border of the thalamus and others that recommend keeping the 20% isodose line medial to the internal capsule. Although these two approaches sometimes overlap, at our institution we utilize preprocedure MRI sequences fused with the in-frame imaging to ensure that the 20% isodose line is kept medial to the internal capsule and superior to white matter tracts.[56]

Since its first report in the early 1990s,[57] several studies have shown safety and efficacy of gamma knife thalamotomy[56,58,59,60] with a few studies suggesting longer term efficacy. Tremor reduction following gamma knife thalamotomy has been reported in 70 to 92% of patients mainly utilizing the FTM scales. The average tremor improvement is reported 51 to 60% at 1-year follow-up. In 2010, Young et al reported that 72% of patients continued to show an average of 58% improvement at a mean follow-up after 58 months.[59] There is usually a delayed reduction in tremor after gamma knife thalamotomy typically occurring over 3 to 6 months and some studies identifying tremor reduction up to a year following therapy.[61]

Adverse events can occur, including motor deficits, paresthesias, or dysarthria; however, the reported adverse event rates (1.6–8.4%) are lower than those in case of DBS. Although small, one prospective, blinded trial reported a 2% incidence of adverse events that were transient in nature.[60] Patients who develop sensory or motor complications following gamma knife thalamotomy have been shown to have larger lesions and/or edema. The perilesional edema has been shown to respond partially or completely to steroids,[62] and several authors have reported resolution of sensory or motor issues with steroids and time in many of those patients who experience these adverse events.

9.8.2 High-Frequency Focused Ultrasound

Although the concept of using ultrasound for neural lesioning was conceived in the 1950s, the practical application of MRI-guided focused ultrasound (MRgFUS) as a noninvasive method for precise lesioning of deep foci in the brain is relatively recent. It is proving to be an important therapeutic option for patients who may poorly tolerate DBS. Cost-effective analysis shows that FUS has higher utility than DBS and is comparable to radiosurgery.[63]

Procedurally, FUS relies on stereotactic targeting similar to radiosurgical techniques. Briefly, upon shaving the patient's head and fixation of a stereotactic head frame to the patient's skull with use of local anesthetic, a diaphragm is placed over the scalp to be filled with water and connected to an ultrasound transducer. The patient is then placed in an MRI-ultrasound system with a high-density high-frequency phased-array transducer and typical stereotactic targeting is performed as done for DBS using AC-PC coordinates. MRI scans are done with FUS targeting temperatures 40 to 45 °C to confirm anatomic targeting. Then, low-power 10 to 20-second therapeutic sonications are delivered while monitoring temperature with MR thermography, targeting

55 to 63 °C.[64] These temperatures result in protein denaturation and eventually necrosis in the targeted thalamus.[64,65]

Pilot studies of FUS in small groups of patients demonstrated that it could be used safely and effectively to create Vim thalamic lesions in ET patients with 75 to 80% reduction in tremor, which has been replicated in more recent cohorts.[64,66,67] The sole double-blind randomized controlled trial of FUS consisted of 76 patients with moderate-to-severe ET refractory to medical therapy that were randomized to unilateral Vim thalamic FUS therapy or sham therapy.[64] FUS therapy resulted in a significant decrease in upper extremity tremor scores, assessed by the FTM tremor rating scale, and a significant improvement the quality of life, assessed with QUEST. Treatment resulted in 76 adverse events, including a 34% alteration in sensation (14% at 1 year), 36% gait disturbance (9% at 1 year), and 5% cerebellar deficits at 1 year. In July 2016, FUS was approved by the Food and Drug Administration for use in ET; research programs are progressing rapidly to further develop the indications and technologies of FUS.[68] The limitations of FUS include MRI compatibility and/or tolerability for patients, inability to affect head/voice/axial tremor symptoms, and inability to achieve targeted lesioning in a small proportion of patients (thought to be due to cranial characteristics).

9.9 Future directions

9.9.1 Image-Guided DBS Based on DTI versus Awake MER-Guided DBS

With the advent of increasingly powerful MRI capabilities, imaging technology has advanced greatly from the days of the pneumocephalogram and AC-PC coordinate-derived targeting of the thalamus. The target for ET, i.e., the Vim is difficult to distinguish from the other thalamic nuclei on current imaging, therefore, indirect targeting using stereotactic coordinates are relied on along with MERs and intraoperative macrostimulation testing. However, some research in rodents has shown that the efficacy of DBS is related to the activation of fiber tracts afferent to different nuclei, such as the STN or in this case, Vim, and not the nuclei themselves.[69]

DTI is a technique that visualizes the white matter tracts using multiple diffusion-weighted images in different gradient directions.[70] It can delineate the fibers of the dentaterubrothalamic tract (DRT). The DRT is thought to be the somatomotor pathway for tremor and runs vertically from the dentate nucleus to the red nucleus and then runs laterally along a horizontal course to the thalamus.[71] The DRT was found to intersect with the three typical stereotactic target nuclei/regions for tremor surgery—the Vim, posterior subthalamic nucleus (STN), and the caudal zona incerta.[72] Bilateral DBS targeting of the middle of the DRT was 90% effective in treating dystonic head tremor in a patient.[72] Another study found that diffusion tractography in DBS patients with significant tremor reduction from Vim stimulation had similar patterns of connectivity in the cerebellum, brainstem, thalamus, and motor cortex.[73] This study highlights the importance of the anatomical network of structural connectivity between the thalamus and the primary motor cortex in tremor generation.[73]

The reliance of direct targeting methods such as DTI or the use of indirect targeting with stereotactic coordinates, while the patients are under general anesthesia, has been challenged by those who use MER and macrostimulation to confirm the stereotactic and functional accuracy of their targets. Proponents who use the former technique argue that the "asleep" method can be performed safely for patients and with minimal stereotactic error. It minimizes the risk of intracranial hemorrhage from multiple passes with the microelectrodes, and has similar outcomes in the reduction of tremor compared to those who underwent "awake" surgery.[74] Susceptibility-weighted images of the basal ganglia and thalamic structures obtained with 7 T MRI offer superior anatomic localization and delineation of the architecture of the DBS targets, making it a useful tool for Vim targeting.[75] Direct image guidance with 7 T MRI, however, is rarely available and cannot be accomplished in the head frame. Having surgery with the patients under general anesthesia is becoming more accepted and can be utilized if required. There are some reports that suggest tremor reduction outcomes in patients are not inferior to those who have undergone the conventional technique.[74,76] Recently, a single-center pilot trial, Deep Brain Stimulation for Tremor Tractographic Versus Traditional (DISTINCT), was commenced to directly compare the techniques of asleep DTI-assisted DBS surgery for ET versus the awake conventional coordinate-based stereotactic surgery with MER and intraoperative testing.[77]

References

[1] Louis ED, Ferreira JJ. How common is the most common adult movement disorder? Update on the worldwide prevalence of essential tremor. Mov Disord. 2010; 25(5):534–541

[2] Putzke JD, Whaley NR, Baba Y, Wszolek ZK, Uitti RJ. Essential tremor: predictors of disease progression in a clinical cohort. J Neurol Neurosurg Psychiatry. 2006; 77(11):1235–1237

[3] Bermejo-Pareja F, Puertas-Martín V. Cognitive features of essential tremor: a review of the clinical aspects and possible mechanistic underpinnings. Tremor Other Hyperkinet Mov (N Y). 2012; 2:02-74-541-1

[4] Jain S, Lo SE, Louis ED. Common misdiagnosis of a common neurological disorder: how are we misdiagnosing essential tremor? Arch Neurol. 2006; 63 (8):1100–1104

[5] di Biase L, Brittain JS, Shah SA, et al. Tremor stability index: a new tool for differential diagnosis in tremor syndromes. Brain. 2017; 140(7):1977–1986

[6] Fahn S. Clinical Rating Scale for Tremor. In: Jankovik J, Tolosa E, eds. Parkinson's and Movement Disorders. In. Baltimore-Munich: Urban and Schwarzenberg; 1988:225–234

[7] Elble R, Comella C, Fahn S, et al. Reliability of a new scale for essential tremor. Mov Disord. 2012; 27(12):1567–1569

[8] Tio M, Tan EK. Genetics of essential tremor. Parkinsonism Relat Disord. 2016; 22 Suppl 1:S176–S178

[9] Bain PG, Findley LJ, Thompson PD, et al. A study of hereditary essential tremor. Brain. 1994; 117(Pt 4):805–824

[10] Lorenz D, Frederiksen H, Moises H, Kopper F, Deuschl G, Christensen K. High concordance for essential tremor in monozygotic twins of old age. Neurology. 2004; 62(2):208–211

[11] Clark LN, Louis ED. Challenges in essential tremor genetics. Rev Neurol (Paris). 2015; 171(6–7):466–474

[12] Gulcher JR, Jónsson P, Kong A, et al. Mapping of a familial essential tremor gene, FET1, to chromosome 3q13. Nat Genet. 1997; 17(1):84–87

[13] Higgins JJ, Lombardi RQ, Pucilowska J, Jankovic J, Tan EK, Rooney JP. A variant in the HS1-BP3 gene is associated with familial essential tremor. Neurology. 2005; 64(3):417–421

[14] Shatunov A, Sambuughin N, Jankovic J, et al. Genomewide scans in North American families reveal genetic linkage of essential tremor to a region on chromosome 6p23. Brain. 2006; 129(Pt 9):2318–2331

[15] Hicks JE, Konidari I, Scott BL, et al. Linkage of familial essential tremor to chromosome 5q35. Mov Disord. 2016; 31(7):1059–1062

[16] Merner ND, Girard SL, Catoire H, et al. Exome sequencing identifies FUS mutations as a cause of essential tremor. Am J Hum Genet. 2012; 91(2):313–319

[17] Stefansson H, Steinberg S, Petursson H, et al. Variant in the sequence of the LIN-GO1 gene confers risk of essential tremor. Nat Genet. 2009; 41(3):277–279

[18] Thier S, Lorenz D, Nothnagel M, et al. Polymorphisms in the glial glutamate transporter SLC1A2 are associated with essential tremor. Neurology. 2012; 79 (3):243–248

[19] Müller SH, Girard SL, Hopfner F, et al. Genome-wide association study in essential tremor identifies three new loci. Brain. 2016; 139(Pt 12):3163–3169

[20] Kuhlenbäumer G, Hopfner F, Deuschl G. Genetics of essential tremor: meta-analysis and review. Neurology. 2014; 82(11):1000–1007

[21] Hopfner F, Deuschl G. Is essential tremor a single entity? Eur J Neurol. 2018

[22] Deuschl G, Raethjen J, Lindemann M, Krack P. The pathophysiology of tremor. Muscle Nerve. 2001; 24(6):716–735

[23] Lamarre Y, Mercier LA. Neurophysiological studies of harmaline-induced tremor in the cat. Can J Physiol Pharmacol. 1971; 49(12):1049–1058

[24] Elble RJ. Physiologic and essential tremor. Neurology. 1986; 36(2):225–231

[25] Rajput A, Robinson CA, Rajput AH. Essential tremor course and disability: a clinicopathologic study of 20 cases. Neurology. 2004; 62(6):932–936

[26] Lenka A, Bhalsing KS, Panda R, et al. Role of altered cerebello-thalamo-cortical network in the neurobiology of essential tremor. Neuroradiology. 2017; 59(2):157–168

[27] Louis ED, Lenka A. The olivary hypothesis of essential tremor: time tolLay this model to rest? Tremor Other Hyperkinet Mov (N Y). 2017; 7:473

[28] Yin W, Lin W, Li W, Qian S, Mou X. Resting state fMRI demonstrates a disturbance of the cerebello-cortical circuit in essential tremor. Brain Topogr. 2016; 29(3):412–418

[29] Louis ED. Twelve clinical pearls to help distinguish essential tremor from other tremors. Expert Rev Neurother. 2014; 14(9):1057–1065

[30] Louis ED, Vonsattel JP, Honig LS, Ross GW, Lyons KE, Pahwa R. Neuropathologic findings in essential tremor. Neurology. 2006; 66(11):1756–1759

[31] Choe M, Cortés E, Vonsattel JP, Kuo SH, Faust PL, Louis ED. Purkinje cell loss in essential tremor: random sampling quantification and nearest neighbor analysis. Mov Disord. 2016; 31(3):393–401

[32] Marin-Lahoz J, Gironell A. Linking essential tremor to the cerebellum: neurochemical evidence. Cerebellum. 2016; 15(3):243–252

[33] Brittain JS, Cagnan H, Mehta AR, Saifee TA, Edwards MJ, Brown P. Distinguishing the central drive to tremor in Parkinson's disease and essential tremor. J Neurosci. 2015; 35(2):795–806

[34] Sharifi S, Nederveen AJ, Booij J, van Rootselaar AF. Neuroimaging essentials in essential tremor: a systematic review. Neuroimage Clin. 2014; 5:217–231

[35] Antonini A, Berto P, Lopatriello S, Tamma F, Annemans L, Chambers M. Cost-effectiveness of 123I-FP-CIT SPECT in the differential diagnosis of essential tremor and Parkinson's disease in Italy. Mov Disord. 2008; 23(15):2202–2209

[36] Cuberas-Borrós G, Lorenzo-Bosquet C, Aguadé-Bruix S, et al. Quantitative evaluation of striatal I-123-FP-CIT uptake in essential tremor and parkinsonism. Clin Nucl Med. 2011; 36(11):991–996

[37] Tolosa E, Borght TV, Moreno E, DaTSCAN Clinically Uncertain Parkinsonian Syndromes Study Group. Accuracy of DaTSCAN (123I-Ioflupane) SPECT in diagnosis of patients with clinically uncertain parkinsonism: 2-year follow-up of an open-label study. Mov Disord. 2007; 22(16):2346–2351

[38] Jia L, Jia-Lin S, Qin D, Qing L, Yan Z. A diffusion tensor imaging study in essential tremor. J Neuroimaging. 2011; 21(4):370–374

[39] Louis ED, Ford B, Wendt KJ, Lee H, Andrews H. A comparison of different bedside tests for essential tremor. Mov Disord. 1999; 14(3):462–467

[40] Elble R, Bain P, Forjaz MJ, et al. Task force report: scales for screening and evaluating tremor: critique and recommendations. Mov Disord. 2013; 28 (13):1793–1800

[41] Ondo W, Hashem V, LeWitt PA, et al. Comparison of the Fahn-Tolosa-Marin Clinical Rating Scale and the Essential Tremor Rating Assessment Scale Movement Disorders Clinical Practice Early View Im Internet: http://onlinelibrary.wiley.com/doi/10.1002/mdc3.12560/abstract

[42] Burke D. Essential Tremor Treatment and Management. In: Medscape; 2016

[43] Zesiewicz TA, Elble RJ, Louis ED, et al. Evidence-based guideline update: treatment of essential tremor: report of the Quality Standards subcommittee of the American Academy of Neurology. Neurology. 2011; 77(19): 1752–1755

[44] Higuchi MA, Topiol DD, Ahmed B, et al. Impact of an Interdisciplinary Deep Brain Stimulation Screening Model on post-surgical complications in essential tremor patients. PLoS One. 2015; 10(12):e0145623

[45] Machado AG, Deogaonkar M, Cooper S. Deep brain stimulation for movement disorders: patient selection and technical options. Cleve Clin J Med. 2012; 79 Suppl 2:S19–S24

[46] Deuschl G, Bain P. Deep brain stimulation for tremor [correction of trauma]: patient selection and evaluation. Mov Disord. 2002; 17 Suppl 3:S102–S111

[47] Munhoz RP, Picillo M, Fox SH, et al. Eligibility criteria for deep brain stimulation in Parkinson's disease, tremor, and dystonia. Can J Neurol Sci. 2016; 43 (4):462–471

[48] Eller JL, Burchiel KJ. Deep Brain Stimulation for Tremor. In: Bakay R, Hrsg. Movment Disorder Surgery, The Essentials: Thieme Medical Publishers; 2009:153–165

[49] Rodriguez RL, Fernandez HH, Haq I, Okun MS. Pearls in patient selection for deep brain stimulation. Neurologist. 2007; 13(5):253–260

[50] Metman LV. Selection of Centers, Diseases, and Patients for Movement Disorder Surgery. In: Bakay R, Hrsg. Movement Disorder Surgery, The Essentials: Thieme Medical Publishers; 2009:48–57

[51] Richter EO, Hamani C, Lozano AM. Efficacy and Complications of Deep Brain Stimulation for Movement Disorders. In: Bakay R, Hrsg. Movement Disorder Surgery, The Essentials: Thieme Medical Publishers; 2009:227–236

[52] Schaeffer EL, Liu DY, Guerin J, Ahn M, Lee S, Asaad WF. A low-cost solution for quantification of movement during DBS surgery. J Neurosci Methods. 2018; 303:136–145

[53] Starr PA. Avoiding Complications and Correcting Errors. In: Bakay, Hrsg

[54] Young R. Stereotactic Radiosurgery for Movement Disorders. In: Starr P, Hrsg. Neurosurgical Operative Atlas. Second. Aufl. New York: Thieme Medical Publishers; 2009:165–168

[55] Elaimy AL, Demakas JJ, Arthurs BJ, et al. Gamma knife radiosurgery for essential tremor: a case report and review of the literature. World J Surg Oncol. 2010; 8:20

[56] Kooshkabadi A, Lunsford LD, Tonetti D, Flickinger JC, Kondziolka D. Gamma knife thalamotomy for tremor in the magnetic resonance imaging era. J Neurosurg. 2013; 118(4):713–718

[57] Guo WY, Lindqvist M, Lindquist C, et al. Stereotaxic angiography in gamma knife radiosurgery of intracranial arteriovenous malformations. AJNR Am J Neuroradiol. 1992; 13(4):1107–1114

[58] Kondziolka D, Ong JG, Lee JY, Moore RY, Flickinger JC, Lunsford LD. Gamma knife thalamotomy for essential tremor. J Neurosurg. 2008; 108(1):111–117

[59] Young RF, Li F, Vermeulen S, Meier R. Gamma knife thalamotomy for treatment of essential tremor: long-term results. J Neurosurg. 2010; 112(6):1311–1317

[60] Witjas T, Carron R, Krack P, et al. A prospective single-blind study of gamma knife thalamotomy for tremor. Neurology. 2015; 85(18):1562–1568

[61] Ohye C, Shibazaki T, Ishihara J, Zhang J. Evaluation of gamma thalamotomy for parkinsonian and other tremors: survival of neurons adjacent to the thalamic lesion after gamma thalamotomy. J Neurosurg. 2000; 93 Suppl 3:120–127

[62] Friedman DP, Goldman HW, Flanders AE, Gollomp SM, Curran WJ, Jr. Stereotactic radiosurgical pallidotomy and thalamotomy with the gamma knife: MR imaging findings with clinical correlation—preliminary experience. Radiology. 1999; 212(1):143–150

[63] Ravikumar VK, Parker JJ, Hornbeck TS, et al. Cost-effectiveness of focused ultrasound, radiosurgery, and DBS for essential tremor. Mov Disord. 2017; 32 (8):1165–1173

[64] Elias WJ, Lipsman N, Ondo WG, et al. A randomized trial of focused ultrasound thalamotomy for essential tremor. N Engl J Med. 2016; 375(8):730–739

[65] Elias WJ, Huss D, Voss T, et al. A pilot study of focused ultrasound thalamotomy for essential tremor. N Engl J Med. 2013; 369(7):640–648

[66] Lipsman N, Schwartz ML, Huang Y, et al. MR-guided focused ultrasound thalamotomy for essential tremor: a proof-of-concept study. Lancet Neurol. 2013; 12(5):462–468

[67] Zaaroor M, Sinai A, Goldsher D, et al. Magnetic resonance-guided focused ultrasound thalamotomy for tremor: a report of 30 Parkinson's disease and essential tremor cases. J Neurosurg. 201 8:202–210

[68] Fishman PS, Frenkel V. Focused ultrasound: an emerging therapeutic modality for neurologic disease. Neurotherapeutics. 2017; 14(2):393–404

[69] Gradinaru V, Mogri M, Thompson KR, Henderson JM, Deisseroth K. Optical deconstruction of parkinsonian neural circuitry. Science. 2009; 324(5925):354–359

[70] Nimsky C. Diffusion Tensor Imaging-Guided Resection. In: al. He, Hrsg. Intraoperative MR-Guided Neurosurgery: Thieme Medical Publishers; 2011:139–149

[71] Schlaier J, Anthofer J, Steib K, et al. Deep brain stimulation for essential tremor: targeting the dentato-rubro-thalamic tract? Neuromodulation. 2015; 18 (2):105–112

[72] Coenen VA, Allert N, Mädler B. A role of diffusion tensor imaging fiber tracking in deep brain stimulation surgery: DBS of the dentato-rubro-thalamic tract (drt) for the treatment of therapy-refractory tremor. Acta Neurochir (Wien). 2011; 153(8):1579–1585, discussion 1585

[73] Klein JC, Barbe MT, Seifried C, et al. The tremor network targeted by successful VIM deep brain stimulation in humans. Neurology. 2012; 78(11):787–795

[74] Chen T, Mirzadeh Z, Chapple K, Lambert M, Dhall R, Ponce FA. "Asleep" deep brain stimulation for essential tremor. J Neurosurg. 2016; 124(6):1842–1849

[75] Abosch A, Yacoub E, Ugurbil K, Harel N. An assessment of current brain targets for deep brain stimulation surgery with susceptibility-weighted imaging at 7 tesla. Neurosurgery. 2010; 67(6):1745–1756, discussion 1756

[76] Chen T, Mirzadeh Z, Ponce FA. "Asleep" deep brain stimulation surgery: a critical review of the literature. World Neurosurg. 2017; 105:191–198

[77] Sajonz BE, Amtage F, Reinacher PC, et al. Deep Brain Stimulation for Tremor Tractographic Versus Traditional (DISTINCT): study protocol of a randomized controlled feasibility trial. JMIR Res Protoc. 2016; 5(4):e244

10 Deep Brain Stimulation for Dystonia—Clinical Review and Surgical Considerations

Ankur Butala, Teresa Wojtasiewicz, Kelly Mills, Taylor E. Purvis, William S. Anderson

Abstract

Dystonia is a heterogeneous and disabling neurological disorder that is often refractory to conventional medical treatments. In this chapter, we will review the clinical manifestation of dystonia, from focal presentations as in cervical dystonia or as a generalized disorder significantly affecting independence and quality of life. A brief historical review explains evolving conceptions of diagnosis, genotype-phenotype correlations, and a unique mechanism to gain insight into the pathophysiology of neurological disease. We review treatment considerations including oral agents and botulinum toxin, which is the mainstay of treatment. However, we focus on surgical considerations regarding pre-, intra-, and postoperative management via deep brain stimulation.

Keywords: dystonia, DYT, torticollis, deep brain stimulation, globus pallidus interna

10.1 Introduction

Dystonia musculorum deformans, or simply "dystonia," is a multifaceted movement disorder, coined as such by Dr. Hermann Oppenheim in 1911 and characterized as "a very peculiar [disorder] … pronounced tonic cramping states … in the neck, head, and the proximal extremities … [with a] 'torqued gait' … representing an inextricable mix of voluntary movements, tic movements, and choreiform movements."[1,2] A syndromic classification rather than an etiological one, dystonia is characterized by intermittent or sustained involuntary muscular contractions or postures of the limbs, often twisted, writhing, or tremulous. The resulting postures lead to difficulties in activities of daily living (ADLs), reduced independence, lost work hours, chronic pain, and an increased risk of eventual irreversible musculoskeletal comorbidities such as scoliosis, limb and axial bony deformities, and contractures. In this chapter, we review relevant clinical considerations of dystonia focusing on neurosurgical pre-, peri-, and postoperative considerations.

10.2 Classification and Examination of Dystonias

Historically an imprecise diagnosis, dystonia was reclassified by an international panel using two major axes: clinical (time of onset: childhood- vs. adult-onset, or anatomical distribution of regions: focal, segmental, hemibody, generalized, or multifocal) and etiological (i.e., primary vs. secondary).[3,4,5,6] We briefly review each axis in semi-isolation. Clinical differentiation is particularly relevant to surgical preassessment and warrants some elaboration. However, it should be noted that despite recent advances in mapping pathophysiology, a consensus regarding phenomenology or globally unifying mechanistic explanation is lacking.[7,8] When more than one region is involved, dystonias may be segmental (contiguous regions), multifocal (noncontiguous), or hemidystonia (hemibody, usually secondary to acquired structural pathology). Dystonias may be "generalized" when involving the trunk and two other regions. These dystonias cause lifelong disability and often necessitate more aggressive intervention, such as deep brain stimulation (DBS).

10.2.1 Axis I—Clinical Considerations

The diagnosis of dystonia remains a bedside one requiring several phenomenological and provocative considerations. At a minimum, a dystonic contraction occurs with the simultaneous activity of muscle agonists and antagonists, such as with forearm flexors and extensors leading to the development of a sustained posture of the hand and fingers. The duration of contractions may vary considerably from brief moments (myoclonus-like durations[9]) to sustained spasms (which may be confused with contractures). Commonly, rhythmic or semirhythmic movements accompany the posture, appearing as a tremor and mistaken as "essential" or rubral tremor. The presence of temporal fluctuations and focal involvement further impede prompt diagnosis and represent an emerging research focus.[8] Focal dystonias may be a *forme fruste* of a later, more generalized dystonia (e.g., lower limb predominance with DYT5 or rostral presentation with ADCY5[10]). When present, a dystonic tremor may briefly abate when the dystonia is fully unopposed (i.e., the complete uncompensated manifestation) in a "null point" which may be thought of as a new, default, "resting state" of the limb.

Dystonic movements may lead to abnormal twisting postures, hence the historical term "torsion dystonia" is also used. Particular attention is paid to the distribution of symptoms, whether involving an isolated region of the body (*focal* dystonia as with the most common manifestation spasmodic torticollis or cervical dystonia), multiple contiguous regions (*segmental* dystonia, formerly *Meige's* syndrome or oromandibular dystonia), or generalized. The presence of comorbid movement phenomena, such as decrementing bradykinesia or resting tremor (Parkinsonism), myoclonus, or cerebellar pathology may implicate an identifiable etiology. Temporal variability is also notable, including diurnal fluctuations or the presence of periods of normality before paroxysmal "storms."

Next, provocative maneuvers or the effect of action should be assessed; many dystonias are now recognized to have exquisite task specificity or be induced by specific actions. Task-specific dystonias may develop in parts of the body that are involved in skilled or repetitive movements such as writing or playing a musical instrument, as in an embouchure dystonia.[11,12] Previously suspected to be mostly functional (i.e., psychogenic), action-induced dystonia may be difficult to clarify phenomenologically. Persons may subconsciously fight against postures by compensatory activation of adjacent or more proximal antagonists. Unfortunately, well-established diagnostic criteria for task-specific dystonias are lacking and remain the subject of study.[8]

Lastly, the presence of subtle exam findings of overflow, mirroring, or *geste antagonistes* can support a dystonia diagnosis. Overflow movements occur when muscles adjacent to those implicated in the dystonia are unconsciously activated either ipsilaterally or contralaterally, usually in concert with provocative maneuvers. In contrast, mirroring occurs when the use of less severely affected or unaffected limb (in the case of a unilateral dystonia) provokes dystonic movements ipsilaterally. These have high positive predictive value to confirm the presence of a task-specific dystonia, though sensitivity may be low.[13]

Special consideration is reserved for alleviating maneuvers (AMs),[14] formerly known as *sensory tricks* or *geste antagonistes*, which implicate emerging sensorimotor circuit inhibition models of dystonia. Classically, a patient might report an improvement of a cervical torticollis by touching his or her cheek or chin,[15] illustrating the most common tactile example of an AM. Prevalence reports vary in literature, but more than 70% of patients with dystonia have an AM of varying efficacy. However, emerging research suggests a broader possibility of sensory, nontactile stimuli[16,17] and interoceptive manifestations[18] that may have an alleviating or exacerbating effect.[19] These maneuvers relieve the dystonic posturing to different degrees both within an individual and among persons with dystonia in general. Converging lines of evidence from blink reflex prepulse inhibition and electromyography[20,21] studies suggest anomalous gating of sensorimotor integration between motoric efferent and sensory afferent systems.[22] As a result, feedback signals, such as by touch (in the case of a tactile AM), briefly normalize a pathological imbalance between cortical facilitation and inhibition.[23]

10.2.2 Axis II—Etiological Considerations

Etiologically, dystonias may be "primary" when they present early in life and cannot be attributed to an acquired cause. Primary (or genetic) dystonias may present in a generalized or focal fashion. The dopa-responsive dystonia (DRD) gene (Segawa Disease, DYT5a-*GCH1*) was sequenced in the early 1990s.[24] Since then, more than 25 monogenic forms have been identified (as of this writing).[25] These may be subdivided as either "isolated" or "combined." Broadly, combined dystonias are associated with myoclonus, Parkinsonism, or hyperkinetic movements. The majority have an autosomal dominant inheritance, albeit variable penetrance. For instance, early-onset generalized dystonias resulting from mutation of *TOR1A* (DYT1) or *THAP1* (DYT6) have a penetrance of 30 to 60%, respectively, despite autosomal dominant inheritance.[26]

In addition, dystonias may fluctuate with anxiety, circadian rhythms, exercise, or fasting. Action specificity implicates a reproducible and consistent relationship with an action and may cause severe disability in persons repeatedly engaging in complex or repetitive movements. Examples include writer's cramp, musician's dystonia, or runner's dystonia.[11]

While the majority of primary dystonias have autosomal dominant inheritance, notable exceptions include X-linked dystonia-parkinsonism (Lubag dystonia, DYT3-*TAF1*, Xq13.1), autosomal recessive variant DRD (DYT5b-*TH*, 11p15.5), or dystonias associated with matrilineal mitochondrial disorders such as Leigh syndrome. Accordingly, dystonia is a global disorder

with a higher preponderance in more genetically homogenous populations, such as persons with Ashkenazi ancestry[27] or from the Faroe Islands.[28] Pooled analysis of multiple population-based studies with a substantial sample (n > 10 million) suggest a combined prevalence of primary dystonia as 16.4 per 1 million persons.[29] The predominant cases were focal dystonias (primarily dominant arm, as in writer's cramp or primary writing tremor) and cervical dystonias, each with a pooled prevalence of 15.4 and 5.0 per 1 million, respectively. These are suspected to be underestimates due to referral bias of the tertiary medical centers driving data collection.

In contrast, the incidence of secondary, acquired dystonias is unknown in the setting of complex genotype–phenotype interactions and often occult environmental triggers. Neoplastic, hemorrhagic, or ischemic insults to the thalamus or basal ganglia may cause focal, segmental, or hemibody dystonias with or without comorbid hyperkinetic movement of chorea-ballism or myoclonus.[30,31] Even dystonia-associated perinatal hypoxic-ischemic damage may manifest well into young adulthood.[32,33] A variety of medications may induce a delayed tardive dystonia, including antipsychotics, antiemetics, antidepressants, and anticonvulsants.[34]

10.2.3 Rating Scales

Given the heterogeneity of primary and secondary dystonias, both regarding phenotypic presentation and etiology, a rigorous systematic approach is necessary to facilitate categorization and further study. For this, several standardized rating scales have been developed and validated over the years relevant to both specific dystonia and the disorder as a whole. A number of different scales are available specific to blepharospasm,[35] cervical dystonia,[36] and focal[37] and generalized dystonias.[38] While a comprehensive review is tangential to the goal of this manuscript, nonetheless, a few scales deemed "recommended" by the Movement Disorders Society Task Force on Rating Scales relevant to preoperative assessment merit further comment. These scales are as follows:

- Toronto Western Spasmodic Torticollis Rating Scale (TWSTRS)[36]: This scale has been in use since 1994 for clinical assessments and is a validated outcome measure in clinical trials of botulinum toxin, pharmacotherapies, and DBS. It has three subscales that measure the clinician-assessed physical severity and response to alleviating maneuvers, as well as patient-informed sections on disability and pain. It is the most widely utilized scale for cervical dystonia with fair interrater reliability, though it may be considered too extensive for routine clinical use.
- Fahn–Marsden Dystonia Rating Scale (FMDRS)[39,40]: The FMDRS is a widely used clinician rating scale assessing generalized dystonia by the regional motor manifestation and degree of disability. It has also been widely utilized to determine DBS outcomes in adults and children, though it was formulated to assess primary dystonia in adults.

10.3 Medical Management

Many patients with dystonia can have adequate control of their symptoms without surgery, though no current therapy can alter the natural history of the disease.[41] Symptomatic management is complex and multifaceted and focuses on the most disabling symptom and mechanism by which dystonia restricts independence or ADLs. Broadly, medical management for dystonia can be divided into three categories: (1) nonpharmacological options, such as physical therapy and bracing, (2) pharmacological treatment, and (3) chemodenervation (botulinum toxin). A selected review of various treatment options follows.

10.3.1 Physical and Supportive Therapy

There are a multitude of nonpharmacological therapies for dystonia, such as biofeedback training, postural exercises, bracing, and behavioral therapies.[41,42,43,44] The majority of investigations of these treatments have been case series, with few clinical trials.[41,42,43,44] Some evidence are promising, particularly recent studies of motor retraining and transcutaneous electrical nerve stimulation (TENS) in focal dystonia such as writer's or musician's cramp. Notably, TENS does not seem to provide a benefit in primary writing dystonia.[45,46,47] Due to the lack of high-quality evidence of the efficacy of physiotherapy in dystonia, these therapies should be adjuvant, not first-line, treatments.[43] Clinical evidence does support the use of physical rehabilitation programs in conjunction with other therapy, such as botulinum toxin injection.[48] Further evidence is needed to delineate what specific physical therapy interventions are useful for patients.

10.3.2 Pharmacological Considerations

There are no established disease-modifying therapies for any dystonia to date, and the management is symptomatic and targeted at areas of maximal disability. Few well-powered blinded clinical trials are investigating pharmacological options in dystonia, and existing recommendations are largely based on empirical observations and open-label studies.

Dopaminergic treatments

A subset of dystonias may be exquisitely sensitive to dopamine, such as DRD (Segawa disease, DYT5a).[49,50] Dopamine is often tried first in a person presenting with an unspecified dystonia to rapidly winnow differential diagnoses. Classically described DRDs are rapidly responsive to low-dose levodopa, though higher amounts may ultimately be necessary. A lack of meaningful response within 3 months suggests revisiting the suspected etiology.

Dopamine antagonists and depleters

Dopamine antagonists, such as clozapine, have been used in the treatment of both acute tardive dystonias and idiopathic dystonias,[51,52,53] though efficacy is equivocal and the side effects (both immediate and long term) are notable. However, dopamine modulation via inhibition of vesicular monoamine transporter 2 (VMAT2; tetrabenazine, valbenazine, and deutetrabenazine) seems to have efficacy for tardive dystonia[54] and idiopathic dystonia.[55] Expensive and difficult to obtain agents in the United States, dopamine modulators are primarily used in conditions when dystonia is an ancillary manifestation along with choreoathetosis, myoclonus, or tics.[56,57,58]

Anticholinergic

Before the Food and Drug Administration approval of botulinum toxin and the advent of surgical interventions, pharmacological treatment of dystonia relied upon anticholinergic agents that have long been observed to improve acute dystonic reactions from antipsychotics.[59,60,61] The earliest observations were largely empirical and anecdotal from the early 20th century. Fahn recognized that the anticholinergic trihexyphenidyl was better tolerated in children than adults, especially with regards to xerostomia, urinary retention, and constipation common to adults at high doses.[62] Early clinical trial data supported this observation,[63] prompting improvements in clinician-rated measures of dystonia severity and disability indices. Similar observations were made with secondary forms of dystonia such as cerebral palsy.[64,65] However, botulinum toxin has consistently demonstrated superior efficacy and tolerability over anticholinergics,[66] consigning them to second- or third-line agents in management. The available evidence is primarily anecdotal in children with little systematic evidence in adults.[67]

Anticonvulsants

Early interest in nootropics and possible disease-modifying treatments suggested the use of pyrrolidone derivatives, piracetam, and levetiracetam in animal models of paroxysmal dystonias.[68] Initially supported by case reports in focal and generalized dystonia,[69,70] a larger open-label prospective study refuted these findings.[71]

10.3.3 Botulinum Injections

Intramuscular injection of botulinum toxin is widely regarded as the first-line treatment for dystonia, with level 1A recommendations by several multidisciplinary societies[42] and national organizations.[72,73,74] Evidence support the use of botulinum injections in primary cranial (excluding oromandibular) dystonia, cervical dystonia, and writer's cramp.[75,76,77] Botulinum is safe in adults as well as pediatric patients.[78] The two serotypes of botulinum toxin available in the United States, onabotulinumtoxinA (type A) and rimabotulinumtoxinB (type B), differ in their pharmacological mechanism of action but both have been shown to be effective in the treatment of dystonia.[79,80]

10.4 Surgical Treatment

Surgical neuromodulation for dystonia increased over the past century. Modern surgical approaches include variations on ablative pallidotomies and thalamotomies, performed since the 1940s to 1960s,[81,82] and DBS.[83,84] Evidence have shown that DBS of the pallidum can provide excellent relief, though the outcomes vary on the basis of patient characteristics.[85,86,87,88,89,90,91] Careful preoperative evaluation and counseling about expected results of surgery are critical to select patients who will have maximum benefit from surgery. Multiple approaches for DBS for dystonia exist. Here we will review both the classical stereotactic frame-based and intraoperative magnetic resonance imaging (MRI)-guided approaches to the internal globus pallidus (GPi).

10.4.1 Deep Brain Stimulation

Pallidal DBS is an accepted treatment for dystonia in many patients resistant to medical therapy and botulinum injections. Long-term follow-up with multiple randomized, controlled trials has shown significant benefit of DBS in primary generalized and cervical dystonia.[85,86,87,88,89,90] There is also evidence that patients with specific secondary forms of dystonia may benefit from DBS.[85] Though DBS is beneficial in many subtypes of dystonia, the outcomes vary based on subtype. Moreover, many other patient factors can affect a patient's response to DBS. Preoperative evaluation by an interdisciplinary team can ensure dystonia patients achieve maximum benefit from intervention. A multidisciplinary team is also helpful for subsequent perioperative care and postoperative optimization and management.

Though the GPi is the most common target for stimulation, other targets have been explored, including cortical and thalamic targets.[92,93,94] More commonly, when significant tremor accompanies dystonia, the thalamic ventralis intermedius nucleus (Vim) DBS may improve both dystonia and tremor features when performed unilaterally,[95,96] bilaterally,[97] or in association with GPi DBS.[94,98,99,100] DBS targeting the posterior region of the ventrolateral nucleus of the thalamus has also been shown in some case series to improve dystonic features.[101]

Clinical observations of subthalamic DBS for Parkinson's disease improving secondary dystonia have prompted an inquiry into subthalamic nucleus (STN) and STN-adjacent targets for dystonia.[93,102] Subsequently, other groups have postulated that nearby regions such as the caudal zona incerta (cZi)[103] or posterior subthalamic area may be a more relevant node to target.[104,105,106] Thus far, the available literature does not strongly support the superiority of one target above another for all patients with dystonia, highlighting the need for head-to-head randomized trials in the future.

Surgical procedure, frame-based DBS

Preoperative workup and counseling, including general medical clearance and evaluation by an interdisciplinary movement disorders team, is performed. In most centers, frame-based targeting requires patients to be awake during the procedure with intravenous sedation administered during the opening. Preoperative counseling to ensure patients will be able to tolerate the awake method is critical. Before surgery, an MRI is obtained to assist with target planning that includes gadolinium-enhanced volumetric T1 imaging as well as T2 volumetric imaging with fast spin-echo, 3D gradient echo, and axial inversion recovery images. The patient is placed in a stereotactic frame set parallel to the Frankfort plane. Computed tomography (CT) is performed using the fiducial localizer box and fused to a preoperative MRI on a computerized planning station. A combination of atlas-based targeting using anterior commissure-posterior commissure (AC-PC) distance and other midline structures (indirect targeting) and MRI-guided targeting (direct targeting) may be performed, using a computerized stereotactic planning station. The trajectory is planned, and the X, Y, Z and arc and ring angle coordinates are obtained. In the operating room, the stereotactic frame is fixed to the operating table to minimize head movement during surgery. The skin incision is made and a burr hole is drilled at each entry point. A DBS electrode fixation device used to anchor the lead at the end of the case is seated securely around each burr hole. An introducer cannula is placed along the intended trajectory using intraoperative X-ray or CT to guide placement. The microelectrode is passed along the trajectory through the cannula and microelectrode recording (MER) proceeds utilizing an arrangement of microelectrodes, for example, two electrodes descending in parallel central and more medial trajectories to assess for tetanic responses. MER techniques may vary among different DBS centers due to differences in electrodes used and the number simultaneously passed simultaneously passed. For a long time, most North American and European DBS centers have been using some form of MER. However, intraoperative image guidance (discussed subsequently) is challenging this paradigm.

To perform MER, a high-impedance platinum-iridium microelectrode is threaded into the cannula which is attached to a microdrive on a head stage above the burr hole. The microelectrode is advanced to within 15 mm of the target, subsequently advanced in step-wise fashion while a physiologist, neurologist, or neurosurgeon monitors the audio and digitized field recording. Relevant grey matter nuclei or sensorimotor regions are confirmed by characteristic firing pattern observed and the presence of a kinesthetic response to passive movement. Regions may be delineated based on patterns of high- or low-frequency activity, the absence thereof (suggesting a white matter bundle), tonic or phasic discharge patterns, and background ambient noise. MER may be followed by macrostimulation at the base of the track and then ascending often using a guard ring electrode mounted above the microelectrode tip. High-frequency stimulation ranging between 0.5 and 5 mA in current may be utilized to test for induced side effects. Patients may be screened for changes in dystonia, though improvements are not commonly seen intraoperatively. More importantly, intraoperative stimulation facilitates earlier detection of visual and somatosensory symptoms, buttressing image-based localization relative to the optic tract, internal capsule, and medial lemniscus.

The initially planned trajectory may be modified based on information gleaned by MER, resulting in the ultimate track in which the DBS electrode will be implanted. Stimulation may be attempted again in bipolar fashion, as opposed to the monopolar stimulation previously performed for side effects or symptomatic benefit using the microelectrode assembly. The DBS lead localization and depth may be confirmed with intraoperative fluoroscopy or CT, which is the final stage at which revisions to lead position are feasible. Leads are then secured with the cranial fixation system and the lead cabling is tunneled under the scalp in preparation for the implantable pulse generator (IPG) placement, which is commonly performed in a second stage procedure at a later date. A final fluoroscopic image is obtained to confirm that the leads have not migrated during tunneling and the incision is closed. Postoperative or intraoperative head CT imaging may also be obtained to compare the actual trajectory against the planned trajectory on the planning station. At a later date, the patient returns for the second stage of the procedure, i.e., implantation of the DBS system pulse generator. The right side is preferred to avoid interfering with any potential future need for a cardiac pacemaker.

Surgical procedure, MRI-guided DBS[107,108]

Intraoperative imaging-guided DBS for dystonia may utilize MRI or CT for real-time verification of lead placement, i.e., iMRI or iCT, respectively. Due to higher resolution of cortical and subcortical anatomy, iMRI guidance may have superior favorability to CT guidance. Due to the author's familiarity with iMRI, we review it here as an illustration of intraoperative imaging in dystonia. For additional consideration of iCT in DBS, the interested reader should refer: Servello et al[109] and Bot et al.[110]

Preoperative evaluation for MRI-guided DBS is similar to considerations for general anesthesia. The patient is brought into the operating room suite for induction for endotracheal general anesthesia, then placed into an MRI-compatible head fixation system (▶ Fig. 10.1 and ▶ Fig. 10.2) and fiducial grids are placed at the estimated scalp entry point for GPi targeting after standard prepping and draping (▶ Fig. 10.3). A standard whole-head 3D T1 volumetric acquisition MRI scan with gadolinium is obtained to formulate an initial entry point. Skin incisions and burr holes are made at each entry point, followed by fixation of alignment bases (▶ Fig. 10.4). Repeat whole-head 3D T1 volumetric scan (without contrast) and high-resolution thin-slice slabs are performed to visualize the relevant anatomical target. These scans are used to align the introducer cannula to achieve less than 1 mm radial error in targeting. Ceramic guidance stylets are inserted through the cannula into the target positions. A 3D T1-weighted volumetric acquisition scan is obtained to confirm good positioning within the GPi and quantify placement error (▶ Fig. 10.5). The stylets are then removed and replaced with two DBS leads after removal from the MRI bore. The DBS leads are secured with the burr hole fixation system and tunneled under the scalp in preparation for the IPG placement. The incision is closed, and the patient returns for implantation of the DBS system pulse generator at a later date.

10.4.2 Postoperative Complications

Though DBS for dystonia is regarded to be safe and effective, the procedure is associated with the same types of complications as DBS for other movement disorders.[111,112,113,114,115,116,117,118,119,120,121,122,123,124,125] Complications due to DBS can be procedure related, hardware related, or stimulation related.

Procedure-related complications

These complications include hemorrhage, postoperative delirium/psychosis, and seizures.[111,112,113,114,115,116,117,118,119,120,121,122,123,124] Many procedure-related complications from DBS, such as postoperative delirium, seizure, vasovagal response, and headache, are self-limited and do not cause permanent deficits.[111,112,113,114,115,116,117,118,119,120,121,122,123,124] However, DBS carries a risk of intracranial hemorrhage that can lead to significant neurological deficits and death.[114,116,118,121,123,126] Fortunately, the rate of hemorrhage after DBS is quite low, ranging from 0.78 to 5%, with approximately half of patients showing symptoms.[114,116,118,121,123,126] Large series of patients undergoing DBS have shown that dystonia does not appear to be associated with higher rates of hemorrhage compared to other diagnoses treated with DBS. Other patient factors, such as older age and hypertension, are correlated with hemorrhage.[123] Some studies found a higher rate of hemorrhage in the GPi DBS than in the STN DBS, but further analysis has not shown an association between anatomic target and risk of hemorrhage.[125,127,128] One particular consideration in dystonia patients is *status dystonicus*, a rare acute exacerbation of dystonic symptoms triggered by changes in therapy, infection, or dehydration. Resulting autonomic instability, respiratory compromise, rhabdomyolysis, or acute renal failure may be life-threatening.[129,130] Management of status dystonicus requires careful observation in a critical care unit with intravenous hydration and other supportive medical therapy such as benzodiazepines and antipyretics.[129,130]

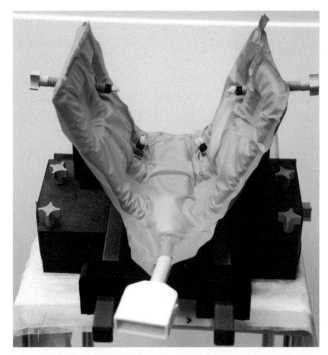

Fig. 10.1 Photograph of intraoperative magnetic resonance imaging coil, with head fixation system.

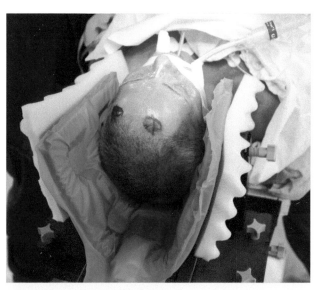

Fig. 10.2 Intubated patient positioned in magnetic resonance imaging coil, supine and neutral position.

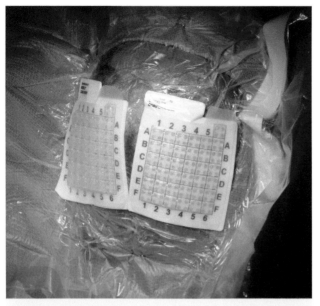

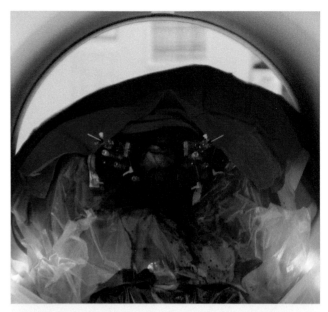

Fig. 10.3 Positioning of navigation grids prior to navigation-protocol magnetic resonance imaging.

Fig. 10.4 Bilateral navigation towers, with patient in an intraoperative magnetic resonance imaging scanner.

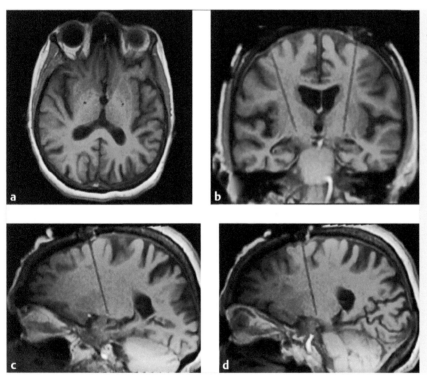

Fig. 10.5 MRI showing lead placement in GPi with intraoperative magnetic resonance imaging -based navigation. (a) axial image, (b) coronal image, (c) left lead, sagittal view, (d) right lead, sagittal view.

Hardware-related complications

Hardware-related complications, including infection, wound breakdown, lead migration, lead fracture, IPG malfunction, and tethering/pain, can plague patients even years after implantation of their devices. Infections, which include both immediate postoperative infections and delayed infections due to wound breakdown, are the most common complications from DBS, occurring in an average of 5 to 6% of patients.[111,114,116,117,118,119, 121,122,131,132,133,134,135,136] The most common site for infections appears to be the IPG site.[111,117,118,122,131,137,138] Superficial infections, or those confined to the IPG pocket, may be amenable to conservative management with antibiotics or removal of the IPG and connections alone.[136,137,139] These conservative approaches allow salvage of part or all of the DBS system in up to 50% of patients.[117,118,136,137,139] Severe infections, or those that have failed conservative management, require removal of the device and antibiotic treatment for several months before consideration of reimplantation. There appears to be no change in infection risk based on diagnostic group, so dystonia does not require special considerations for infection prevention.[111,114,116, 117,118,119,121,122,131,132,133,134,135,136] However, dystonia patients may develop status dystonicus that is triggered by the physiologic stress of infection or the abrupt cessation in therapy from hardware removal. Lead-related complications, including lead fracture or another hardware failure, can also result in abrupt cessation of therapy delivery. If a lead fracture or failure is suspected, the initial evaluation includes checking DBS system impedance and current with subsequent X-ray imaging.[140] The risk of lead fracture appears to be higher in patients with dystonia compared to other movement disorders, with up to 5.6% of patients experiencing a lead fracture.[111,117,131,133,141,142] Cervical tension from dystonic postures may explain this higher rate of lead fracture.[111,117,131,133,141,142]

10.4.3 Stimulation Side Effects

DBS can be associated with neurological side effects specifically related to the anatomical target, in the absence of hemorrhage or lead malposition. Stimulation of the GPi, the most common target for treatment of dystonia, is relatively well tolerated.

Patients with dystonia do not appear to develop significant cognitive decline after GPi DBS, and many psychiatric outcomes show improvement in overall markers of mood after surgery.[143,144,145] Dysarthria is the most common stimulation-related effect in dystonia patients, occurring in 4 to 11% of patients, and can theoretically be improved or reversed with programming. However, some patients may have persistent symptoms even after reprogramming.[119,131,146] Stimulation in the GPi is also associated with stimulation-induced bradykinesia and "freezing" of gait with varying degrees of severity.[132,147,148,149] The incidence of bradykinesia is difficult to assess as there is some indication of slowed motor responses after DBS even in patients who do not report symptomatic bradykinesia.[90,150]

10.5 Outcomes and DBS Programming (▶ Fig. 10.6)

10.5.1 Primary Generalized Dystonia

Primary generalized dystonias have been the focus of most of the studies among dystonia subtypes. Early case series of bilateral GPi implantation showed Burke–Fahn–Marsden Dystonia Rating Scale (BFMDRS) motor score improvements between 22 and 86% over follow-up periods of up to 66 months.[101,152,153,154, 155,156,157] These encouraging results prompted several prospective controlled trials of GPi DBS in primary generalized

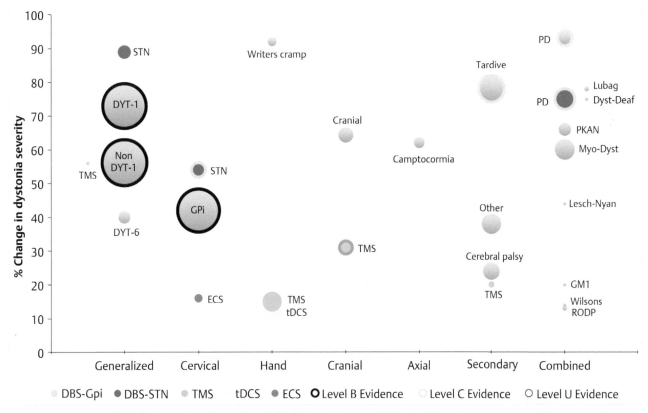

Fig. 10.6 Evidence of efficacy for brain stimulation in dystonia (from Fox and Alterman[151]). Each bubble represents the evidence that a particular type of brain stimulation is effective for a particular type of dystonia. The position of the bubble along the y axis reflects the average improvement in dystonia severity, the size of the bubble reflects the number of patients studied, and the bubble outline reflects the quality of the evidence assessed by American Academy of Neurology criteria (level B: black outline, level C: grey outline, level U: no outline). Treatments with the best evidence of efficacy have larger bubbles higher on the graph and outlined by darker lines.

dystonia. In one of the first seminal prospective studies of high-frequency GPi stimulation, Vidailhet et al showed robust, more than 50% improvements in objective motor scores and disabilities domains of BMFDRS 12 months after implantation, with a minority of subjects showing up to 75% improvement.[89] Similarly, Krupsh et al reported randomized, sham-controlled data showing that after 3 months, patients with bilateral GPi DBS had 39.9% improvement in BFMDRS motor score compared to 4.5% improvement in BFMDRS motor score with sham stimulation.[90] After 12 months, patients had 45% improvement in BFMDRS motor score compared to baseline.[90] In 2010, another multicenter prospective trial showed 43.8% improvement in BFMDRS motor score after 12 months compared to preoperative baseline.[158] Follow-up of patients with primary generalized dystonia after GPi DBS placement show that the benefit of DBS is long lasting. Most patients tend to exhibit progressive improvement from preoperative baseline with time, with 58 to 76% patients showing long-term improvement from preoperative baseline (based on BFMDRS-motor score), with long-term follow-up ranging from 3 to 20 years.[119,133,134,159,160,161] Importantly, despite a higher-than-expected population prevalence of psychiatric comorbidity in this cohort, GPi DBS does not appear to significantly affect neuropsychiatric outcomes.[162]

These clinical observations have implicated that genetically characterized primary dystonia (in contrast to secondary dystonias reviewed later) may be more responsive to DBS. Panov et al followed 47 patients with DYT1 dystonia for up to 10 years, demonstrating sustained improvements (<30% baseline preoperative scores) of motor function and disability, with several subjects able to discontinue medication.[133]

10.5.2 Focal Dystonia/Cervical Dystonia

In contrast to primary dystonias, focal dystonias, such as cervical dystonia, have more variable treatment results. Medication- and neurotoxin-refractory idiopathic cervical dystonia have been most rigorously studied with several retrospective, non-blinded series showing surgical outcomes comparable to those with primary generalized dystonia.[91] Krauss et al demonstrated that there is a wider but still significant effect size after surgery with 28 to 70.2% improvements in TWSTRS severity scores.[141, 146,163,164,165,166,167] Benefits accrue over time, with 3-month postoperative TWSTRS severity, disability, and pain scores improving until 20 months postoperatively (severity 38 to 63%, disability 54 to 69%, and pain 38 to 50%).[141] In contrast, other reports postulate the bulk of symptomatic improvement occurs within 1 year with relatively stable scores thereafter.[87,167,168] Nonetheless, long-term follow-up shows that, like primary generalized dystonia, the initial improvement in outcomes persists with 47.6% improvement from baseline TWSTRS score after an average 7.7 years of follow-up. Clinician-rated improvements in dystonia severity may be dissociated from patient-reported measures such as pain or disability with ADLs.[163]

Idiopathic craniocervical dystonia (Meige's syndrome), a segmental dystonia involving the periorbital, facial, bucco-oral, and cervical muscles, is often refractory to pharmacotherapy and chemodenervation, the latter often limited by adverse effects. Bilateral GPi DBS has also been demonstrated by Ostrem et al to induce 4–5 point improvements on the relevant eye and facial BMFDRS motor subscores, with associated improvements in

functional disability more than 6 months after implantation.[169] Similar to response rates in cervical and generalized dystonia, up to 80% improvement in BFMDRS cranial and cervical subscales have been reported up to 10 years post implantation in case reports and small case series.[170,171,172,173] In a recent large-scale review of 69 bilateral GPi DBS and 6 bilateral STN DBS patients, there was a mean improvement of 66.9% in motor scales and 56% in disability scales, without evidence that age impacted the outcomes at onset or disease duration.[174] Additional parameters, such as higher voltages (>3.0 V) and pulse widths (>185 millisecond) are not uncommon in the treatment of dystonia.

10.5.3 Secondary Dystonia

Secondary dystonias are a heterogeneous group of pathologies with dystonic symptoms that have shown varied responses to DBS.[175] Certain subtypes of secondary dystonia appear to be particularly amenable to DBS. The majority of evidence supporting the use of DBS in secondary dystonia is derived from case reports and case series, rather than the blinded, controlled studies that have been performed in primary generalized and cervical dystonias. Tardive dystonia is a severe, intractable form of dystonia resulting from a side effect of dopaminergic antagonist medications that seem to show a good response to DBS, reporting a wide range of 20 to 100% improvement in symptoms (based on BFMDRS motor score). Most patients experience approximately 50 to 70% improvement in symptoms over at least 6 months.[86,93,176,177,178,179,180,181] Cerebral palsy patients have more modest improvements in classic scales of dystonia symptoms after DBS, ranging from 23.6 to 49.5%.[182,183,184,185] Some studies have shown that despite a lack of improvement in the BFMDRS score, the overall improvement in the quality of life is significant.[184] For these patients, even though the effect size is not as large as the effect for other subtypes of dystonia, the possibility of modest benefits from surgery may be enough to proceed.[184,185] Anecdotal evidence suggest that DBS may be effective for a range of other types of secondary dystonia, including multiple sclerosis, Lesch–Nyhan syndrome, and dystonia after stroke.

10.5.4 Postulates on Mechanism of Action

A brief discussion of evolving perspectives on the mechanism of action of DBS may serve as a segue to practical considerations regarding postoperative programming. Historically, the primary impetus for DBS was as a replacement for ablative procedures, informing the use of high-frequency stimulation to induce a "depolarization block" in a cell population, thus mimicking a lesion.[186] However, early intraoperative observations demonstrated that STN-stimulation could induce muscular tetanic contraction rather than paresis (as would be assumed if a functional lesion was dominant). These clinical observations were supported by in vivo electrophysiological study of pallidal neuron firing rates[187] and elevated synaptic glutamate found via microdialysis.[188] Since initial observation, a variety of putative mechanisms of action relevant to dystonia have been proposed, as succinctly summarized by Murrow: regularization of neuronal activity,[189] disruption of pathologic corticostriatothalamic beta-band oscillations,[190] and increased inhibitory GABA release via pallidal afferents.[191] Additionally, emerging computational informatics models of dystonia and other brain disorders view pathophysiology through a lens of disordered information transmission.[192,193] In sum, interventional DBS techniques have not only provided a therapeutic opportunity but also enabled new insight into disease pathogenesis allowing for better treatments in the future.

10.5.5 DBS Programming and Stimulation Parameters

Initial programming is traditionally performed 4 weeks postoperatively in a medication-OFF state allowing microlesional effects to subside and total expression of physical symptoms to occur. Rarely, earlier activation may be advisable, for example, during an acute dystonic crisis.[130,194] Contemporary DBS systems are "open-loop," in which a clinician programmer modifies stimulation based on serial examination. These permit a wide degree of flexibility in adjusting parameters that include: current (mA) or voltage (V) amplitude, pulse width (millisecond), frequency (Hz), and case or lead contact(s) polarity (cathode-anode position). By extension, stimulation parameter adjustment may increase or decrease the size and intensity of volume of tissue activation (VTA). The general guiding principle of DBS programming is: improving motor symptoms while minimizing adverse sensorimotor effects. Programming in dystonia may be challenging as some phasic components, such as tremor, may transiently improve initially, but maximal global dystonia improvement may require several months of continuous stimulation (▶ Fig. 10.7).

To date, there is no broad consensus of "ideal" DBS settings specifically for dystonia, though numerous approaches have been suggested with congruent imperatives of maximizing motor benefit and minimizing adverse effects.[194,195,196] Since a clinical benefit may not be immediately evident, the initial program consists of activating each lead contact in monopole (case as an anode, contact as a cathode) and gradually increasing stimulus intensity, voltage or current amplitude,[197,198] until transient or sustained side effects are observed. Considering both GPi and STN targets, adverse effects may include muscular contractions of the upper or lower limb, dysarthria, paresthesias, neuropsychiatric features, diplopia, or phosphenes.

Stimulation of contact(s) within the posterolateral GPi seems to result in the maximum motor benefit. The contact immediately dorsal to that, which induces phosphenes, usually localizes to ventral GPi.[199,200,201] Bipolar or double monopolar configurations are often necessary to maximize VTA. Conservative initial parameters, similar to those used for Parkinson's disease, may be a moderate-high frequency (130 Hz) and narrow pulse width (60–90 millisecond). However, multiple alternative approaches have also been considered, including high pulse width[155,202] or frequency modulation.[153,155,166,191,203] Heterogenous stimulation responses to low or high frequency have been reported for focal dystonias versus generalized dystonias. Given the lack of clear evidence of the superiority of settings, parameters are tempered by net current delivery to promote battery longevity. In the absence of a clear clinical biomarker of response, patients may leave at the highest stimulus amplitude tolerated or counseled to increase stimulus intensity over several weeks rapidly. Quarterly follow-up visits using standardized rating scales are

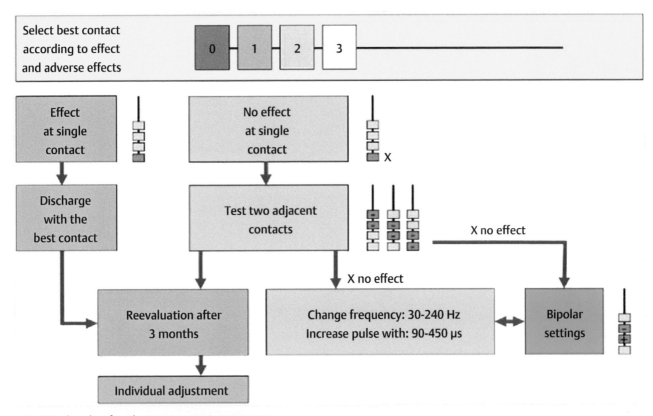

Fig. 10.7 Flow chart for selecting programming parameters.

required to evaluate the delayed efficacy and optimize settings. After maximizing VTA, many groups favor increasing pulse width incrementally up to 450 milliseconds. Low-frequency stimulation (< 60 Hz) may be an option if all the other options fail.

Dystonia DBS programming highlights limitations of open-loop devices and current programming approaches. Emerging lines of inquiry into optimizing treatment of dystonia include modification of the traditional rectangular DBS waveform from passive to active charge balancing[204] and lower frequency phase-specific stimulation.[205] Perhaps most intriguing fact is that a wider appreciation of cerebellar contributions to modulating basal ganglia activity is opening new treatment avenues and novel targets of stimulation.[206,207,208,209,210]

10.6 Conclusion

In this chapter, we provide an overview of clinical features and management considerations focusing on DBS for dystonia. DBS offers a single method for dramatically improving quality of life for patients, regardless of the distribution of symptoms or genetic, and in some cases, acquired etiology. In addition, DBS illustrates a way in which in vivo real-time physiological monitoring provides insight into the pathology of dystonia. Moreover, as dystonia circuit dynamics are broadly postulated as mechanisms of approach to other neuropsychiatric disorders, the efficacy of DBS in dystonia offers hope that previously debilitating disorders may be conquered and highlights the enduring relevance of circuit models of disease.

References

[1] Klein C, Fahn S. Translation of Oppenheim's 1911 paper on dystonia. Mov Disord. 2013; 28(7):851–862

[2] Oppenheim H. Über eine eigenartige Krampfkrankheit des kindlichen und jugendlichen Alters (Dysbasia lordotica progressiva, Dystonia musculorum deformans). Neurologisches Centralblatt. 1911; 30:1090–1107

[3] Marsden CD. Dystonia: the spectrum of the disease. Res Publ Assoc Res Nerv Ment Dis. 1976; 55:351–367

[4] Albanese A, Bhatia K, Bressman SB, et al. Phenomenology and classification of dystonia: a consensus update. Mov Disord. 2013; 28(7):863–873

[5] Morgan VL, Rogers BP, Abou-Khalil B. Segmentation of the thalamus based on BOLD frequencies affected in temporal lobe epilepsy. Epilepsia. 2015; 56 (11):1819–1827

[6] Morgante F, Klein C. Dystonia. Continuum (Minneap Minn). 2013; 19 5 Movement Disorders:1225–1241

[7] Albanese A. How many dystonias? Clinical evidence. Front Neurol. 2017; 8:18

[8] Pirio Richardson S, Altenmüller E, Alter K, et al. Research priorities in limb and task-specific dystonias. Front Neurol. 2017; 8:170

[9] Obeso JA, Rothwell JC, Lang AE, Marsden CD. Myoclonic dystonia. Neurology. 1983; 33(7):825–830

[10] Carapito R, Paul N, Untrau M, et al. A de novo ADCY5 mutation causes early-onset autosomal dominant chorea and dystonia. Mov Disord. 2015; 30(3): 423–427

[11] Torres-Russotto D, Perlmutter JS. Task-specific dystonias: a review. Ann N Y Acad Sci. 2008; 1142:179–199

[12] Frucht SJ, Fahn S, Greene PE, et al. The natural history of embouchure dystonia. Mov Disord. 2001; 16(5):899–906

[13] Sitburana O, Wu LJ, Sheffield JK, Davidson A, Jankovic J. Motor overflow and mirror dystonia. Parkinsonism Relat Disord. 2009; 15(10):758–761

[14] Patel N, Hanfelt J, Marsh L, Jankovic J, members of the Dystonia Coalition. Alleviating manoeuvres (sensory tricks) in cervical dystonia. J Neurol Neurosurg Psychiatry. 2014; 85(8):882–884

[15] Broussolle E, Laurencin C, Bernard E, Thobois S, Danaila T, Krack P. Early illustrations of geste antagoniste in cervical and generalized dystonia. Tremor Other Hyperkinet Mov (N Y). 2015; 5:332

[16] Lee CN, Eun MY, Kwon DY, Park MH, Park KW. "Visual sensory trick" in patient with cervical dystonia. Neurol Sci. 2012; 33(3):665–667

[17] Stojanovic M, Kostic V, Stankovic P, Sternic N. Improvement in laryngeal dystonia with background noise. Mov Disord. 1997; 12(2):249–250

[18] Greene PE, Bressman S. Exteroceptive and interoceptive stimuli in dystonia. Mov Disord. 1998; 13(3):549–551

[19] Asmus F, von Coelln R, Boertlein A, Gasser T, Mueller J. Reverse sensory geste in cervical dystonia. Mov Disord. 2009; 24(2):297–300

[20] Gómez-Wong E, Martí MJ, Tolosa E, Valls-Solé J. Sensory modulation of the blink reflex in patients with blepharospasm. Arch Neurol. 1998; 55(9): 1233–1237

[21] Peterson DA, Sejnowski TJ. A dynamic circuit hypothesis for the pathogenesis of blepharospasm. Front Comput Neurosci. 2017; 11:11

[22] Abbruzzese G, Berardelli A. Sensorimotor integration in movement disorders. Mov Disord. 2003; 18(3):231–240

[23] Ramos VF, Karp BI, Hallett M. Tricks in dystonia: ordering the complexity. J Neurol Neurosurg Psychiatry. 2014; 85(9):987–993

[24] Ozelius L, Kramer PL, Moskowitz CB, et al. Human gene for torsion dystonia located on chromosome 9q32-q34. Neuron. 1989; 2(5):1427–1434

[25] Klein C. Genetics in dystonia. Parkinsonism Relat Disord. 2014; 20 Suppl 1: S137–S142

[26] Phukan J, Albanese A, Gasser T, Warner T. Primary dystonia and dystonia-plus syndromes: clinical characteristics, diagnosis, and pathogenesis. Lancet Neurol. 2011; 10(12):1074–1085

[27] Inzelberg R, Hassin-Baer S, Jankovic J. Genetic movement disorders in patients of Jewish ancestry. JAMA Neurol. 2014; 71(12):1567–1572

[28] Joensen P. High prevalence of primary focal dystonia in the Faroe Islands. Acta Neurol Scand. 2016; 133(1):55–60

[29] Steeves TD, Day L, Dykeman J, Jetté N, Pringsheim T. The prevalence of primary dystonia: a systematic review and meta-analysis. Mov Disord. 2012; 27(14):1789–1796

[30] Hawker K, Lang AE. Hypoxic-ischemic damage of the basal ganglia. Case reports and a review of the literature. Mov Disord. 1990; 5(3):219–224

[31] Lee MS, Marsden CD. Movement disorders following lesions of the thalamus or subthalamic region. Mov Disord. 1994; 9(5):493–507

[32] Burke RE, Fahn S, Gold AP. Delayed-onset dystonia in patients with "static" encephalopathy. J Neurol Neurosurg Psychiatry. 1980; 43(9):789–797

[33] Saint Hilaire MH, Burke RE, Bressman SB, Brin MF, Fahn S. Delayed-onset dystonia due to perinatal or early childhood asphyxia. Neurology. 1991; 41 (2 (Pt 1)):216–222

[34] Zádori D, Veres G, Szalárdy L, Klivényi P, Vécsei L. Drug-induced movement disorders. Expert Opin Drug Saf. 2015; 14(6):877–890

[35] Jankovic J, Kenney C, Grafe S, Goertelmeyer R, Comes G. Relationship between various clinical outcome assessments in patients with blepharospasm. Mov Disord. 2009; 24(3):407–413

[36] Consky E, Lang A. Clinical assessments of patients with cervical dystonia. In: Jankovic J, Hallett M, eds. Therapy with botulinum toxin. Vol. 25. New York, NY: Marcel Dekker; 1994:211–237

[37] Müller J, Wissel J, Kemmler G, et al. Craniocervical dystonia questionnaire (CDQ-24): development and validation of a disease-specific quality of life instrument. J Neurol Neurosurg Psychiatry. 2004; 75(5):749–753

[38] Comella CL, Leurgans S, Wuu J, Stebbins GT, Chmura T, Dystonia Study Group. Rating scales for dystonia: a multicenter assessment. Mov Disord. 2003; 18(3):303–312

[39] Krystkowiak P, du Montcel ST, Vercueil L, et al. SPIDY Group. Reliability of the Burke-Fahn-Marsden scale in a multicenter trial for dystonia. Mov Disord. 2007; 22(5):685–689

[40] Burke RE, Fahn S, Marsden CD, Bressman SB, Moskowitz C, Friedman J. Validity and reliability of a rating scale for the primary torsion dystonias. Neurology. 1985; 35(1):73–77

[41] Jankovic J. Medical treatment of dystonia. Mov Disord. 2013; 28(7):1001–1012

[42] Albanese A, Asmus F, Bhatia KP, et al. EFNS guidelines on diagnosis and treatment of primary dystonias. Eur J Neurol. 2011; 18(1):5–18

[43] Delnooz CC, Horstink MW, Tijssen MA, van de Warrenburg BP. Paramedical treatment in primary dystonia: a systematic review. Mov Disord. 2009; 24 (15):2187–2198

[44] De Pauw J, Van der Velden K, Meirte J, et al. The effectiveness of physiotherapy for cervical dystonia: a systematic literature review. J Neurol. 2014; 261 (10):1857–1865

[45] Espay AJ, Hung SW, Sanger TD, Moro E, Fox SH, Lang AE. A writing device improves writing in primary writing tremor. Neurology. 2005; 64(9):1648–1650

[46] Meunier S, Bleton JP, Mazevet D, et al. TENS is harmful in primary writing tremor. Clin Neurophysiol. 2011; 122(1):171–175

[47] Tinazzi M, Farina S, Bhatia K, et al. TENS for the treatment of writer's cramp dystonia: a randomized, placebo-controlled study. Neurology. 2005; 64(11):1946–1948

[48] Tassorelli C, Mancini F, Balloni L, et al. Botulinum toxin and neuromotor rehabilitation: an integrated approach to idiopathic cervical dystonia. Mov Disord. 2006; 21(12):2240–2243

[49] Nygaard TG, Marsden CD, Duvoisin RC. Dopa-responsive dystonia. Adv Neurol. 1988; 50:377–384

[50] Segawa M, Hosaka A, Miyagawa F, Nomura Y, Imai H. Hereditary progressive dystonia with marked diurnal fluctuation. Adv Neurol. 1976; 14:215–233

[51] Karp BI, Goldstein SR, Chen R, Samii A, Bara-Jimenez W, Hallett M. An open trial of clozapine for dystonia. Mov Disord. 1999; 14(4):652–657

[52] Jankovic J. Tardive syndromes and other drug-induced movement disorders. Clin Neuropharmacol. 1995; 18(3):197–214

[53] Shapleske J, Mickay AP, Mckenna PJ. Successful treatment of tardive dystonia with clozapine and clonazepam. Br J Psychiatry. 1996; 168(4):516–518

[54] Simpson GM. The treatment of tardive dyskinesia and tardive dystonia. J Clin Psychiatry. 2000; 61 Suppl 4:39–44

[55] Jankovic J, Beach J. Long-term effects of tetrabenazine in hyperkinetic movement disorders. Neurology. 1997; 48(2):358–362

[56] Chen JJ, Ondo WG, Dashtipour K, Swope DM. Tetrabenazine for the treatment of hyperkinetic movement disorders: a review of the literature. Clin Ther. 2012; 34(7):1487–1504

[57] Jankovic J. Treatment of hyperkinetic movement disorders with tetrabenazine: a double-blind crossover study. Ann Neurol. 1982; 11(1):41–47

[58] Jankovic J, Orman J. Tetrabenazine therapy of dystonia, chorea, tics, and other dyskinesias. Neurology. 1988; 38(3):391–394

[59] Boyer WF, Bakalar NH, Lake CR. Anticholinergic prophylaxis of acute haloperidol-induced acute dystonic reactions. J Clin Psychopharmacol. 1987; 7(3):164–166

[60] Holloman LC, Marder SR. Management of acute extrapyramidal effects induced by antipsychotic drugs. Am J Health Syst Pharm. 1997; 54(21):2461–2477

[61] Stern TA, Anderson WH. Benztropine prophylaxis of dystonic reactions. Psychopharmacology (Berl). 1979; 61(3):261–262

[62] Fahn S. High dosage anticholinergic therapy in dystonia. Neurology. 1983; 33(10):1255–1261

[63] Burke RE, Fahn S, Marsden CD. Torsion dystonia: a double-blind, prospective trial of high-dosage trihexyphenidyl. Neurology. 1986; 36(2):160–164

[64] Sanger TD, Bastian A, Brunstrom J, et al. Child Motor Study Group. Prospective open-label clinical trial of trihexyphenidyl in children with secondary dystonia due to cerebral palsy. J Child Neurol. 2007; 22(5):530–537

[65] van den Heuvel CNAM, Tijssen MA, van de Warrenburg BPC, Delnooz C. The symptomatic treatment of acquired dystonia: a systematic review. Mov Disord Clin Pract. 2016; 3(6):548–558

[66] Brans JW, Lindeboom R, Snoek JW, et al. Botulinum toxin versus trihexyphenidyl in cervical dystonia: a prospective, randomized, double-blind controlled trial. Neurology. 1996; 46(4):1066–1072

[67] Albanese A, Barnes MP, Bhatia KP, et al. A systematic review on the diagnosis and treatment of primary (idiopathic) dystonia and dystonia plus syndromes: report of an EFNS/MDS-ES Task Force. Eur J Neurol. 2006; 13(5):433–444

[68] Löscher W, Richter A. Piracetam and levetiracetam, two pyrrolidone derivatives, exert antidystonic activity in a hamster model of paroxysmal dystonia. Eur J Pharmacol. 2000; 391(3):251–254

[69] Sullivan KL, Hauser RA, Louis ED, Chari G, Zesiewicz TA. Levetiracetam for the treatment of generalized dystonia. Parkinsonism Relat Disord. 2005; 11(7):469–471

[70] Zesiewicz TA, Louis ED, Sullivan KL, Menkin M, Dunne PB, Hauser RA. Substantial improvement in a Meige's syndrome patient with levetiracetam treatment. Mov Disord. 2004; 19(12):1518–1521

[71] Hering S, Wenning GK, Seppi K, Poewe W, Mueller J. An open trial of levetiracetam for segmental and generalized dystonia. Mov Disord. 2007; 22(11):1649–1651

[72] Hallett M, Albanese A, Dressler D, et al. Evidence-based review and assessment of botulinum neurotoxin for the treatment of movement disorders. Toxicon. 2013; 67:94–114

[73] Simpson DM, Hallett M, Ashman EJ, et al. Practice guideline update summary: Botulinum neurotoxin for the treatment of blepharospasm, cervical dystonia, adult spasticity, and headache: Report of the Guideline Development Subcommittee of the American Academy of Neurology. Neurology. 2016; 86(19):1818–1826

[74] Simpson DM, Blitzer A, Brashear A, et al. Therapeutics and Technology Assessment Subcommittee of the American Academy of Neurology. Assessment: Botulinum neurotoxin for the treatment of movement disorders (an evidence-based review): report of the Therapeutics and Technology Assessment Subcommittee of the American Academy of Neurology. Neurology. 2008; 70(19):1699–1706

[75] Kruisdijk JJ, Koelman JH, Ongerboer de Visser BW, de Haan RJ, Speelman JD. Botulinum toxin for writer's cramp: a randomised, placebo-controlled trial and 1-year follow-up. J Neurol Neurosurg Psychiatry. 2007; 78(3):264–270

[76] Bentivoglio AR, Fasano A, Ialongo T, Soleti F, Lo Fermo S, Albanese A. Fifteen-year experience in treating blepharospasm with Botox or Dysport: same toxin, two drugs. Neurotox Res. 2009; 15(3):224–231

[77] Truong D, Duane DD, Jankovic J, et al. Efficacy and safety of botulinum type A toxin (Dysport) in cervical dystonia: results of the first US randomized, double-blind, placebo-controlled study. Mov Disord. 2005; 20(7):783–791

[78] Albavera-Hernández C, Rodríguez JM, Idrovo AJ. Safety of botulinum toxin type A among children with spasticity secondary to cerebral palsy: a systematic review of randomized clinical trials. Clin Rehabil. 2009; 23(5):394–407

[79] Pappert EJ, Germanson T, Myobloc/Neurobloc European Cervical Dystonia Study Group. Botulinum toxin type B vs. type A in toxin-naïve patients with cervical dystonia: Randomized, double-blind, noninferiority trial. Mov Disord. 2008; 23(4):510–517

[80] Duarte GS, Castelão M, Rodrigues FB, et al. Botulinum toxin type A versus botulinum toxin type B for cervical dystonia. Cochrane Database Syst Rev. 2016; 10:CD004314

[81] Cooper IS. Clinical and physiologic implications of thalamic surgery for disorders of sensory communication. 2. Intention tremor, dystonia, Wilson's disease and torticollis. J Neurol Sci. 1965; 2(6):520–553

[82] Cooper IS. 20-year follow-up study of the neurosurgical treatment of dystonia musculorum deformans. Adv Neurol. 1976; 14:423–452

[83] Gildenberg PL. Evolution of basal ganglia surgery for movement disorders. Stereotact Funct Neurosurg. 2006; 84(4):131–135

[84] Cif L, Hariz M. Seventy years with the globus pallidus: pallidal surgery for movement disorders between 1947 and 2017. Mov Disord. 2017; 32(7):972–982

[85] Pretto TE, Dalvi A, Kang UJ, Penn RD. A prospective blinded evaluation of deep brain stimulation for the treatment of secondary dystonia and primary torticollis syndromes. J Neurosurg. 2008; 109(3):405–409

[86] Damier P, Thobois S, Witjas T, et al. French Stimulation for Tardive Dyskinesia (STARDYS) Study Group. Bilateral deep brain stimulation of the globus pallidus to treat tardive dyskinesia. Arch Gen Psychiatry. 2007; 64(2):170–176

[87] Kiss ZH, Doig-Beyaert K, Eliasziw M, Tsui J, Haffenden A, Suchowersky O, Functional and Stereotactic Section of the Canadian Neurosurgical Society, Canadian Movement Disorders Group. The Canadian multicentre study of deep brain stimulation for cervical dystonia. Brain. 2007; 130(Pt 11):2879–2886

[88] Diamond A, Shahed J, Azher S, Dat-Vuong K, Jankovic J. Globus pallidus deep brain stimulation in dystonia. Mov Disord. 2006; 21(5):692–695

[89] Vidailhet M, Vercueil L, Houeto JL, et al. French Stimulation du Pallidum Interne dans la Dystonie (SPIDY) Study Group. Bilateral deep-brain stimulation of the globus pallidus in primary generalized dystonia. N Engl J Med. 2005; 352(5):459–467

[90] Kupsch A, Benecke R, Müller J, et al. Deep-Brain Stimulation for Dystonia Study Group. Pallidal deep-brain stimulation in primary generalized or segmental dystonia. N Engl J Med. 2006; 355(19):1978–1990

[91] Moro E, LeReun C, Krauss JK, et al. Efficacy of pallidal stimulation in isolated dystonia: a systematic review and meta-analysis. Eur J Neurol. 2017; 24(4):552–560

[92] Romito LM, Franzini A, Perani D, et al. Fixed dystonia unresponsive to pallidal stimulation improved by motor cortex stimulation. Neurology. 2007; 68(11):875–876

[93] Sun B, Chen S, Zhan S, Le W, Krahl SE. Subthalamic nucleus stimulation for primary dystonia and tardive dystonia. Acta Neurochir Suppl (Wien). 2007; 97(Pt 2):207–214

[94] Woehrle JC, Blahak C, Kekelia K, et al. Chronic deep brain stimulation for segmental dystonia. Stereotact Funct Neurosurg. 2009; 87(6):379–384

[95] Racette BA, Dowling J, Randle J, Mink JW. Thalamic stimulation for primary writing tremor. J Neurol. 2001; 248(5):380–382

[96] Minguez-Castellanos A, Carnero-Pardo C, Gómez-Camello A, et al. Primary writing tremor treated by chronic thalamic stimulation. Mov Disord. 1999; 14(6):1030–1033

[97] Kuncel AM, Turner DA, Ozelius LJ, Greene PE, Grill WM, Stacy MA. Myoclonus and tremor response to thalamic deep brain stimulation parameters in a patient with inherited myoclonus-dystonia syndrome. Clin Neurol Neurosurg. 2009; 111(3):303–306

[98] Hedera P, Phibbs FT, Dolhun R, et al. Surgical targets for dystonic tremor: considerations between the globus pallidus and ventral intermediate thalamic nucleus. Parkinsonism Relat Disord. 2013; 19(7):684–686

[99] Morishita T, Foote KD, Haq IU, Zeilman P, Jacobson CE, Okun MS. Should we consider Vim thalamic deep brain stimulation for select cases of severe refractory dystonic tremor. Stereotact Funct Neurosurg. 2010; 88(2):98–104

[100] Fasano A, Bove F, Lang AE. The treatment of dystonic tremor: a systematic review. J Neurol Neurosurg Psychiatry. 2014; 85(7):759–769

[101] Vercueil L, Pollak P, Fraix V, et al. Deep brain stimulation in the treatment of severe dystonia. J Neurol. 2001; 248(8):695–700

[102] Ostrem JL, San Luciano M, Dodenhoff KA, et al. Subthalamic nucleus deep brain stimulation in isolated dystonia: a 3-year follow-up study. Neurology. 2017; 88(1):25–35

[103] Plaha P, Khan S, Gill SS. Bilateral stimulation of the caudal zona incerta nucleus for tremor control. J Neurol Neurosurg Psychiatry. 2008; 79(5):504–513

[104] Buhmann C, Moll CK, Zittel S, Münchau A, Engel AK, Hamel W. Deep brain stimulation of the ventrolateral thalamic base and posterior subthalamic area in dystonic head tremor. Acta Neurochir Suppl (Wien). 2013; 117:67–72

[105] Blomstedt P, Fytagoridis A, Tisch S. Deep brain stimulation of the posterior subthalamic area in the treatment of tremor. Acta Neurochir (Wien). 2009; 151(1):31–36

[106] Blomstedt P, Sandvik U, Fytagoridis A, Tisch S. The posterior subthalamic area in the treatment of movement disorders: past, present, and future. Neurosurgery. 2009; 64(6):1029–1038, discussion 1038–1042

[107] Anderson WS, Lenz FA. Surgery insight: deep brain stimulation for movement disorders. Nat Clin Pract Neurol. 2006; 2(6):310–320

[108] Starr PA, Turner RS, Rau G, et al. Microelectrode-guided implantation of deep brain stimulators into the globus pallidus internus for dystonia: techniques, electrode locations, and outcomes. Neurosurg Focus. 2004; 17(1):E4

[109] Servello D, Zekaj E, Saleh C, Pacchetti C, Porta M. The pros and cons of intraoperative CT scan in evaluation of deep brain stimulation lead implantation: A retrospective study. Surg Neurol Int. 2016; 7 Suppl 19:S551–S556

[110] Bot M, van den Munckhof P, Bakay R, Stebbins G, Verhagen Metman L. Accuracy of intraoperative computed tomography during deep brain stimulation procedures: comparison with postoperative magnetic resonance imaging. Stereotact Funct Neurosurg. 2017; 95(3):183–188

[111] Jitkritsadakul O, Bhidayasiri R, Kalia SK, Hodaie M, Lozano AM, Fasano A. Systematic review of hardware-related complications of deep brain stimulation: do new indications pose an increased risk? Brain Stimul. 2017; 10(5):967–976

[112] Brüggemann N, Kühn A, Schneider SA, et al. Short- and long-term outcome of chronic pallidal neurostimulation in monogenic isolated dystonia. Neurology. 2015; 84(9):895–903

[113] Romito LM, Zorzi G, Marras CE, Franzini A, Nardocci N, Albanese A. Pallidal stimulation for acquired dystonia due to cerebral palsy: beyond 5 years. Eur J Neurol. 2015; 22(3):426–e32

[114] Beric A, Kelly PJ, Rezai A, et al. Complications of deep brain stimulation surgery. Stereotact Funct Neurosurg. 2001; 77(1–4):73–78

[115] Burdick AP, Fernandez HH, Okun MS, Chi YY, Jacobson C, Foote KD. Relationship between higher rates of adverse events in deep brain stimulation using standardized prospective recording and patient outcomes. Neurosurg Focus. 2010; 29(2):E4

[116] Chen T, Mirzadeh Z, Chapple K, Lambert M, Ponce FA. Complication rates, lengths of stay, and readmission rates in "awake" and "asleep" deep brain simulation. J Neurosurg. 2017; 127(2):360–369

[117] Constantoyannis C, Berk C, Honey CR, Mendez I, Brownstone RM. Reducing hardware-related complications of deep brain stimulation. Can J Neurol Sci. 2005; 32(2):194–200

[118] Fenoy AJ, Simpson RK, Jr. Risks of common complications in deep brain stimulation surgery: management and avoidance. J Neurosurg. 2014; 120(1):132–139

[119] Isaias IU, Alterman RL, Tagliati M. Deep brain stimulation for primary generalized dystonia: long-term outcomes. Arch Neurol. 2009; 66(4):465–470

[120] Kaminska M, Perides S, Lumsden DE, et al. Complications of deep brain stimulation (DBS) for dystonia in children: the challenges and 10 year experience in a large paediatric cohort. Eur J Paediatr Neurol. 2017; 21(1):168–175

[121] Patel DM, Walker HC, Brooks R, Omar N, Ditty B, Guthrie BL. Adverse events associated with deep brain stimulation for movement disorders: analysis of 510 consecutive cases. Neurosurgery. 2015; 11 Suppl 2:190–199

[122] Sillay KA, Larson PS, Starr PA. Deep brain stimulator hardware-related infections: incidence and management in a large series. Neurosurgery. 2008; 62(2):360–366, discussion 366–367

[123] Zrinzo L, Foltynie T, Limousin P, Hariz MI. Reducing hemorrhagic complications in functional neurosurgery: a large case series and systematic literature review. J Neurosurg. 2012; 116(1):84–94

[124] Buhmann C, Huckhagel T, Engel K, et al. Adverse events in deep brain stimulation: A retrospective long-term analysis of neurological, psychiatric and other occurrences. PLoS One. 2017; 12(7):e0178984

[125] Gorgulho A, De Salles AA, Frighetto L, Behnke E. Incidence of hemorrhage associated with electrophysiological studies performed using macroelectrodes and microelectrodes in functional neurosurgery. J Neurosurg. 2005; 102(5):888–896

[126] Park CK, Jung NY, Kim M, Chang JW. Analysis of delayed intracerebral hemorrhage associated with deep brain stimulation surgery. World Neurosurg. 2017; 104:537–544

[127] Binder DK, Rau GM, Starr PA. Risk factors for hemorrhage during microelectrode-guided deep brain stimulator implantation for movement disorders. Neurosurgery. 2005; 56(4):722–732, discussion 722–732

[128] Xiaowu H, Xiufeng J, Xiaoping Z, et al. Risks of intracranial hemorrhage in patients with Parkinson's disease receiving deep brain stimulation and ablation. Parkinsonism Relat Disord. 2010; 16(2):96–100

[129] Allen NM, Lin JP, Lynch T, King MD. Status dystonicus: a practice guide. Dev Med Child Neurol. 2014; 56(2):105–112

[130] Termsarasab P, Frucht SJ. Dystonic storm: a practical clinical and video review. J Clin Mov Disord. 2017; 4(10):10

[131] Kenney C, Simpson R, Hunter C, et al. Short-term and long-term safety of deep brain stimulation in the treatment of movement disorders. J Neurosurg. 2007; 106(4):621–625

[132] Meoni S, Fraix V, Castrioto A, et al. Pallidal deep brain stimulation for dystonia: a long-term study. J Neurol Neurosurg Psychiatry. 2017; 88(11):960–967

[133] Panov F, Gologorsky Y, Connors G, Tagliati M, Miravite J, Alterman RL. Deep brain stimulation in DYT1 dystonia: a 10-year experience. Neurosurgery. 2013; 73(1):86–93, discussion 93

[134] Sobstyl M, Kmieć T, Ząbek M, Szczałuba K, Mossakowski Z. Long-term outcomes of bilateral pallidal stimulation for primary generalised dystonia. Clin Neurol Neurosurg. 2014; 126:82–87

[135] Tagliati M, Krack P, Volkmann J, et al. Long-term management of DBS in dystonia: response to stimulation, adverse events, battery changes, and special considerations. Mov Disord. 2011; 26 Suppl 1:S54–S62

[136] Piacentino M, Pilleri M, Bartolomei L. Hardware-related infections after deep brain stimulation surgery: review of incidence, severity and management in 212 single-center procedures in the first year after implantation. Acta Neurochir (Wien). 2011; 153(12):2337–2341

[137] Fenoy AJ, Simpson RK, Jr. Management of device-related wound complications in deep brain stimulation surgery. J Neurosurg. 2012; 116(6):1324–1332

[138] Umemura A, Jaggi JL, Hurtig HI, et al. Deep brain stimulation for movement disorders: morbidity and mortality in 109 patients. J Neurosurg. 2003; 98(4):779–784

[139] Bhatia S, Zhang K, Oh M, Angle C, Whiting D. Infections and hardware salvage after deep brain stimulation surgery: a single-center study and review of the literature. Stereotact Funct Neurosurg. 2010; 88(3):147–155

[140] Fernández FS, Alvarez Vega MA, Antuña Ramos A, Fernández González F, Lozano Aragoneses B. Lead fractures in deep brain stimulation during long-term follow-up. Parkinsons Dis. 2010; 2010(409356):409356

[141] Krauss JK, Loher TJ, Pohle T, et al. Pallidal deep brain stimulation in patients with cervical dystonia and severe cervical dyskinesias with cervical myelopathy. J Neurol Neurosurg Psychiatry. 2002; 72(2):249–256

[142] Yianni J, Nandi D, Shad A, Bain P, Gregory R, Aziz T. Increased risk of lead fracture and migration in dystonia compared with other movement disorders following deep brain stimulation. J Clin Neurosci. 2004; 11(3):243–245

[143] Jahanshahi M, Czernecki V, Zurowski AM. Neuropsychological, neuropsychiatric, and quality of life issues in DBS for dystonia. Mov Disord. 2011; 26 Suppl 1:S63–S78

[144] Hälbig TD, Gruber D, Kopp UA, Schneider GH, Trottenberg T, Kupsch A. Pallidal stimulation in dystonia: effects on cognition, mood, and quality of life. J Neurol Neurosurg Psychiatry. 2005; 76(12):1713–1716

[145] de Gusmao CM, Pollak LE, Sharma N. Neuropsychological and psychiatric outcome of GPi-deep brain stimulation in dystonia. Brain Stimul. 2017; 10 (5):994–996

[146] Volkmann J, Mueller J, Deuschl G, et al. DBS study group for dystonia. Pallidal neurostimulation in patients with medication-refractory cervical dystonia: a randomised, sham-controlled trial. Lancet Neurol. 2014; 13(9):875–884

[147] Schrader C, Capelle HH, Kinfe TM, et al. GPi-DBS may induce a hypokinetic gait disorder with freezing of gait in patients with dystonia. Neurology. 2011; 77(5):483–488

[148] Blahak C, Capelle HH, Baezner H, Kinfe TM, Hennerici MG, Krauss JK. Micrographia induced by pallidal DBS for segmental dystonia: a subtle sign of hypokinesia? J Neural Transm (Vienna). 2011; 118(4):549–553

[149] Berman BD, Starr PA, Marks WJ, Jr, Ostrem JL. Induction of bradykinesia with pallidal deep brain stimulation in patients with cranial-cervical dystonia. Stereotact Funct Neurosurg. 2009; 87(1):37–44

[150] Huebl J, Brücke C, Schneider GH, Blahak C, Krauss JK, Kühn AA. Bradykinesia induced by frequency-specific pallidal stimulation in patients with cervical and segmental dystonia. Parkinsonism Relat Disord. 2015; 21(7):800–803

[151] Fox MD, Alterman RL. Brain stimulation for torsion dystonia. JAMA Neurol. 2015; 72(6):713–719

[152] Yianni J, Bain PG, Gregory RP, et al. Post-operative progress of dystonia patients following globus pallidus internus deep brain stimulation. Eur J Neurol. 2003; 10(3):239–247

[153] Kupsch A, Klaffke S, Kühn AA, et al. The effects of frequency in pallidal deep brain stimulation for primary dystonia. J Neurol. 2003; 250(10):1201–1205

[154] Katayama Y, Fukaya C, Kobayashi K, Oshima H, Yamamoto T. Chronic stimulation of the globus pallidus internus for control of primary generalized dystonia. Acta Neurochir Suppl (Wien). 2003; 87:125–128

[155] Coubes P, Cif L, El Fertit H, et al. Electrical stimulation of the globus pallidus internus in patients with primary generalized dystonia: long-term results. J Neurosurg. 2004; 101(2):189–194

[156] Vayssiere N, van der Gaag N, Cif L, et al. Deep brain stimulation for dystonia confirming a somatotopic organization in the globus pallidus internus. J Neurosurg. 2004; 101(2):181–188

[157] Eltahawy HA, Saint-Cyr J, Giladi N, Lang AE, Lozano AM. Primary dystonia is more responsive than secondary dystonia to pallidal interventions: outcome after pallidotomy or pallidal deep brain stimulation. Neurosurgery. 2004; 54 (3):613–619, discussion 619–621

[158] Valldeoriola F, Regidor I, Mínguez-Castellanos A, et al. Grupo ESpañol para el EStudio de la EStimulación PALidal en la DIStonía. Efficacy and safety of pallidal stimulation in primary dystonia: results of the Spanish multicentric study. J Neurol Neurosurg Psychiatry. 2010; 81(1):65–69

[159] Vidailhet M, Vercueil L, Houeto JL, et al. French SPIDY Study Group. Bilateral, pallidal, deep-brain stimulation in primary generalised dystonia: a prospective 3 year follow-up study. Lancet Neurol. 2007; 6(3):223–229

[160] Loher TJ, Capelle HH, Kaelin-Lang A, et al. Deep brain stimulation for dystonia: outcome at long-term follow-up. J Neurol. 2008; 255(6):881–884

[161] Volkmann J, Wolters A, Kupsch A, et al. DBS study group for dystonia. Pallidal deep brain stimulation in patients with primary generalised or segmental dystonia: 5-year follow-up of a randomised trial. Lancet Neurol. 2012; 11 (12):1029–1038

[162] Meoni S, Zurowski M, Lozano AM, et al. Long-term neuropsychiatric outcomes after pallidal stimulation in primary and secondary dystonia. Neurology. 2015; 85(5):433–440

[163] Cacciola F, Farah JO, Eldridge PR, Byrne P, Varma TK. Bilateral deep brain stimulation for cervical dystonia: long-term outcome in a series of 10 patients. Neurosurgery. 2010; 67(4):957–963

[164] Hung SW, Hamani C, Lozano AM, et al. Long-term outcome of bilateral pallidal deep brain stimulation for primary cervical dystonia. Neurology. 2007; 68(6):457–459

[165] Krauss JK, Pohle T, Weber S, Ozdoba C, Burgunder JM. Bilateral stimulation of globus pallidus internus for treatment of cervical dystonia. Lancet. 1999; 354(9181):837–838

[166] Moro E, Piboolnurak P, Arenovich T, Hung SW, Poon YY, Lozano AM. Pallidal stimulation in cervical dystonia: clinical implications of acute changes in stimulation parameters. Eur J Neurol. 2009; 16(4):506–512

[167] Yamada K, Hamasaki T, Hasegawa Y, Kuratsu J. Long disease duration interferes with therapeutic effect of globus pallidus internus pallidal stimulation in primary cervical dystonia. Neuromodulation. 2013; 16(3):219–225, discussion 225

[168] Walsh RA, Sidiropoulos C, Lozano AM, et al. Bilateral pallidal stimulation in cervical dystonia: blinded evidence of benefit beyond 5 years. Brain. 2013; 136(Pt 3):761–769

[169] Ostrem JL, Marks WJ, Jr, Volz MM, Heath SL, Starr PA. Pallidal deep brain stimulation in patients with cranial-cervical dystonia (Meige syndrome). Mov Disord. 2007; 22(13):1885–1891

[170] Inoue N, Nagahiro S, Kaji R, Goto S. Long-term suppression of Meige syndrome after pallidal stimulation: a 10-year follow-up study. Mov Disord. 2010; 25(11):1756–1758

[171] Sako W, Morigaki R, Mizobuchi Y, et al. Bilateral pallidal deep brain stimulation in primary Meige syndrome. Parkinsonism Relat Disord. 2011; 17(2): 123–125

[172] Lyons MK, Birch BD, Hillman RA, Boucher OK, Evidente VG. Long-term follow-up of deep brain stimulation for Meige syndrome. Neurosurg Focus. 2010; 29(2):E5

[173] Reese R, Gruber D, Schöenecker T, et al. Long-term clinical outcome in meige syndrome treated with internal pallidum deep brain stimulation. Mov Disord. 2011; 26(4):691–698

[174] Wang X, Zhang C, Wang Y, et al. Deep brain stimulation for craniocervical dystonia (Meige syndrome): a report of four patients and a literature-based analysis of its treatment effects. Neuromodulation. 2016; 19(8):818–823

[175] Vidailhet M, Jutras MF, Grabli D, Roze E. Deep brain stimulation for dystonia. J Neurol Neurosurg Psychiatry. 2013; 84(9):1029–1042

[176] Chang EF, Schrock LE, Starr PA, Ostrem JL. Long-term benefit sustained after bilateral pallidal deep brain stimulation in patients with refractory tardive dystonia. Stereotact Funct Neurosurg. 2010; 88(5):304–310

[177] Sako W, Goto S, Shimazu H, et al. Bilateral deep brain stimulation of the globus pallidus internus in tardive dystonia. Mov Disord. 2008; 23(13): 1929–1931

[178] Trottenberg T, Volkmann J, Deuschl G, et al. Treatment of severe tardive dystonia with pallidal deep brain stimulation. Neurology. 2005; 64(2):344–346

[179] Gruber D, Trottenberg T, Kivi A, et al. Long-term effects of pallidal deep brain stimulation in tardive dystonia. Neurology. 2009; 73(1):53–58

[180] Capelle HH, Blahak C, Schrader C, et al. Chronic deep brain stimulation in patients with tardive dystonia without a history of major psychosis. Mov Disord. 2010; 25(10):1477–1481

[181] Spindler MA, Galifianakis NB, Wilkinson JR, Duda JE. Globus pallidus interna deep brain stimulation for tardive dyskinesia: case report and review of the literature. Parkinsonism Relat Disord. 2013; 19(2):141–147

[182] Marks WA, Honeycutt J, Acosta F, Jr, et al. Dystonia due to cerebral palsy responds to deep brain stimulation of the globus pallidus internus. Mov Disord. 2011; 26(9):1748–1751

[183] Vidailhet M, Yelnik J, Lagrange C, et al. French SPIDY-2 Study Group. Bilateral pallidal deep brain stimulation for the treatment of patients with dystonia-choreoathetosis cerebral palsy: a prospective pilot study. Lancet Neurol. 2009; 8(8):709–717

[184] Gimeno H, Tustin K, Selway R, Lin JP. Beyond the Burke-Fahn-Marsden Dystonia Rating Scale: deep brain stimulation in childhood secondary dystonia. Eur J Paediatr Neurol. 2012; 16(5):501–508

[185] Koy A, Hellmich M, Pauls KA, et al. Effects of deep brain stimulation in dyskinetic cerebral palsy: a meta-analysis. Mov Disord. 2013; 28(5):647–654

[186] Magariños-Ascone C, Pazo JH, Macadar O, Buño W. High-frequency stimulation of the subthalamic nucleus silences subthalamic neurons: a possible cellular mechanism in Parkinson's disease. Neuroscience. 2002; 115(4): 1109–1117

[187] Hashimoto T, Elder CM, Okun MS, Patrick SK, Vitek JL. Stimulation of the subthalamic nucleus changes the firing pattern of pallidal neurons. J Neurosci. 2003; 23(5):1916–1923

[188] Windels F, Bruet N, Poupard A, et al. Effects of high frequency stimulation of subthalamic nucleus on extracellular glutamate and GABA in substantia nigra and globus pallidus in the normal rat. Eur J Neurosci. 2000; 12(11): 4141–4146

[189] Dorval AD, Kuncel AM, Birdno MJ, Turner DA, Grill WM. Deep brain stimulation alleviates parkinsonian bradykinesia by regularizing pallidal activity. J Neurophysiol. 2010; 104(2):911–921

[190] Kühn AA, Kempf F, Brücke C, et al. High-frequency stimulation of the subthalamic nucleus suppresses oscillatory beta activity in patients with Parkinson's disease in parallel with improvement in motor performance. J Neurosci. 2008; 28(24):6165–6173

[191] Liu LD, Prescott IA, Dostrovsky JO, Hodaie M, Lozano AM, Hutchison WD. Frequency-dependent effects of electrical stimulation in the globus pallidus of dystonia patients. J Neurophysiol. 2012; 108(1):5–17

[192] Johnson MD, Miocinovic S, McIntyre CC, Vitek JL. Mechanisms and targets of deep brain stimulation in movement disorders. Neurotherapeutics. 2008; 5 (2):294–308

[193] Grill WM, Snyder AN, Miocinovic S. Deep brain stimulation creates an informational lesion of the stimulated nucleus. Neuroreport. 2004; 15(7):1137–1140

[194] Kupsch A, Tagliati M, Vidailhet M, et al. Early postoperative management of DBS in dystonia: programming, response to stimulation, adverse events, medication changes, evaluations, and troubleshooting. Mov Disord. 2011; 26 Suppl 1:S37–S53

[195] Picillo M, Lozano AM, Kou N, Munhoz RP, Fasano A. Programming deep brain stimulation for tremor and dystonia: the Toronto Western Hospital Algorithms. Brain Stimul. 2016; 9(3):438–452

[196] Isaias IU, Fadil H, Tagliati M, Marks WJ Jr. Managing dystonia patients treated with deep brain stimulation. In: Marks Jr. WJ, ed. Deep Brain Stimulation Management. Cambridge University Press; 2015:108–117

[197] Beaulieu-Boire I, Fasano A. Current or voltage? Another Shakespearean dilemma. Eur J Neurol. 2015; 22(6):887–888

[198] Bronstein JM, Tagliati M, McIntyre C, et al. The rationale driving the evolution of deep brain stimulation to constant-current devices. Neuromodulation. 2015; 18(2):85–88, discussion 88–89

[199] Pinsker MO, Volkmann J, Falk D, et al. Deep brain stimulation of the internal globus pallidus in dystonia: target localisation under general anaesthesia. Acta Neurochir (Wien). 2009; 151(7):751–758

[200] Cheung T, Noecker AM, Alterman RL, McIntyre CC, Tagliati M. Defining a therapeutic target for pallidal deep brain stimulation for dystonia. Ann Neurol. 2014; 76(1):22–30

[201] Hamani C, Moro E, Zadikoff C, Poon YY, Lozano AM. Location of active contacts in patients with primary dystonia treated with globus pallidus deep brain stimulation. Neurosurgery. 2008; 62(3) Suppl 1:217–223, discussion 223–225

[202] Vercueil L, Houeto JL, Krystkowiak P, et al. Spidy GROUP (French Pallidal stimulation Group for dystonia). Effects of pulse width variations in pallidal stimulation for primary generalized dystonia. J Neurol. 2007; 254 (11):1533–1537

[203] Bereznai B, Steude U, Seelos K, Bötzel K. Chronic high-frequency globus pallidus internus stimulation in different types of dystonia: a clinical, video, and MRI report of six patients presenting with segmental, cervical, and generalized dystonia. Mov Disord. 2002; 17(1):138–144

[204] Almeida L, Martinez-Ramirez D, Ahmed B, et al. A pilot trial of square biphasic pulse deep brain stimulation for dystonia: the BIP dystonia study. Mov Disord. 2017; 32(4):615–618

[205] Cagnan H, Pedrosa D, Little S, et al. Stimulating at the right time: phase-specific deep brain stimulation. Brain. 2017; 140(1):132–145

[206] Bologna M, Berardelli A. Cerebellum: an explanation for dystonia? Cerebellum Ataxias. 2017; 4:6

[207] Calderon DP, Fremont R, Kraenzlin F, Khodakhah K. The neural substrates of rapid-onset Dystonia-Parkinsonism. Nat Neurosci. 2011; 14(3):357–365

[208] Chen CH, Fremont R, Arteaga-Bracho EE, Khodakhah K. Short latency cerebellar modulation of the basal ganglia. Nat Neurosci. 2014; 17(12):1767–1775

[209] Shakkottai VG, Batla A, Bhatia K, et al. Current opinions and areas of consensus on the role of the cerebellum in dystonia. Cerebellum. 2017; 16(2):577–594

[210] Shaikh AG, Zee DS, Crawford JD, Jinnah HA. Cervical dystonia: a neural integrator disorder. Brain. 2016; 139(Pt 10):2590–2599

11 Deep Brain Stimulation for Obsessive Compulsive Disorder

Garrett P. Banks, Pranav Nanda, Ruchit V. Patel, Sameer A. Sheth

Abstract

Since its first application for obsessive-compulsive disorder (OCD) in 1999, deep brain stimulation (DBS) has emerged as a viable option of treatment for patients with severe and refractory forms of this disorder. The evidence base for this therapy ranges from several open-label studies to a few randomized, double-blind, sham-controlled trials. These studies have reported response rates in the range of 50 to 80%, which is particularly notable given the highly severe and refractory nature of these patients' symptoms. Multicenter trials demonstrate that this therapy can be effectively standardized and adopted for general use. Although one study yielded positive results with a subthalamic nucleus (STN) target, the ventral capsule/ventral striatum (VC/VS) region has emerged as the most common and most robustly substantiated target for DBS for OCD. The preponderance of evidence now suggests that the effective target in this region is not a gray matter nucleus, but rather white matter fiber bundles. The tracts coursing through this white matter target connect the thalamus with ventromedial and orbitofrontal cortices, underscoring the importance of these cortico-basal ganglia-thalamocortical (CBTC) regions in OCD and suggesting the value of modulating CBTC circuits to alleviate OCD symptoms. These findings support the theory that DBS operates not only by influencing a local region but also by affecting more widespread and diffuse networks. Various trials coupling this network approach with novel designs and devices are imminent, and they promise to leverage diverse teams of clinicians, neuroscientists, and engineers to uncover further insights into the application of DBS for the treatment of severe and refractory OCD.

Keywords: deep brain stimulation, obsessive-compulsive disorder, ventral capsule, ventral striatum, neuromodulation, anxiety disorder, psychiatric neurosurgery

11.1 Introduction

Obsessive-compulsive disorder (OCD) produces recurrent thoughts, images, feelings, and behaviors that persist despite attempts to eliminate them and are accompanied by marked and often overwhelming anxiety.[1] The disorder leads to significant and dramatic impairment in social and occupational functioning. OCD has a lifetime prevalence of 2 to 3%, and it is estimated that 1.2% of the population has suffered from OCD symptoms in the last year.[2] Current first-line treatment consists of a combination of behavioral therapy and pharmacological agents; however, even with access to best available medication and behavioral therapy, 10 to 20% of patients will remain severely disabled by the disorder. This statistic is worsened further by the fact that even when properly treated, many patients stop their medication due to unwanted side effects.[3] Thus despite advances in pharmacotherapy and behavioral therapy, a large number of individuals still suffer from severe and undertreated OCD. Therefore, patients with severe and refractory OCD may benefit from consideration of surgical intervention.

11.2 Development of Stereotactic Neurosurgery for OCD

The first stereotactic neurosurgical procedure in humans, a medial thalamotomy, was performed for psychiatric/behavioral reasons. Neurologist Ernst Spiegel and neurosurgeon Henry Wycis modified the Horsley–Clarke apparatus, devised four decades prior for targeting specific regions within animal brains, to create a human stereotactic system. They reported the technique and a brief description of the indications and results in one patient with "emotional reactivity" in their landmark 1947 monograph.[4] The next two decades witnessed the development of other lesion procedures for psychiatric indications, including the capsulotomy, cingulotomy, and subcaudate tractotomy.

Following on the heels of the Spiegel and Wycis report, psychiatrist/neurosurgeon Jean Talairach stereotactically targeted the anterior limb of the internal capsule (ALIC), thereby performing the first capsulotomy.[5] Talairach's capsulotomy, like Wycis's thalamotomy, was created by surgically introducing a radiofrequency electrode into the target and thermocoagulating the tissue. A few years later, neurosurgeon Lars Leksell performed the first capsulotomy using stereotactically targeted radiation, thereby creating the field of stereotactic radiosurgery.[6] The capsulotomy is thought to exert its effect by altering communication between thalamic nuclei and prefrontal cortical (PFC) regions, especially orbital and medial PFC. Specialized centers continue to perform capsulotomy procedures to this day, with response rates (≥ 35% decrease in Yale–Brown Obsessive-Compulsive Scale [YBOCS]) ranging from 40 to 70%.[7,8,9]

Cingulotomy involves the creation of a lesion in the dorsal anterior cingulate cortex and cingulum bundle. Foltz and White first described the procedure in 1962,[10] and Ballantine subsequently performed and studied it extensively.[11,12] The rationale for targeting this region was based on the work of Papez, in which he described a circuit from the hippocampus to the mammillary bodies, including the cingulate cortex that was important for processing emotion and anxiety.[13] Recent series of cingulotomy for OCD have demonstrated response rates of 30 to 50%.[14,15]

The subcaudate tractotomy consists of creating a lesion in the frontal white matter inferior to the caudate head, designed to disrupt frontothalamic connections. Knight first performed these procedures in the early 1960s using stereotactic placement of ytrrium-90 radioactive seeds to produce a focal lesion.[16] There has been little outcome data from this procedure in the era of YBOCS measurements (> 1990), and in modern practice it is rarely performed as a standalone procedure.

The combination of cingulotomy and subcaudate tractotomy is termed the limbic leucotomy, and was introduced by Kelly in the early 1970s.[17] This procedure may be performed as a single surgery[18] or as a staged procedure, where the subcaudate tractotomy is performed on patients not responsive to cingulotomy.[14,19]

Since the early days of human stereotactic neurosurgery, brain stimulation existed side by side with lesion procedures as another tool for treating psychiatric disorders, but did not gain traction for the first few decades due to limitation in device technology. In 1954, Pool described implanting an electrode and stimulating the caudate nucleus of a patient with severe depression, leading to an improvement in appetite and mood.[20] Deep brain stimulation (DBS) in its modern form was developed in the 1980s by Benabid[21] and became an extremely valuable addition to the neurosurgical armamentarium for treating movement disorders. It was first applied for psychiatric disorders in 1999, when Nuttin reported the first cases of DBS for OCD, finding that three of four implanted patients demonstrated clinical response to stimulation of the ALIC.[22] Although at that time DBS was widely considered to operate as a functional lesion, later research has indicated a more complex effect of stimulation,[23,24,25] calling this putative mechanism of action into question.

11.3 OCD Pathophysiology

The mid 1980s witnessed the development of key insights into the organization of cortical and subcortical circuitry, as well as their integration for the regulation of behavior. These theories proposed the existence of cortical-basal ganglia-thalamocortical (CBTC) circuits that pass information along loops involving cortex, striatum, pallidum, subthalamic nucleus, and thalamus.[26] These distinct but overlapping circuits regulate control over motor actions as well as emotion, mood, and decision-making behaviors. Dysfunction in these circuits can lead to alteration of these behaviors, manifesting as various neuropsychiatric disorders. The important corollary notion is that the identification of the dysfunction opens the door for targeted interventions (such as DBS) to attempt to restore functionality and treat the disorders. Perhaps best understood are the CBTC circuits regulating movement, as evidenced by the success of DBS for movement disorders. Several other circuits encompass regions of the brain governing behaviors that are perturbed due to psychiatric disease, including prefrontal regions such as orbitofrontal cortex (OFC), dorsolateral prefrontal (dlPFC), and anterior cingulate cortex (ACC).

The current prevailing theory regarding the pathophysiology of OCD is based on this CBTC theory and dysfunction within prefrontal circuits.[20] One of the implicated circuit loops involves the OFC and the ventromedial caudate and is thought to mediate how a person responds to emotionally salient stimuli. As with all CBTC circuits, it comprises an excitatory direct pathway and an inhibitory indirect pathway that exist in equilibrium in healthy individuals. However, the direct pathway is thought to be pathologically hyperactive in OCD patients, thereby generating an unchecked positive feedback loop in this first circuit.[20] This hyperactivity, which has been observed robustly and consistently in OCD patients in functional imaging studies,[27,28,29] has been proposed to manifest as exaggerated attention to

perceived threat, thereby contributing to the obsessions of OCD.[30] Compulsions may then develop as a means to handle these obsessions, and the temporary relief attained by these compulsions leads to their reinforcement and the entrenchment of the stereotypical behaviors of OCD. Indeed, optogenetic studies in mouse models have demonstrated that chronic activation of pathways between OFC and striatum generates OCD-like repetitive behaviors.[31]

Another implicated CBTC circuit involves the dlPFC and dorsolateral caudate.[22] This pathway underpins executive function and facilitates cognitive flexibility. It appears to be hypoactive in OCD patients leading to cognitive inflexibility and rendering them unable to deviate from ritualistic compulsions.[32,33] Along with the aforementioned aberrant CBTC loop, pathologic activity in these circuits generates anxiety-provoking obsessions, abnormal compulsive behaviors transiently relieving this anxiety, and a lack of flexibility needed to abandon these rigid behavioral patterns.[34]

The ACC has also been implicated in the pathophysiology of OCD. As a hub for cognitive control functions, the dACC integrates with various other involved frontal regions.[35] It has extensive reciprocal cortical connections with the dlPFC, and plays a major role in modulating cognitive flexibility and executive function.[36,37] In addition, the ACC has projections to the primary, premotor, and supplementary motor cortices, which theoretically help govern behavior execution and cessation.[27,38] Abnormal activity levels have been seen in the ACC of OCD patients in both resting-state and symptom-provocation functional imaging studies.[39,40,41,42] Moreover, the involvement of ACC in OCD pathophysiology is further supported by the efficacy of cingulotomy in alleviating OCD symptoms.[15]

11.4 Development of Targets for DBS for OCD

A variety of targets have been developed for DBS for OCD (▶ Fig. 11.1). The first and most commonly used target was chosen as a direct extension of the capsulotomy experience, targeting the ALIC.[28] Targets within the vicinity of this region have been defined with different names. ALIC refers to the entire white matter structure, as the original capsulotomy studies targeted this entire region. Another widely used targeting term is the ventral capsule/ventral striatum (VC/VS), referring to the ventral most portion of the ALIC and the underlying gray matter of the VS immediately below it. Referring to the target as the ALIC or VC/VS emphasizes the idea that the target may actually be a white matter target, such that the goal of stimulation is to influence the fibers coursing through this region. By targeting these fibers, stimulation can influence the regions they connect, i.e., PFC and subcortical regions, via the CBTC circuit. The emphasis on white matter targeting is becoming the prevailing view in this field.[43,44] Nonetheless, some of the older studies have emphasized the gray matter as the actual surgical target, referring to it as the VS or nucleus accumbens (NAc).

The therapeutic mechanism of DBS within this target region likely extends beyond the creation of a reversible lesion that partially impedes information transfer.[45,46] DBS may also affect white matter pathways by generating consistent axonal activation through supra-threshold stimulation.[23] In addition, stimulation

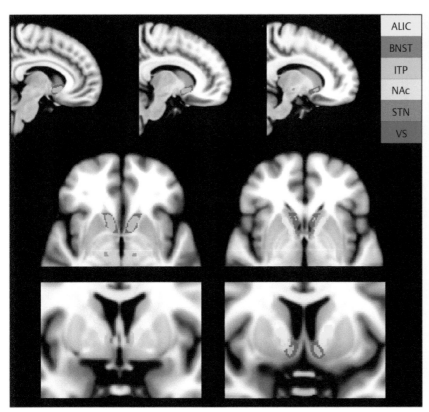

ALIC
BNST
ITP
NAc
STN
VS

Fig. 11.1 Regions historically targeted for DBS for OCD. The figure presents the portions of respective regions targeted by published studies of DBS for OCD. ALIC, anterior limb of the internal capsule (*yellow*); BNST, bed nucleus of the stria terminalis (*green*); ITP, inferior thalamic peduncle (*salmon*); NAc, nucleus accumbens (*cyan*); STN, subthalamic nucleus (*red*); VS, ventral striatum (*royal blue*).

likely affects adjacent gray matter structures such as the striatum; recently it has been posited that VC/VS stimulation effects on the bed nucleus of the stria terminalis may be crucial to the target's efficacy.[47]

The subthalamic nucleus (STN) has also been utilized as a target for DBS for OCD. The STN is an essential component of the indirect pathway of CBTC circuits.[48] It has multiple subdivisions, including a motor territory (which is a target for DBS for Parkinson's disease), an oculomotor territory, an associative territory, and a limbic territory.[49] While the mechanism is only partially understood, electrical stimulation of the limbic territory is thought to modify the STN interaction with the CBTC circuits implicated in OCD and thereby decrease symptom severity.[50]

11.5 Criteria for Candidacy

Candidacy for DBS for OCD follows essentially the same criteria as those adopted for lesion procedures decades ago. The main categories of criteria are diagnosis, chronicity, severity, and refractoriness. The primary diagnosis should be OCD. Additional common diagnoses are mood disorder, anxiety, eating disorders, and others, but these should not be the primary diagnoses. Some comorbidities are exclusions, as exemplified below. Typical chronicity criteria are ≥ 5 years since diagnosis. Some groups also adopt a minimum duration of severe symptoms. Severity is usually measured with the Yale Brown Obsessive Compulsive Scale (YBOCS), a measure of disease severity in OCD.[51] Most groups use a minimum score of approximately 28, or approximately 14 if only obsessions or only compulsions are present. Refractoriness is measured relative to pharmacological and cognitive behavioral therapy. Typical requirements are at least

three trials of ≥ 12 weeks of maximum tolerated doses of serotonin reuptake inhibitors (selective or not), including one trial with clomipramine, at least two augmentation strategies such as the use of antipsychotic or tricyclic antidepressant drugs, and at least 20 hours of expert OCD-specific exposure/response prevention (ERP) therapy (although shorter participation may be allowed if nonadherence is due to intolerance of therapy). Other typical inclusion criteria are age (18 to 75 years), ability to provide informed consent, and demonstrating appropriate expectations from surgical outcome. Exclusion criteria include comorbid psychiatric disorders with the potential to interfere with treatment, clinically significant conditions affecting brain function or structure, extremely low cognitive ability, current substance use disorder, and recent suicide attempt or active, formed suicidal ideation.

11.6 Efficacy of DBS for OCD

Nuttin reported the first patient series on the efficacy of DBS for OCD in 1999.[28] Bilateral electrodes were implanted in the ALIC of four patients with severe OCD. The study reported beneficial effects in three of the four patients, with a self-reported 90% decrease in compulsive and ritualistic behaviors in one patient. The reported results were descriptive, not incorporating measurements using the standard symptom scale, the YBOCS.[51] Nevertheless, it demonstrated the safety and potential viability of DBS for the alleviation of OCD symptoms.

Since this initial report, there have been a number of studies on DBS for OCD, ranging from uncontrolled case series to randomized, blinded trials. Here we highlight results from studies with cohorts of at least six patients (▶ Table 11.1). We

Table 11.1 DBS for OCD studies

First author	Target	N	Design	Findings	Response rate
Nuttin et al.[28]	ALIC	4	Open-label	Exploratory study showing that stimulation at VC/VS can produce symptomatic alleviation of OCD symptoms	N/A
Mallet et al.[50]	STN	17	Double-blind, randomized, active versus sham crossover	Activity stimulation versus sham was significantly different, with the average patient with sham stimulation having a YBOCS of 28 and the average stimulation patient having a YBOCS of 19	N/A
Huff et al.[54]	Right NAc	10	Double-blind, randomized, active versus sham crossover	No difference was seen between active and sham stimulation. At 12 months, the average YBOCS of the cohort dropped seven points. Only 1 of 10 demonstrated 35% or greater reduction in YBOCS	1/10 (10%)
Denys et al.[55]	NAc	16	Open-label, optimization followed by double-blind, randomized, active versus sham crossover	When comparing stimulation to sham, a reduction of 8.3 points in YBOCS was seen. At approximately 2-year follow-up, 9 of 16 patients were responders	9/16 (56%)
Goodman et al.[56]	VC/VS	6	Double-blind, randomized, staggered onset	No difference between active stim and sham stimulation for the small cohort. At 1 year, 4 of 6 patients were responders	4/6 (66%)
Greenberg et al.[57]	VC/VS	26	Open label	At long-term follow-up, 16 of 26 patients were considered responders to DBS	16/26 (62%)
Jimenez et al.[29]	ITP	6	Open label	All 6 of 6 patients were responders to stimulation at 1 year out. On average, the group YBOCS decreased to half that of baseline	6/6 (100%)
Luyten et al.[47]	ALIC/BNST	24	Open-label, optimization followed by double-blind, randomized, active versus sham crossover	Median decrease was 37% comparing stim to sham. For the 17 of 24 patients still using DBS 4 years after implant, a median 66% decrease was seen and 15 of 24 were still implanted and demonstrating response at last follow-up. The authors also claim vicinity to the BNST improved outcomes	15/24 (63%)
Tyagi et al.[58]	STN + VC/VS	6	Double-blind, randomized, active versus sham crossover	Short stimulation trials of 3 months duration showed that better results are obtained by stimulating VC/VS compared to STN, and the combination of the two produces slightly better outcomes in YBOCS scores	5/6 (83%)

Abbreviations: ALIC, anterior limb of the internal capsule; BNST, bed nucleus of the stria terminalis; DBS, deep brain stimulation; ITP, inferior thalamic peduncle; N/A, not available; NAc, nucleus accumbens; STN, subthalamic nucleus; VC/VS, ventral capsule/ventral striatum; YBOCS, Yale–Brown Obsessive-Compulsive Scale.

excluded studies whose results are included in a later publication,[52,53] in order to avoid duplication. To date, a total of eight studies have met these criteria.[28,29,47,50,54,55,56,57] One study used unilateral DBS[54] and the other seven used bilateral implantation strategies. Six of the eight studies implanted electrodes in the regions of the ALIC or VC/VS, albeit with a variety of nominal target names, including the NAc,[54,55] VC/VS,[56,57] bed nucleus of the stria terminalis (BNST),[47] and inferior thalamic peduncle (ITP).[29] One study targeted the STN,[50] and the most recent study targeted both VC/VS and STN regions in order to compare efficacy in the two locations.[58]

In 2008, a French consortium published their results studying the effects of STN stimulation in a crossover, double-blind, multicenter study of 16 patients treated with stimulation of the anterior territory of the STN.[50] After a 2-month postimplantation recovery phase, investigators tested a range of stimulation parameters across all contacts to establish the optimal parameter set for each individual. Patients were then randomized 1:1 to receive either active stimulation or sham (DBS off) for 3 months, using the individualized parameter set as a starting point. There was then a 1-month washout period (DBS off for both groups), followed by another 3-month period in which each patient crossed over to the other treatment. Thus eight patients were in the on-off group, and the other eight were in the off-on group, with each patient serving as his/her own control. Clinical response was measured at the end of each crossover phase. Of note, the YBOCS criterion for response was a decrease of 25%, a lower threshold than the typical 35% reduction criterion used in most DBS studies. The primary outcome measure of the study was the change in YBOCS score at the end of the stimulation compared to the sham period. The study did indeed meet its primary endpoint, as YBOCS scores were significantly lower (i.e., symptoms were less severe) after active stimulation than they were after sham stimulation (19 vs. 28, respectively, $p = 0.01$). As secondary assessments, the global assessment of functioning and clinical global impression were also significantly improved during active stimulation, suggesting a significant improvement in both symptom severity and quality of life. Neuropsychological, depression, and anxiety measures did not change significantly with active stimulation. Thus, this trial provides Level I evidence that active stimulation of the STN reduces OCD symptoms.[59]

Two years later, the group from Cologne, Germany reported their single-institution results using a double-blind crossover design with unilateral stimulation of the right ALIC and NAc in 10 patients.[54] Patients were implanted with a single right-sided DBS electrode with its two distal contacts in the NAc and two proximal contacts in the ventral ALIC. Patients were then randomized to 3 months of either active or sham stimulation, before crossing over to the other group for the second 3-month period. There was no intervening washout period between the two stimulation periods. This double-blind portion was then followed by an open-label extension period of 12 months post surgery.

The primary outcome measure was YBOCS score change at 12 months. At this time point, only one patient (10%) had achieved a full response (using the standard $\geq 35\%$ reduction criterion), but the overall change in YBOCS score compared to presurgical baseline was significant (32.2–25.4, $p = 0.012$). Four additional patients (40%) had achieved a partial response (25–34%

reduction). Limiting the analysis to the blinded crossover period, there was a significant difference between baseline and on-stimulation (32.2 vs. 27.9, respectively, $p = 0.033$), but no difference between off-stimulation and on-stimulation (31.1 vs. 27.9, respectively, $p = 0.205$). Thus, despite the eventual significant decrease in YBOCS score during the open-label phase, the lack of difference between active and sham stimulation periods provides insufficient evidence to support unilateral ALIC/NAc DBS.[59]

Three other studies published in 2010 described the effects of bilateral stimulation of the VC/VS region. The Amsterdam, Netherlands group implanted bilateral DBS electrodes targeting the NAc in 16 patients.[55] The trial consisted of three phases. Following implantation, patients first underwent open-label stimulation for 8 months. Approximately 2 months into this phase, OCD-focused exposure therapy was added to the DBS. After the open phase, patients underwent a 4-week double-blind, sham-controlled phase. They were randomly assigned to either active or sham stimulation for 2 weeks and then crossed over to the other arm for 2 weeks with no intervening washout period. The third "maintenance" phase consisted of open-label stimulation.

During the open-label phase, YBOCS scores across the cohort decreased by 46% ($p < 0.001$), and 9 out of 16 patients (56%) achieved response criteria (using the standard $\geq 35\%$ reduction criterion). During the blinded crossover phase, there was a difference in response pattern between the on-off group (first on stimulation, then off) compared to the off-on group. The former did not show a significant change (i.e., 25.8 on stimulation to 30.7 off stimulation, $p = 0.18$), possibly driven by concern about the potential withdrawal of stimulation during blinding (nocebo effect) leading to higher YBOCS scores during the first arm of the crossover. In contrast, the off-on group showed a significant change (i.e., 29.5 off stimulation to 17.6 on stimulation, $p = 0.009$). When pooled across the entire cohort, the active stimulation group achieved a significantly greater YBOCS score reduction than the sham group (8.3 points, 25% reduction, $p = 0.004$). YBOCS scores decreased significantly during the final open-label maintenance phase also as compared to preoperative baseline (17.5 points, 52% reduction, $p = 0.001$). Depression and anxiety measures also decreased significantly with active stimulation. In terms of targeting, the beneficial effects were primarily seen when using contacts at the border between the shell of the NAc and the white matter of the capsule, rather than within the core of the NAc. Limitations of this trial are its single center design, the short blinded phase, and the presence of a long open-label phase prior to blinding which may have provided patients a clue about their blinded assignment. This trial provides Level II evidence supporting bilateral NAc/ALIC DBS.[59]

A multi-institutional U.S. group centered at the University of Florida in Gainesville, FL reported results from a double-blind staggered-onset study of VC/VS DBS in six patients.[56] After implantation, three patients had the device turned on at 30 days, and the other three had device turned on at 60 days, in double-blind fashion. Blinding was discontinued at 120 days and followed by open-label stimulation. There was no significant difference between the early and delayed onset groups at month 2, although the study was limited by being relatively underpowered to observe such a difference and by a relatively short stagger. On the other hand, there was a significant decrease in YBOCS score over the 12-month duration of the trial (15.7 points, p = 0.0392), and 4 out of 6 (67%) patients were responders (defined as ≥ 35% decrease and YBOCS score ≤ 16) by month 12. Over the course of the study, depression symptoms were also found to improve significantly. This trial provides Level III evidence supporting bilateral VC/VS DBS.

In one more study in 2010, Greenberg et al from Brown University in Providence, RI reported their international, multi-center experience of DBS for OCD.[57] This cohort consisted of 26 patients treated across four centers in Belgium and the United States using an open-label design, targeting the VC/VS region. After 1 month of stimulation, seven patients (28%) had achieved response criterion (≥ 35% YBOCS score decrease). By 3 months, the response rate was 50%, and the average YBOCS score across the cohort had decreased from 34.0 at the preoperative baseline to 21.0 (38%). At last follow-up at an average of 31.4 months post surgery, the response rate was 61.5%. This evolving improvement over time is typical of DBS for OCD studies and likely relates to the search for optimal stimulation parameters and to the slow induction of plasticity in the targeted neurologic circuit, among other factors.

In addition to including multiple institutions, this study also spanned nearly a decade. Across all four centers, patients with more recently implanted electrodes achieved better symptomatic outcomes. Because patient selection was similar throughout, this improvement over time likely reflects refinement of surgical targeting. The anatomical target evolved over the course of study, primarily moving posteriorly. Earlier, patients were implanted several millimeters anterior to the anterior commissure (AC) in the vicinity of the area traditionally targeted during capsulotomy procedures. Later patients were implanted more posteriorly, approximately even with the AC. The stimulation target also moved slightly medially in order to stay within the ALIC. Due to this movement of the target, a reduction in stimulation voltage required was observed along with improved responses, suggesting that the more posteromedial location was closer to the optimal target. Importantly, the results from this study prompted the U.S. Food and Drug Administration (FDA) to grant limited approval to DBS for OCD in 2009 in the form of a Humanitarian Device Exemption (HDE).

In 2013, a group from Mexico City reported the results of their open-label study targeting the ITP in a cohort of six patients.[29] As described by the authors, this target was chosen in recognition of the importance of the fibers it contains connecting the thalamus and OFC. The authors targeted the ITP a few millimeters lateral to the fornix and approximately 4 mm posterior to the AC, a location only a few millimeters posterior to the final target of the Greenberg et al report.[57] Thus the ITP target may also be considered within the family of targets in the ALIC region. There was a steady decrease in YBOCS scores over the course of the 36-month follow-up period. At 12 months, median YBOCS score had decreased from presurgical baseline of 35.8 to 17.5, a statistically significant change, and all six patients had reduction of ≥ 40%. By 24 months, however, three patients had dropped out, so even though the remaining three patients still had improved scores, statistical power was too low to show a significant change. This study provides Level III evidence in favor of ITP DBS with promising results in need of confirmation with a larger cohort and controlled design.

The Belgian group that first introduced DBS for OCD subsequently conducted a larger trial in 24 patients.[47] Results were published in 2015, but the study covered implants that occurred over a 12-year period from 1998 to 2010. The group initially targeted the ALIC, approximately 15 mm anterior to the AC, but moved progressively more posteriorly over the course of the study. The last several patients were implanted using a target just posterior to the AC. The deepest contact was placed in the gray matter of the BNST, a small nucleus slightly lateral to the fornices and septal nuclei, posterior to the NAc, and approximately even in anteroposterior direction with the AC. Similar to the study by Greenberg et al,[57] this evolution was driven by clinical observations of improved outcome with the more posterior target.

Following implantation, patients were optimized in open-label fashion for a few months. They then entered a double-blind, randomized crossover phase in which they were either on or off stimulation for up to 3 months, and then were crossed over to the other arm. A total of 17 patients completed the crossover portion of the study. During the crossover phase, patients exhibited a significant improvement in YBOCS score (median 37%) during active stimulation relative to sham stimulation. Similarly, significant improvements were observed in measures of depression, anxiety, and global functioning during active stimulation. At 4 years post implantation and at last follow-up, patients' YBOCS scores improved significantly (median 45%), and 16 of the 24 patients (67%) were responders.

The authors additionally stratified the 24 patients based on anatomical target: primarily in the ALIC (n = 6), primarily in the BNST (n = 15), or comparably within both (n = 3). Using this classification, 1 out of 6 patients of the ALIC subgroup, 12 out of 15 patients of BNST subgroup, and all 3 patients of the ALIC/BNST subgroup were responders at last follow-up, suggesting that either BNST stimulation or stimulation of the ALIC near the BNST provided superior and long-term results. This study provides compelling evidence that DBS in the region of the BNST is effective for OCD. Of note, the BNST is not a classic component of CBTC circuitry. Animal studies have described its role in regulating fear and anxiety,[60] but its function in humans is not well described. This trial raises the question that whether stimulation of this nucleus per se is critical to symptomatic response, or whether it is a useful marker for surrounding white matter tracts that are actually the critical target.

Most recently, the Oxford, U.K. group completed a trial inspired by previous works in both STN and VC/VS targets.[58] Results were published in abstract form in 2017, with full manuscript publication pending at the time of this writing. The group simultaneously implanted six patients in both STN and VC/VS targets and used a double-blind crossover protocol with 12 weeks in each arm to compare their relative efficacy. Response rate was 3/6 with STN stimulation alone (mean YBOCS score reduction 42%), 5/6 with VC/VS stimulation alone (mean reduction 53%), and 5/6 with both targets stimulated (mean reduction 62%). The authors concluded that VC/VS stimulation was more effective than STN stimulation. They also found that the most effective VC/VS contacts were in the ventral white matter of the capsule and not in the gray matter of the VS. The study's sample size is small and the lack of a sham arm precludes accounting for placebo confounds, but the head-to-head target comparison is an important contribution.

A final trial requiring mention has not yet reported results at the time of this writing. The group at Brown University is conducting a double-blind, randomized, sham-controlled trial for deep brain stimulation of the VC/VS in 27 patients with up-front randomization a few weeks after implantation (NCT00640133). Patients receive either active or sham stimulation for 3 months, followed by open-label stimulation. As of this writing, enrollment is complete, but results have not yet been released.

11.7 Adverse Events

Adverse events associated with DBS for OCD can be categorized as being the result of the surgical procedure, the result of the implanted device, or the result of stimulation or stimulation cessation. The most notable procedure-related adverse events involve intracerebral hemorrhage (ICH) and superficial wound infections. Of the 98 patients in studies of DBS for OCD that report serious adverse events,[47,50,54,55,56,57] 5 had an ICH during implantation, all of which were asymptomatic other than 1 resulting in a permanent finger palsy and another resulting in transient apathy. Five patients experienced wound infections which sometimes necessitated device removal. Patients also experienced transient headaches and discomfort at their surgical sites. Device-related adverse events entailed three patients with broken leads and four patients with faulty extensions, all of which required replacement.

Several patients experienced stimulation-related adverse effects on their mood. A lowering of mood was occasionally observed during acute titration. During chronic VC/VS stimulation, 6 of 58 patients experienced increased depression or episodes of suicidal ideation, and another 3 attempted suicide. In the study of BNST stimulation, 12 out of 24 patients were reported to experience suicidal thoughts, although these were identified as unlikely to be stimulation-induced. Worsened mood or increased anxiety were generally the first symptoms experienced by patients whose device failed, either due to inadvertent shutoff or battery depletion abruptly stopping the stimulation. These symptoms typically resolved with the restoration of stimulation, leading the centers to estimate battery life in order to preemptively replace batteries prior to total depletion.

Patients also occasionally reported transient manic symptoms (e.g., disinhibition, elevated mood, hyperactivity, logorrhea, and increased libido). Of the 98 patients in studies describing adverse events, 26 temporarily met criteria for hypomania which dissipated either spontaneously or with stimulation parameter tuning. In addition, stimulation-related changes in weight and sleep patterns were endorsed by multiple patients.

Upon stimulation, patients sometimes describe subjective neuropsychological changes (e.g., memory changes, "clouding," and concentration difficulty).[47,54,55,57] However, objective evaluations using neuropsychological batteries have not yielded significant patterns of change.[56,57] For instance, the group centered at the University of Florida reported that, at 1 year post implantation, 7.1% of patients' neuropsychological comparisons to baseline demonstrated decline from baseline whereas 15.5% demonstrated improvement.[56]

11.8 Summary of Studies

The studies described above provide several important insights into DBS therapy for OCD. First, the region of the ALIC or VC/VS has by far emerged as the most common region targeted. The multicenter French study provided support for the STN target, but used a lower threshold for defining response. Subsequent laudable work using the VC/VS target has reinforced its efficacy, and recent data directly comparing the two targets suggest an advantage for the VC/VS.

Second, empirical evidence over more than a decade has exerted pressure to target the VC/VS region further posteriorly. DBS targeting initially replicated targeting for capsulotomy that, in the 1990s, aimed 10 to 15 mm anterior to the AC. The most recent DBS studies have targeted closer to the AC or even just posterior to it. At the same time, several analyses of the location of effective contacts provide support that this target is a white matter target not a gray matter target. Fibers in this region of the capsule connect the thalamus with ventromedial cortices and OFCs,[44] suggesting that modulating these CBTC regions is critical to reversing the pathophysiology of OCD. Although nomenclature varies across studies (ALIC, VC/VS, ITP, BNST), this premise appears reproducible.

Finally, building from the previous point, the available data supports the idea that DBS is effective through its influence on a network broader than just the region of stimulation. Modulation of a white matter tract allows the influence of the intervention to reach widespread regions connected by the tract's fibers. This conclusion is not surprising, given the CBTC theory of OCD dysfunction. This disorder does not localize to a single brain region, but rather to a diffuse network. Consequently, inclusion of the broader network within the sphere of influence of the therapy should prove most effective. The latency of weeks to months between initiation of stimulation and noticeable improvement observed in these studies is consistent with this network theory. It stands to reason that stimulation-induced changes in the influence of different network regions and communication between them take time to develop. The few existing studies using functional imaging to track changes induced by DBS for OCD are also consistent with this network interpretation.[61,62]

11.9 Considerations for Trial Design

Research into DBS for OCD faces challenges particularly regarding study design. DBS for movement disorders such as Parkinson's disease or essential tremor has the advantage of fairly immediate symptomatic feedback after turning on the stimulation. During a 1- to 1.5-hours initial programing session, the clinician can survey the electrode contacts and have a good idea of the most effective contacts. In the case of OCD, symptom improvement can take weeks to months to manifest fully. This temporal lag presents a challenge to the programmer. In addition, medication adjustments, life events, and natural variation in symptoms can occur in the intervening lag period, presenting further confounds that cannot be controlled easily. These factors make it difficult to attribute direct causality between a programming adjustment and symptomatic change.

Investigators designing clinical trials of DBS for OCD have had to recognize and contend with these effects. Trials that randomize patients to active versus sham stimulation must make each arm long enough in duration to allow differences to emerge, typically at least 3 months. As an example of this pitfall, too short a randomized period may have factored into the lack of difference observed in recent trials of DBS for depression.[63,64,65] Longer studies are of course more expensive thus, cost and funding constraints are a further challenge.

Another question is whether to randomize up-front[50,54,58] or follow an open-label optimization period.[47,55] There are limitations to both strategies. With up-front randomization, there is often limited ability to explore the parameter space and identify optimal stimulation parameters. Despite the long time period since DBS for OCD was first introduced in 1999 and the FDA HDE approval in 2009, experience with this therapy is still relatively limited. Finding optimal parameters in individual patients can therefore take time. Up-front randomization risks comparing nonoptimized active stimulation to sham, potentially reducing differences between the groups. This risk is further increased given the 10 to 20% improvement seen with sham stimulation, which may be attributable to placebo effect and/or insertional/microlesion effect (both confounding effects are thought to be most potent immediately after surgery). Inclusion of a delay period after surgery and/or blinded staggered onset[56] may help partially alleviate the sham-related effects.

These concerns with up-front randomization have led some to adopt an open-label optimization followed by randomization.[47,55] This strategy mitigates the concern of unexplored parameter space, but introduces other confounds. Patients can often discern whether stimulation is on or off after experiencing it for several months. Turning the device off in such a design risks unblinding the patient and, therefore, artificially increasing the chance of observing a change. Ramping stimulation on or off over 1 to 2 weeks may mitigate this concern. Another factor is the possibility of nocebo effect, in which a patient may worsen given the prospect of being turned off during the randomized period. This effect would occur at the point of randomization and therefore be particularly notable in the arm randomized to active then sham, as it would produce worsened symptoms despite continued active stimulation.[55] Staggering entry into the randomization period may help alleviate this effect. Finally, the prospect of therapy withdrawal can certainly lead to patient dropout from the trial. Thus, both strategies, up-front randomization and randomization following an optimization period, present challenges. Certain design features may mitigate the respective limitations, but each additional feature adds complexity (with associated costs and potential for mistakes) to the trial. These considerations must be evaluated carefully when designing trials of DBS for OCD.

11.10 Future Directions

A number of trials have presented high-level evidence supporting the efficacy of DBS for OCD, and the FDA has granted an HDE providing limited approval of the therapy. Nevertheless, a number of challenges stand in the way of widespread adoption of this technique. Significant practical issues include lack of awareness in the psychiatric community, reluctance to refer patients to experienced centers for evaluation, and hesitation of patients to undergo brain surgery, however minimally invasive.

Access is also challenging, as only a few centers around the world or the United States have sufficient experience to adequately evaluate patients, appropriately discuss alternatives, perform the procedure, and manage the device. Finally, once a patient has navigated these issues, insurance coverage is a challenge. With the FDA approval, local Centers for Medicare and Medicaid Services (CMS) should provide coverage for patients with Medicare and Medicaid in the United States, but the process can be difficult.[66] Whether private insurers reciprocate and provide coverage is also unpredictable.[67]

Beyond addressing practical challenges, future work will need to address important knowledge gaps. Two of the most salient points are optimizing the physiological basis of the therapy itself, and identifying patients who will most likely respond. The trials described above have made progress in identifying the circuit subcomponents that should be targeted. Consensus is building that stimulation of white matter bundles in the ventral most portion of the ALIC in the superior-inferior dimension and close to the AC in the anterior-posterior dimension produces better outcomes. For the most part, however, previous studies have limited the exploration of stimulation parameter space to a range similar to DBS for movement disorders. Exploring a wider range of frequencies and pulse widths will help understand the response properties of the circuit. Additionally, alternative metrics will likely be required as standard clinical scales such as the YBOCS are neither sensitive to subtle changes, nor designed to be administered multiple times in one day. Real-time, objective measures such as facial expressions[68] or physiological responses would provide much needed granularity.

Perhaps the most promising method of detecting physiological responses would be measurements taken from other circuit regions using intracranial recordings. This approach will be tested in a number of trials that have commenced very recently, with support from the U.S. federally funded BRAIN initiative. Two such trials will use intracranial recordings from the DBS electrode itself, along with cortical recordings from distant network sites, in combination with a next-generation DBS device that can chronically record and stimulate (NCT03184454, NCT03457675). These investigators hypothesize that intracranial physiological recordings will be more sensitive than clinical ratings. Feeding these real-time data into appropriately trained computational models, which may eventually reside onboard the device, will allow more effective adjustments of stimulation parameters in a closed-loop fashion, as has been recently demonstrated for other pathologies.[69,70,71] Another approach used in a recently launched DBS for depression trial also uses intracranial recordings, but pairs them with a DBS device capable of directionally "steering" current (NCT03437928). These investigators hope to tailor network stimulation on an individual basis using the physiological recordings, thereby choosing stimulation strategies that are optimized for each patient. Such strategies will hopefully improve efficacy of the therapy and identify patients and physiological signatures that are most amenable to treatment with DBS.

11.11 Conclusion

The first two decades of experience with DBS for OCD have made steady strides. A number of well-conducted trials, using randomized, double-blind, sham-controlled designs, have demonstrated the benefit of active stimulation. Response rates remain in the 50 to 80% range, which is a remarkable achievement considering the severity and refractoriness of the patients in these trials whose response to other therapies had been minimal. Multicenter trials have demonstrated that best practices can be generalized and adopted by several sites. The U.S. FDA has provided approval in the form of an HDE, making OCD the fourth and only psychiatric disorder approved indication for DBS. Several trials with novel designs and next-generation devices are on the horizon promising to shed light into the intricacies of the underlying brain circuits. Clinical teams of psychiatrists, psychologists, and neurosurgeons are working with engineers, computational neuroscientists, and statisticians to extract meaningful information from the tremendous volume of data that will be derived from these novel trials. Although a number of significant challenges remain, the clinical and scientific communities continue to face them with ever-increasing resolve, armed with new approaches and better tools.

References

[1] Greenberg BD, Price LH, Rauch SL, et al. Neurosurgery for intractable obsessive-compulsive disorder and depression: critical issues. Neurosurg Clin N Am. 2003; 14(2):199–212

[2] Ruscio AM, Stein DJ, Chiu WT, Kessler RC. The epidemiology of obsessive-compulsive disorder in the National Comorbidity Survey Replication. Mol Psychiatry. 2010; 15(1):53–63

[3] Eisen JL, Goodman WK, Keller MB, et al. Patterns of remission and relapse in obsessive-compulsive disorder: a 2-year prospective study. J Clin Psychiatry. 1999; 60(5):346–351, quiz 352

[4] Spiegel EA, Wycis HT, Marks M, Lee AJ. Stereotaxic apparatus for operations on the human brain. Science. 1947; 106(2754):349–350

[5] Talairach J, Hecaen H, David M. Lobotomie préfrontale limitée par électrocoagulation des fibres thalamo-frontales à leur émergence du bras antérieur de la capsule interne. Rev Neurol. 1949; 83:59

[6] Leksell L, Herner T, Liden K. Stereotactic radiosurgery of the brain: report of a case. Kungl Fysiograf Sällsk Lund Förh. 1955; 25:142

[7] Sheehan JP, Patterson G, Schlesinger D, Xu Z. γ knife surgery anterior capsulotomy for severe and refractory obsessive-compulsive disorder. J Neurosurg. 2013; 119(5):1112–1118

[8] Kondziolka D, Flickinger JC, Hudak R. Results following gamma knife radiosurgical anterior capsulotomies for obsessive compulsive disorder. Neurosurgery. 2011; 68(1):28–32, discussion 23–3

[9] Lopes AC, Greenberg BD, Canteras MM, et al. Gamma ventral capsulotomy for obsessive-compulsive disorder: a randomized clinical trial. JAMA Psychiatry. 2014; 71(9):1066–1076

[10] Foltz EL, White LE, Jr. Pain "relief" by frontal cingulumotomy. J Neurosurg. 1962; 19:89–100

[11] Ballantine HT, Jr, Bouckoms AJ, Thomas EK, Giriunas IE. Treatment of psychiatric illness by stereotactic cingulotomy. Biol Psychiatry. 1987; 22(7):807–819

[12] Ballantine HT, Jr, Cassidy WL, Flanagan NB, Marino R, Jr. Stereotaxic anterior cingulotomy for neuropsychiatric illness and intractable pain. J Neurosurg. 1967; 26(5):488–495

[13] Papez JW. A proposed mechanism of emotion. Arch Neurol Psychiatry. 1937; 38(4):725–743

[14] Sheth SA, Neal J, Tangherlini F, et al. Limbic system surgery for treatment-refractory obsessive-compulsive disorder: a prospective long-term follow-up of 64 patients. J Neurosurg. 2013; 118(3):491–497

[15] Dougherty DD, Baer L, Cosgrove GR, et al. Prospective long-term follow-up of 44 patients who received cingulotomy for treatment-refractory obsessive-compulsive disorder. Am J Psychiatry. 2002; 159(2):269–275

[16] Knight G. Stereotactic tractotomy in the surgical treatment of mental illness. J Neurol Neurosurg Psychiatry. 1965; 28:304–310

[17] Kelly D, Richardson A, Mitchell-Heggs N, Greenup J, Chen C, Hafner RJ. Stereotactic limbic leucotomy: a preliminary report on forty patients. Br J Psychiatry. 1973; 123(573):141–148

[18] Montoya A, Weiss AP, Price BH, et al. Magnetic resonance imaging-guided stereotactic limbic leukotomy for treatment of intractable psychiatric disease. Neurosurgery. 2002; 50(5):1043–1049, discussion 1049–1052

[19] Bourne SK, Sheth SA, Neal J, et al. Beneficial effect of subsequent lesion procedures after nonresponse to initial cingulotomy for severe, treatment-refractory obsessive-compulsive disorder. Neurosurgery. 2013; 72(2):196–202, discussion 202

[20] McGovern RA, Sheth SA. Role of the dorsal anterior cingulate cortex in obsessive-compulsive disorder: converging evidence from cognitive neuroscience and psychiatric neurosurgery. J Neurosurg. 2017; 126(1):132–147

[21] Benabid AL, Pollak P, Louveau A, Henry S, de Rougemont J. Combined (thalamotomy and stimulation) stereotactic surgery of the VIM thalamic nucleus for bilateral Parkinson disease. Appl Neurophysiol. 1987; 50(1–6):344–346

[22] Saxena S, Rauch SL. Functional neuroimaging and the neuroanatomy of obsessive-compulsive disorder. Psychiatr Clin North Am. 2000; 23(3):563–586

[23] Lujan JL, Chaturvedi A, McIntyre CC. Tracking the mechanisms of deep brain stimulation for neuropsychiatric disorders. Front Biosci. 2008; 13:5892–5904

[24] McIntyre CC, Savasta M, Kerkerian-Le Goff L, Vitek JL. Uncovering the mechanism(s) of action of deep brain stimulation: activation, inhibition, or both. Clin Neurophysiol. 2004; 115(6):1239–1248

[25] McIntyre CC, Savasta M, Walter BL, Vitek JL. How does deep brain stimulation work? Present understanding and future questions. J Clin Neurophysiol. 2004; 21(1):40–50

[26] Alexander GE, DeLong MR, Strick PL. Parallel organization of functionally segregated circuits linking basal ganglia and cortex. Annu Rev Neurosci. 1986; 9: 357–381

[27] Paus T, Tomaiuolo F, Otaky N, et al. Human cingulate and paracingulate sulci: pattern, variability, asymmetry, and probabilistic map. Cereb Cortex. 1996; 6 (2):207–214

[28] Nuttin B, Cosyns P, Demeulemeester H, Gybels J, Meyerson B. Electrical stimulation in anterior limbs of internal capsules in patients with obsessive-compulsive disorder. Lancet. 1999; 354(9189):1526

[29] Jiménez F, Nicolini H, Lozano AM, Piedimonte F, Salín R, Velasco F. Electrical stimulation of the inferior thalamic peduncle in the treatment of major depression and obsessive compulsive disorders. World Neurosurg. 2013; 80 (3–4):S30.e17–30.e25

[30] Pauls DL, Abramovitch A, Rauch SL, Geller DA. Obsessive-compulsive disorder: an integrative genetic and neurobiological perspective. Nat Rev Neurosci. 2014; 15(6):410–424

[31] Ahmari SE, Spellman T, Douglass NL, et al. Repeated cortico-striatal stimulation generates persistent OCD-like behavior. Science. 2013; 340(6137):1234–1239

[32] Gu BM, Park JY, Kang DH, et al. Neural correlates of cognitive inflexibility during task-switching in obsessive-compulsive disorder. Brain. 2008; 131(Pt 1): 155–164

[33] van den Heuvel OA, Veltman DJ, Groenewegen HJ, et al. Frontal-striatal dysfunction during planning in obsessive-compulsive disorder. Arch Gen Psychiatry. 2005; 62(3):301–309

[34] van den Heuvel OA, van der Werf YD, Verhoef KM, et al. Frontal-striatal abnormalities underlying behaviours in the compulsive-impulsive spectrum. J Neurol Sci. 2010; 289(1–2):55–59

[35] Seeley WW, Menon V, Schatzberg AF, et al. Dissociable intrinsic connectivity networks for salience processing and executive control. J Neurosci. 2007; 27 (9):2349–2356

[36] MacDonald AW, III, Cohen JD, Stenger VA, Carter CS. Dissociating the role of the dorsolateral prefrontal and anterior cingulate cortex in cognitive control. Science. 2000; 288(5472):1835–1838

[37] Brewer JA, Worhunsky PD, Gray JR, Tang YY, Weber J, Kober H. Meditation experience is associated with differences in default mode network activity and connectivity. Proc Natl Acad Sci USA. 2011; 108(50):20254–20259

[38] Paus T. Primate anterior cingulate cortex: where motor control, drive and cognition interface. Nat Rev Neurosci. 2001; 2(6):417–424

[39] Breiter HC, Rauch SL, Kwong KK, et al. Functional magnetic resonance imaging of symptom provocation in obsessive-compulsive disorder. Arch Gen Psychiatry. 1996; 53(7):595–606

[40] Koch K, Wagner G, Schachtzabel C, et al. Aberrant anterior cingulate activation in obsessive-compulsive disorder is related to task complexity. Neuropsychologia. 2012; 50(5):958–964

[41] Perani D, Colombo C, Bressi S, et al. [18F]FDG PET study in obsessive-compulsive disorder. A clinical/metabolic correlation study after treatment. Br J Psychiatry. 1995; 166(2):244–250

[42] Swedo SE, Schapiro MB, Grady CL, et al. Cerebral glucose metabolism in childhood-onset obsessive-compulsive disorder. Arch Gen Psychiatry. 1989; 46(6): 518–523

[43] van den Munckhof P, Bosch DA, Mantione MH, Figee M, Denys DA, Schuurman PR. Active stimulation site of nucleus accumbens deep brain stimulation in obsessive-compulsive disorder is localized in the ventral internal capsule. Acta Neurochir Suppl (Wien). 2013; 117:53–59

[44] Nanda P, Banks GP, Pathak YJ, Sheth SA. Connectivity-based parcellation of the anterior limb of the internal capsule. Hum Brain Mapp. 2017; 38(12): 6107–6117

[45] Agnesi F, Connolly AT, Baker KB, Vitek JL, Johnson MD. Deep brain stimulation imposes complex informational lesions. PLoS One. 2013; 8(8):e74462

[46] Grill WM, Snyder AN, Miocinovic S. Deep brain stimulation creates an informational lesion of the stimulated nucleus. Neuroreport. 2004; 15(7):1137–1140

[47] Luyten L, Hendrickx S, Raymaekers S, Gabriëls L, Nuttin B. Electrical stimulation in the bed nucleus of the stria terminalis alleviates severe obsessive-compulsive disorder. Mol Psychiatry. 2016; 21(9):1272–1280

[48] Parent A, Hazrati LN. Functional anatomy of the basal ganglia. II. The place of subthalamic nucleus and external pallidum in basal ganglia circuitry. Brain Res Brain Res Rev. 1995; 20(1):128–154

[49] Benarroch EE. Subthalamic nucleus and its connections: Anatomic substrate for the network effects of deep brain stimulation. Neurology. 2008; 70(21): 1991–1995

[50] Mallet L, Polosan M, Jaafari N, et al. STOC Study Group. Subthalamic nucleus stimulation in severe obsessive-compulsive disorder. N Engl J Med. 2008; 359 (20):2121–2134

[51] Goodman WK, Price LH, Rasmussen SA, et al. The Yale-Brown Obsessive Compulsive Scale. I. Development, use, and reliability. Arch Gen Psychiatry. 1989; 46(11):1006–1011

[52] Greenberg BD, Malone DA, Friehs GM, et al. Three-year outcomes in deep brain stimulation for highly resistant obsessive-compulsive disorder. Neuropsychopharmacology. 2006; 31(11):2384–2393

[53] Nuttin BJ, Gabriëls LA, Cosyns PR, et al. Long-term electrical capsular stimulation in patients with obsessive-compulsive disorder. Neurosurgery. 2003; 52 (6):1263–1272, discussion 1272–1274

[54] Huff W, Lenartz D, Schormann M, et al. Unilateral deep brain stimulation of the nucleus accumbens in patients with treatment-resistant obsessive-compulsive disorder: Outcomes after one year. Clin Neurol Neurosurg. 2010; 112 (2):137–143

[55] Denys D, Mantione M, Figee M, et al. Deep brain stimulation of the nucleus accumbens for treatment-refractory obsessive-compulsive disorder. Arch Gen Psychiatry. 2010; 67(10):1061–1068

[56] Goodman WK, Foote KD, Greenberg BD, et al. Deep brain stimulation for intractable obsessive compulsive disorder: pilot study using a blinded, staggered-onset design. Biol Psychiatry. 2010; 67(6):535–542

[57] Greenberg BD, Gabriels LA, Malone DA, Jr, et al. Deep brain stimulation of the ventral internal capsule/ventral striatum for obsessive-compulsive disorder: worldwide experience. Mol Psychiatry. 2010; 15(1):64–79

[58] Tyagi H, Zrinzo L, Akram H, et al. A randomised controlled trial of deep brain stimulation in obsessive compulsive disorder: a comparison of ventral capsule/ventral striatum and subthalamic nucleus targets. J Neurol Neurosurg Psychiatry. 2017; 88(8):A8.2–A9

[59] Hamani C, Pilitsis J, Rughani AI, et al. American Society for Stereotactic and Functional Neurosurgery, Congress of Neurological Surgeons, CNS and American Association of Neurological Surgeons. Deep brain stimulation for obsessive-compulsive disorder: systematic review and evidence-based guideline sponsored by the American Society for Stereotactic and Functional Neurosurgery and the Congress of Neurological Surgeons (CNS) and endorsed by the CNS and American Association of Neurological Surgeons. Neurosurgery. 2014; 75(4):327–333, quiz 333

[60] Walker DL, Toufexis DJ, Davis M. Role of the bed nucleus of the stria terminalis versus the amygdala in fear, stress, and anxiety. Eur J Pharmacol. 2003; 463(1–3):199–216

[61] Dougherty DD, Chou T, Corse AK, et al. Acute deep brain stimulation changes in regional cerebral blood flow in obsessive-compulsive disorder. J Neurosurg. 2016; 125(5):1087–1093

[62] Figee M, Luigjes J, Smolders R, et al. Deep brain stimulation restores frontostriatal network activity in obsessive-compulsive disorder. Nat Neurosci. 2013; 16(4):386–387

[63] Dougherty DD, Rezai AR, Carpenter LL, et al. A Randomized Sham-Controlled Trial of Deep Brain Stimulation of the Ventral Capsule/Ventral Striatum for Chronic Treatment-Resistant Depression. Biol Psychiatry. 2015; 78(4):240–248

[64] Holtzheimer PE, Husain MM, Lisanby SH, et al. Subcallosal cingulate deep brain stimulation for treatment-resistant depression: a multisite, randomised, sham-controlled trial. Lancet Psychiatry. 2017; 4(11):839–849

[65] Bari AA, et al. Charting the road forward in psychiatric neurosurgery: proceedings of the 2016 American Society for Stereotactic and Functional Neurosurgery workshop on neuromodulation for psychiatric disorders. J Neurol Neurosurg Psychiatry. 2018; 89(8):886–896

[66] Deeb W, et al. Proceedings of the Fourth Annual Deep Brain Stimulation Think Tank: A Review of Emerging Issues and Technologies. Front Integr Neurosci. 2016; 10:38

[67] Vora AK, Ward H, Foote KD, Goodman WK, Okun MS. Rebound symptoms following battery depletion in the NIH OCD DBS cohort: clinical and reimbursement issues. Brain Stimul. 2012; 5(4):599–604

[68] Girard JM, Cohn JF, Jeni LA, Sayette MA, De la Torre F. Spontaneous facial expression in unscripted social interactions can be measured automatically. Behav Res Methods. 2015; 47(4):1136–1147

[69] Herron JA, Thompson MC, Brown T, Chizeck HJ, Ojemann JG, Ko AL. Chronic electrocorticography for sensing movement intention and closed-loop deep brain stimulation with wearable sensors in an essential tremor patient. J Neurosurg. 2017; 127(3):580–587

[70] Molina R, et al. Report of a patient undergoing chronic responsive deep brain stimulation for Tourette syndrome: proof of concept. J Neurosurg. 201 8; 129: 308–314

[71] Chang EF, Englot DJ, Vadera S. Minimally invasive surgical approaches for temporal lobe epilepsy. Epilepsy Behav. 2015; 47:24–33

12 Deep Brain Stimulation in Epilepsy

Alexander Ksendzovsky, Kareem A. Zaghloul

Abstract

Deep brain stimulation (DBS) has become a promising new treatment for epilepsy. Over the years, several targets have been investigated for stimulation through animal models and clinical trials. These targets include the cerebellum, thalamus, basal ganglia, and hippocampus. However, it is still unclear which is the optimal location for each seizure type, what the optimal stimulation parameters are, or what the underlying mechanisms are. In this chapter, we review each putative target for DBS stimulation.

Keywords: deep brain stimulation, epilepsy, cerebellum, anterior nucleus thalamus, centromedian nucleus thalamus, basal ganglia, hippocampus

12.1 Introduction

Epilepsy impacts approximately 70 million patients worldwide.[1] Thirty percent of patients continue to have seizures despite medical therapy. In this group, continued seizures and polypharmacy have been associated with poor quality of life.[2] In 2001, Wiebe et al established surgery as a viable treatment option for medically refractory epilepsy.[3] Since then, many patients with uncontrolled seizures have undergone surgery with good outcomes. Unfortunately, approximately 75% of patients who have persistent seizures on anti-epileptic medications are not candidates for resective surgery.[4,5] This group includes patients with seizures that arise from eloquent cortex, patients with multiple seizure foci, or patients with generalized epilepsy. For these patients, in addition to the ongoing medical management, other treatment options include vagus nerve stimulation (VNS) and responsive neurostimulation (RNS). However, these options have limited efficacy as only 8% of patients achieve freedom from seizures with multiple medications,[3] 7% with VNS,[6] and 20% with RNS.[7] Thus, novel treatment strategies for medically refractory epilepsy are needed.

Recently, several authors have investigated deep brain stimulation (DBS) as a potential surgical option for patients with medically refractory epilepsy. DBS has gained widespread acceptance as a safe and effective treatment option for movement disorders.[8] However, it's efficacy in treating medically refractory epilepsy is yet to be determined. This is partly because, unlike in Parkinson's disease, the neural circuitry in epilepsy is not well defined. Moreover, at present, there is no current consensus on questions such as why stimulation works, which location to stimulate, which stimulation paradigms to use, or which seizure types respond to stimulation.

Because of its promise in modulating neural circuits, there have been a number of studies researching the use of DBS in several locations. In this chapter, we review the major DBS studies that describe the relevant circuitry, and preclinical and clinical trials related to epilepsy. Surgical targets include the cerebellum, thalamus, basal ganglia, and hippocampus.

12.2 Cerebellum

The cerebellum was the first target for DBS in epilepsy in humans. Originally, this target was chosen because of the general inhibitory nature of Purkinje cells that send projections to deep cerebellar nuclei.[7] It was hypothesized that inhibition of Purkinje cells through stimulation would potentiate the inhibitory effect that the deep cerebellar nuclei have on the thalamus, thereby causing a decrease in the predominantly excitatory outputs from the thalamus to the cortex[9,10] Cerebellar stimulation has been divided into two potential targets: the cerebellar cortex and the deep cerebellar nuclei.

12.2.1 Cerebellar Cortex Stimulation

Previous studies have revealed phase-locked oscillations in the cerebellar cortex, deep cerebellar nuclei, and thalamus[11,12,13] during seizures. Along with the known inhibitory function of the Purkinje cells, this has made the cerebellar cortex an attractive target for DBS experiments.[14] Cerebellar DBS was first investigated in early animal studies that began in the middle of the 20th century. In 1955, Cooke et al showed that cerebellar cortical stimulation decreased seizures in kindled cats.[15] In 1976, Hablitz et al published their results using vermian cortical stimulation in cats to treat generalized epilepsy. In these experiments, both high- and low-frequency cortical stimulation led to a reduction in the number and amplitude of general cortical discharges.[16]

However, later animal experiments proved to be inconsistent. In 1980, Ebner et al used an aluminum gel primate model to characterize the impact of cerebellar stimulation on the activity of neurons within the seizure focus. They failed to find any statistically significant changes.[17] Similarly, Hablitz and Myers et al failed to show any effect on penicillin-induced animal models.[16,18]

Similar to animal trials, human trials for cerebellar cortex stimulation also failed to show consistency. In the early 1970s, Irving Cooper and his colleagues implanted cortical cerebellar electrodes in 32 patients with varying seizure etiologies. They showed more than 50% seizure reduction in 56.2% of patients that sustained for an average of 18 months.[19,20,21] Meanwhile, one year later, another group reported on cerebellar cortical stimulation in six patients. Five out of the six patients had decreased seizure frequency after stimulation.[22] In a separate study, however, stimulating patients with generalized seizures showed significant reduction in only two of six patients.[23] Krauss et al summarized the results of the subsequent two decades worth of open-label human trials. They showed that out of the 36 patients enrolled in these various trials, 91.6% has some seizure reduction but only 12 patients achieved seizure freedom.[24]

Despite this fluctuating data in animal and open-label human trials, several double-blind trials were attempted. Velasco et al studied five patients with heterogeneous seizure semiology. Cortical cerebellar electrodes were placed and were "ON" in three and "OFF" in two patients. In this study, there was only a 33% decrease in seizure activity in patients receiving stimulation compared to those not receiving stimulation.[25] Three smaller, blinded studies also showed limited success. Of the total 14 patients receiving stimulation only two had any benefit.[26,27,28]

The past 40 years of cerebellar cortical stimulation question this technique as a means of treating epilepsy. It seems that mechanistically, the initial hypothesis that DBS stimulation of Purkinje cells would reduce the inhibitory drive on downstream deep cerebellar nuclei that would then effectively reduce seizure activity may be more complicated than anticipated. Indeed, several studies performed on sampled cerebellar tissue in epilepsy patients have demonstrated Purkinje cell degeneration. Such degeneration would suggest that the overall decrease in Purkinje cell volume may confound any effects of direct cerebellar stimulation on downstream nuclei.[24]

12.2.2 Deep Cerebellar Nuclei

Few studies have been performed examining the efficacy of deep cerebellar nucleus stimulation, and as with cortical stimulation, there are conflicting results. The deep cerebellar nuclei are directly connected to the thalamus, and are thus better positioned to modulate thalamic outflow. The deep cerebellar nuclei are divided into three functional and anatomical groups that project to distinct nuclei within the thalamus, which in turn project to distinct cortical regions (▶ Fig. 12.1). The three cerebellar nuclei are the lateral nuclei (dentate), interposed nuclei (globose and emboliform), and fastigial nuclei. The lateral nuclei project preferentially to the parafascicular (Pf) and ventral lateral thalamic (VL) nuclei. The interposed nuclei project primarily to the posterior thalamic nuclear complex (Po) along with VL. The fastigial nuclei send projections on to ventral medial thalamus (VM) and Pf. These projections are even more

complicated as each set of deep cerebellar nuclei has some, though not preferential, projections to all the major thalamic nuclei along with the connections mentioned above.[24] The thalamus in turn has broad projections to several areas of the cortex. VL projects primarily to the primary motor and sensory cortex while the Pf and Po target wide cortical areas including prefrontal cortex, primary sensory and motor cortices, cingulate gyrus, temporal lobe, frontal cortex, and the amygdala. Lastly, VM also projects widely to primary sensory and motor cortices, cingulate gyrus, temporal lobe, frontal cortex, and the amygdala. Despite these direct connections, however, the complexity of this network and redundant pathways likely account for the inconsistent results observed with deep cerebellar stimulation that is described below.

In the earliest animal study that used deep cerebellar stimulation, Dow et al demonstrated inhibition of cortical bursting activity in a focal cortical cobalt rat model of epilepsy.[29] In 1972, Hutton et al directly compared cortical and deep cerebellar stimulation in a cat penicillin focal epilepsy model. They showed seizure reduction with both cortical and deep nuclear stimulation.[30] Subsequently, Babb et al showed a decrease in seizure frequency and seizure duration in a cobalt model of hippocampal epilepsy[31] with deep nuclear stimulation. Finally, a recent study in 2004 showed equivocal results with stimulation of the superior cerebellar peduncle (SCP) in amygdala-kindled rats. The investigators found that SCP stimulation potentiated limbic seizure initiation but decreased secondary generalization.[32]

The literature on deep cerebellar stimulation in humans is scarce, describes heterogenous seizure types, and is slightly conflicting as well. In 1976, Sramka et al reported on four patients with focal, generalized motor and myoclonic seizures that underwent dentate nucleus stimulation at 10 and 100 Hz. These four patients had a moderate improvement in seizure frequency, but the improvement was noted to be only temporary.[33]

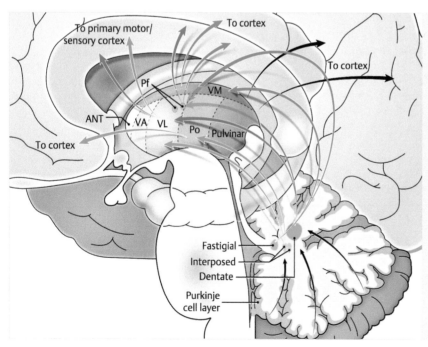

Fig. 12.1 Cerebellar projections to the thalamus and beyond. *Green:* The dentate nucleus projects to the parafascicular (Pf) and ventral lateral thalamic (VL) nuclei. VL projects to the motor and sensory cortex and Pf has wide cortical projections. *Blue:* The interposed nuclei project to the posterior thalamic nuclear complex (Po) and to VL. VL projects to the motor and sensory cortex and Po has wide cortical projections. *Orange:* The fastigial nucleus projects to the ventral medial thalamus (VM) and Pf. Vm and Pf have wide cortical projections.

12.3 The Thalamus

The thalamus has widespread cortical connections. It is the relay site for all sensory information except olfaction which has direct inputs to the cortex.[7] The thalamus also modulates information from the cerebellum, basal ganglia, and limbic systems. Every thalamic nucleus except the reticular nucleus sends reciprocal cortical projections.[26] For this reason, the thalamus has become a target for stimulation in epilepsy. Clinical trials have focused on the centromedian nucleus of the thalamus (CMT) and the anterior nucleus of the thalamus (ANT), and animal studies have focused on their mammalian equivalent, as detailed below.

12.3.1 Centromedian Nucleus

The CMT is part of the nonspecific thalamic system which consists of the intralaminar, paralaminar, and midline nuclei.[34,35,36] The CMT is the largest of these nuclei and is located at the level of the posterior commissure.[37] The nonspecific thalamic nuclei receive inputs from the reticular formation and are thought to play an important role in arousal.[37] They have diffuse projections to other thalamic nuclei, the basal ganglia, and cerebral cortex (▶ Fig. 12.2). The CMT has been implicated in epilepsy from as early as 1951[38] and its larger size makes it amenable to surgical targeting.[37]

There is no direct animal corollary to CMT. However, the murine thalamic reticular nucleus (TRN)[39] has similar projections to and from the reticular system and has been used as a surrogate for the CMT. The TRN houses mainly gamma-aminobutyric acid (GABA)ergic neurons that are thought to be a relay between the corticothalamic and thalamocortical projections.[40,41] Cortical and thalamic neurons send glutamatergic axons to the TRN while the TRN send GABAergic projections to other thalamic nuclei.[40,42,43]

Most animal and human trials have investigated the effect of CMT stimulation on multifocal, generalized focal motor and non-motor seizures. Pantoja-Jimenez et al investigated TRN stimulation in a pentylenetetrazol (PTZ) rat model of generalized epilepsy. High-frequency stimulation prolonged latency to tonic–clonic seizures and status epilepticus. Although the mechanism is not completely clear, Jiminez et al showed that modification of seizure-induced corticothalamic synchrony may play a role in the observed antiepileptic effects of TRN stimulation.[39]

In human subjects, much of the clinical evidence supporting CMT stimulation for epilepsy was pioneered by Velasco and colleagues. In 1987, Velasco et al reported on the first five patients with CMT stimulation for either generalized or multifocal refractory seizures. They showed 80% reduction in generalized tonic–clonic seizures and 60% reduction in generalized nonmotor seizures. One patient was seizure free and three patients were able to reduce medication.[44] In an attempt to replicate these results, a separate group led by Fisher et al in 1992 performed a double-blind crossover trial of electrode implantation in CMT in seven patients. Unlike their predecessors, they did not show significant treatment differences.[45] However, in an open-label follow-up study by the same group, half of the patients had 50% reduction in seizure frequency.[45]

In a larger study, Velasco et al reported on 15 patients who underwent CMT stimulation and were followed for 41.2 months. All patients had long-standing intractable seizures and were not good candidates for resective surgery. They divided the patient cohort into two groups: Lennox–Gastaut (LG) syndrome group and focal seizures with secondary generalization group. Patients in the LG group had 81.6% reduction in seizure frequency while patients in the second group had an overall reduction of 57.3% in

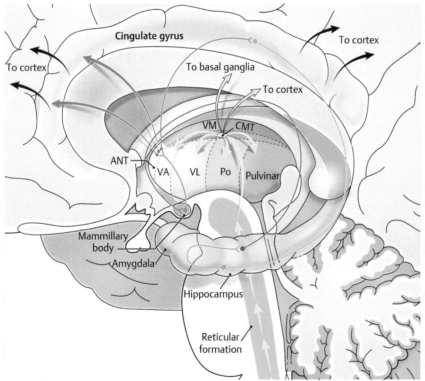

Fig. 12.2 Reticular formation and Papez circuit. *CMT modulates seizures through the reticular formation (yellow):* CMT receives inputs from the reticular formation and has diffuse projections to other thalamic nuclei, the basal ganglia and cerebral cortex *ANT modulates seizures through the Papez circuit:* The mammillary bodies project to the anterior nucleus of the thalamus via the mamillothalamic tract (*red*). The ANT projects to the cingulate gyrus through the thalamocortical fibers (*blue*) which then send projections to the parahippocampal gyrus and to the entorhinal cortex via the cingulum (*orange*) which finally projects back to the hippocampus through the perforant pathway (*pink*). The hippocampus sends projections to the mammillary bodies via the fornix (*purple*). The cingulate gyrus sends projections to various higher cortical structures.

seizure frequency.[46] In a follow-up study specifically probing CMT stimulation for LG, Velasco et al again demonstrated an 80% overall seizure reduction rate at 18 months in 13 LG patients.[47] Further analysis revealed that incorrect lead placement was associated with worsening seizure control. Patients with adequate lead placement enjoyed a seizure reduction of more than 87%, further validating CMT as a target for LG.[47]

Since these trials, there have been several attempts to replicate these results in patients with generalized epilepsy. In 2013, Valentin et al reported on 11 patients treated with CMT DBS for primary generalized and frontal lobe epilepsy refractory to medication or surgical resection. The trial was designed with 3 months of sham treatment, 3 months of stimulation, and 6 months of unblinded stimulation. Overall, all six patients with generalized seizures had more than 50% seizure reduction while blinded and five out of six patients had more than 50% reduction thereafter. In the frontal lobe epilepsy group, only one patient had more than 50% reduction during blinding and three had a therapeutic response after the blinding period was over.[48]

Taken together, these studies suggest that CMT DBS may be beneficial for patients with LG syndrome. Furthermore, investigation on stimulation of the CMT for generalized seizures involving the reticular system or thalamus may be more specifically considered for future trials.

12.3.2 Anterior Nucleus of the Thalamus

The ANT is located at a central point within the circuit of Papez.[49] Papez circuit relays information from the hippocampus and subiculum to the mammillary bodies via the fornix. The mammillary bodies project to the ANT via the mammillothalamic tract. The ANT then projects to the cingulate gyrus which further sends projections to the parahippocampal gyrus and to the entorhinal cortex which finally project back to the hippocampus through the perforant pathway (▶ Fig. 12.2).[50] The cingulate gyrus also sends projections to various higher cortical structures.[7]

Given that seizures frequently originate in the mesial temporal structures, and given the widespread connections between the cingulate and cortical regions, Papez circuit has been implicated in seizure propagation throughout the rest of the brain.[50,51] Abnormalities such as magnetic resonance signal change and sclerosis were found within the components of Papez circuit in patients[51] and in animal models of epilepsy.[52] For these reasons, the ANT has become a promising target for DBS and has been studied in generalized, focal, and temporal lobe epilepsies.

The impact of ANT DBS on generalized epilepsy was evaluated in the pilocarpine and PTZ rat models of epilepsy. This data, however, was tested with inconsistent stimulation parameters, which may account for some of the discordant results observed later in human trials. Hamani et al used the pilocarpine rat model to compare anterior thalamotomy to high-frequency ANT stimulation. Rats in the stimulation group still developed status epilepticus but its latency was significantly prolonged. Interestingly, the thalamotomy group never developed seizures.[53] In a follow-up study, in order to characterize necessary stimulation parameters, the same group showed that stimulation current, not frequency, was related to seizure latency change.[54] Furthermore, Mirski et al showed that high-frequency stimulation (100 Hz) was necessary to raise the seizure threshold in PTZ rats, while low-frequency stimulation (8 Hz) actually lowered it.[55] This lack of consistency in the literature regarding stimulation parameters for generalized epilepsy necessitated its exploration even further. Conovolan et al explored ANT stimulation parameters in chronically seizing pilocarpine rats. High-frequency (130 Hz) stimulation at 100 µA reduced seizures by 52% while higher current (500 µA) at the same frequency increased seizure activity 5.1 times compared to sham.[56] This study further suggested that stimulation current was responsible for ANT-mediated seizure control in animal models.

Similarly, human trials for generalized epilepsy were performed with varying stimulation parameters that resulted in inconsistent outcomes. In 2002, Hodaie et al showed a seizure reduction of 54% after bilateral ANT stimulation with a follow-up of 14.9 months. In these patients, periods of ON and OFF stimulation (up to 2 months) did not change the seizure frequency, raising the possibility that the overall reductions in seizure activity may be related simply to the placement of the leads. Indeed, seizure reduction was seen prior to stimulation in most patients.[57] Several years later, the same group reported long-term outcomes (average 5-year follow-up) in this patient cohort. After long-term stimulation, five patients had more than 50% seizure reduction.[58] The following year, in 2007, Lim et al showed seizure reduction in four heterogeneous patients who also had a lesional effect. Unfortunately, they could not discern whether stimulation of the lesions were responsible for seizure reduction.[59]

Few studies have explored ANT stimulation in temporal lobe epilepsy (TLE). Zhong et al used an amygdala-kindled rat model to evaluate ANT stimulation. Bilateral low-frequency stimulation reduced the incidence of seizures and seizure severity.[60] Given the uncertainties regarding stimulation frequency in previous trials, Stypulkowski et al evaluated ANT stimulation parameters in a penicillin sheep model of TLE. Only stimulation above 80 Hz reduced seizure activity and the activity returned after stimulation was turned off.[61] This suggested that high-frequency stimulation was required for seizure control. Only one study assessed ANT stimulation in patients with TLE. Osorio et al showed an impressive 75.6% seizure reduction in TLE over the course of 36 months of ANT stimulation. This seizure reduction was associated with improved quality of life.[62]

Most of the successes observed with ANT stimulation were found in patients with focal epilepsies with and without generalization. The murine kainic acid model was used to explore the efficacy of ANT stimulation in focal cortical epilepsy. In a study by Takebayashi et al in 2007, unilateral high-frequency ANT stimulation significantly reduced seizure frequency and bilateral stimulation completely eliminated seizures.[63] Unfortunately, these results were not replicated by Lado et al in chronic epileptic rats (after kainic acid-induced status epilepticus) where the results showed an increase in seizure frequency after high-frequency ANT stimulation.[64] Despite this, human trials for focal epilepsies showed promising results. The first clinical trial for DBS in ANT was performed in 1987 in patients with focal cortical seizures by Upton et al. In this study, four out of six patients showed a statistically significant reduction in seizures after DBS lead placement.[65] Furthermore, a separate group reported data in five patients with focal seizures with and without generalization. After 6 to 36 months of monitoring, four out of five patients had reduced seizure severity and reduced generalization, while only one patient had reduced seizure frequency.[66]

These promising results led to the first multicenter, randomized controlled trial for DBS in epilepsy. The Stimulation of the Anterior Nucleus of the Thalamus for Epilepsy (SANTE) trial was set in several institutions and enrolled 110 patients with medically refractory epilepsy (focal cortical seizures with generalization). Patients received bilateral ANT electrode placement and were randomized either to stimulation or no stimulation. The same stimulation parameters were used at all institutions (5 V, 90 μs pulses, and 145 pulses/second). The overall median seizure frequency at the end of the 3-month blinded period decreased by 14.5% in the control group and 40.4% in the treated group. After the blinding period ended, there was an overall seizure reduction of 56% over 2 years and 54% of patients had at least 50% decline in seizure frequency. Fourteen patients were seizure free at 6 months. Interestingly, patients with temporal lobe onset had better seizure reduction than patients with onsets in the parietal or frontal lobes. There was no significant change in mortality and the most common morbidity was surgical site infection (9.1%).[67] Recently, a 5-year follow-up on the SANTE patients was reported. At 5 years, the mean seizure reduction increased from 43% at 1 year to 68% and 16% of the patients were seizure free. A significant improvement in quality of life was also seen at 5 years, when compared to 1 year after stimulation.[68]

After the initial optimistic 2-year results, regulatory bodies in Europe and Canada approved the use of ANT DBS for epilepsy. In the United States, however, the Food and Drug Administration (FDA) was more hesitant and required more compelling efficacy data. In addition, the FDA raised concerns related to individual participants in the SANTE trial who experienced significant increases in seizure activity and the relatively high infection rate.[69] Given the long-term 5-year follow-up data, resubmission to the FDA for approval is currently being considered.[70] The SANTE trial was a step in a positive direction for the use of DBS in epilepsy. As with SANTE, future trials should remain blinded, include a large cohort of patients, and maintain the same stimulation parameters in order to get a more accurate assessment of the efficacy of DBS.

12.4 Basal Ganglia

The caudate and subthalamic nucleus (STN) have recently emerged as targets for stimulation in epilepsy. The role of the basal ganglia, and in particular these two nuclei, in epilepsy stemmed from several decades of investigations exploring caudate and STN connectivity. Overall, these studies showed connections between the basal ganglia and superior colliculus that are thought to regulate cortical activity and epileptic discharges.[71] These pathways and their modulation of cortical activity is known as the nigral control theory.[71] The first two studies investigating this mechanism examined basal ganglia projections and provided context for how the basal ganglia could modulate seizures. Gale and Iadorola showed that the GABAergic projections to the substantia nigra originate from the striatum.[72] In the context of epilepsy, these nigral projections are believed to play a role in GABA-mediated anticonvulsant activity.[72,73] Subsequent studies found that the substantia nigra pars reticulata (SNpr) plays a central role in nigral control and maintains inhibitory control of a group of neurons described as the dorsal midbrain anticonvulsive zone (DMAZ) which is adjacent to the superior colliculus. These neurons have widespread projections to the cortex and are thus thought to modulate cortical activity.[71] SNpr tonically inhibits the DMAZ via GABAergic inhibitory projections. When the SNpr is deactivated there is increased activity within DMAZ which leads to inhibition of epileptogenic cortical areas.[72,74,75,76,77,78,79,80,81] Thus, by taking advantage of this pathway, one possibility would be that modulating DMAZ inhibition through the SNpr by stimulating the caudate within the dorsal striatum would lead to seizure control (▶ Fig. 12.3).

The SNpr also receives tonic excitatory input from the STN[82,83,84] and phasic inhibitory input from the globus pallidus pars externa (GPe).[83,85] Thus theoretically, inhibition of STN and phasic activation of GPe could activate nigral control of epilepsy through the DMAZ. Since this original discovery, several lesioning and activation studies of STN, striatum, GPe, and SNpr have

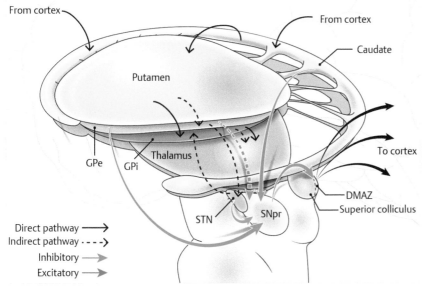

Fig. 12.3 Basal Ganglia circuitry and the nigral control theory. *Striatal pathway:* The caudate sends inhibitory projections to substantia nigra pars reticulata (SNpr). SNpr then tonically (*solid arrows*) inhibits the dorsal midbrain anticonvulsive zone (DMAZ). DMAZ has wide cortical projections. When the SNpr is deactivated there is increased activity within the DMAZ which leads to inhibition of epileptogenic cortical area. *Subthalamic nucleus (STN),* Caudate nuclues (CN) and Globus pallidus pars externa (GPe) pathway: The STN sends tonic excitatory input to SNpr. CN sends tonic inhibitory (*red solid arrow*) to the SNpr. GPe sends phasic inhibitory (*red dotted arrow*) projections to SNpr. Inhibition of STN, activation of CN and phasic activation of GPe can modulate DMAZ through SNpr. *Other connections of the basal ganglia (black thin arrow).*

directly shown that modulation of the DMAZ suppresses epileptic activity.[71]

12.4.1 Subthalamic Nucleus

The role of STN in seizure modulation was initially explored through pharmacological and ablative measures. Inhibition of STN with N-methyl-D-aspartate (NMDA) antagonists[82] and GABA agonists[86,87] has been shown to suppress seizure activity in animal epilepsy models. Furthermore, lesioning of STN led to decreased SNpr neuronal activation with downstream disinhibition of DMAZ.[88] Given the above data, the STN became a natural target for high-frequency stimulation in animal models and in small clinical trials.

In 1998, Vercueli et al showed seizure reduction in a generalized, nonconvulsive epilepsy rat model with bilateral high-frequency (130 Hz) STN stimulation.[89] The following year, the same group also showed decreased focal motor seizures in a kainic acid rat model with unilateral and bilateral STN stimulation.[89] Recently, Prabhu et al reduced seizures with high-frequency STN stimulation in two primates who underwent motor cortex penicillin injection.[90]

Over the years, the above data and the extensive safety data seen with DBS in movement disorders has made STN stimulation an attractive option for epilepsy management. Alim Benabid showed seizure control with STN stimulation in the first patient, a young girl with medically and surgically refractory focal cortical dysplasia.[91] Since then, several small-scale trials have examined the utility of STN stimulation for seizure control. In 2002, Chabardes et al stimulated the STN in five patients with heterogeneous seizure onset and showed 64% reduction in seizure frequency in four of five patients.[92] Furthermore, Handforth et al showed seizure frequency reduction in two patients with bilateral STN stimulation, also with heterogeneous disease.[93] In 2011, Wille et al implanted STN DBS electrodes in five patients with progressive myoclonic epilepsy and followed them for 12 to 42 months. They had a reduction of seizures from 30 to 100% and all had improved quality of life.[94]

Although clinically encouraging, human trials do not provide any concrete evidence that the nigral pathway is responsible for seizure control. A cortico-subthalamic pathway has been described in humans[95] and animals[96] connecting frontal motor areas,[97] somatosensory areas,[98] and the insular cortex[97] to the STN. Hence, it is possible that the retrograde activation of inhibitory neurons within these cortical areas may actually be responsible for the antiepileptic properties of STN activation.[99]

12.4.2 Caudate Nucleus

As was the case for the STN, the initial basis for caudate nucleus (CN) stimulation was the cortico-striato-thalamic network, specifically through the nigral control pathway. Unlike projections from STN, however, the caudate sends GABAergic inhibitory efferent fibers to the SNpr. Therefore, activation (as opposed to inhibition) of the CN theoretically inhibits SNpr, thereby releasing tonic inhibition of the superior colliculus DMAZ neurons (▶ Fig. 12.3).[71]

There have been few animal studies examining CN stimulation. In early 1969 Mutani et al performed CN stimulation in 10 cats with cobalt-induced focal seizures. The authors were able

to prevent seizures from occurring with CN stimulation.[100] Several years later, Wagner et al showed decreased focal epileptic activity with CN stimulation in the penicillin-hippocampus cat model.[101] Oakley and Ojemann investigated CN stimulation in a chronic, aluminum primate model of focal cortical epilepsy. They showed decreased seizure frequency with low-frequency stimulation and increased seizure frequency with high-frequency stimulation, supporting the nigral control theory for caudate stimulation.[102] These results support the idea that CN activation releases inhibitory control from SNpr to DMAZ, thus potentiating antiepileptic activity.

To a certain degree, human trials of CN stimulation support the animal trials and thus the nigral control theory as well. Starting shortly after the first animal trials, several studies confirmed a potential benefit of low-frequency CN stimulation.[103] In 1997, Chkhenkeli et al placed a variety of permanent and externalized electrodes into the CN, as well as other places, in 57 patients. Low-frequency stimulation (4–6 Hz) led to decreased activity and epileptic discharges within temporal epileptic foci. Furthermore, low-frequency stimulation stopped the spread of these seizures after they formed. High-frequency stimulation at 50 to 100 Hz had the opposite effect.[104] In a follow-up study in 2004, the same group tested stimulation of stereoelectroencephalography (SEEG) electrodes on epileptiform activity and seizure frequency in a large number of monitored patients. Again, they showed that low-frequency stimulation at the CN decreased interictal discharges and epileptic discharges in mesial and cortical structures. Epileptiform activity was enhanced with high-frequency stimulation (50–100 Hz).[105]

Despite the limited data and heterogeneous patient populations, both the STN and CN remain targets for further study. The efficacy of low-frequency CN stimulation taken together with high-frequency STN stimulation lends credence to the nigral control theory of epilepsy, suggesting that this pathway may provide several potential targets for mechanistic and therapeutic investigation.

12.5 Hippocampus

Stimulating the seizure focus to control epilepsy has recently been investigated as a possible approach for directly aborting seizure activity.[7] Most studies of direct control have been performed by directly stimulating mesial structures during temporal lobe seizures. Given its role as a seizure generator in TLE and its widespread cortical connections, the hippocampus is a promising target for direct stimulation trials. Briefly, the major hippocampal outputs travel through the fornix and entorhinal cortex. The fornix connects the hippocampal formation to the cingulate gyrus through Papez circuit, as outlined above. The cingulate gyrus then projects to the temporal cortex, frontal cortex, and the olfactory cortex. In a second path, the hippocampus connects to the entorhinal cortex through the subiculum and amygdala. From here, these structures connect to vast cortical regions. Furthermore, the hippocampus' afferents come from diffuse inputs including the entorhinal cortex, cingulate, temporal and orbital cortex, and olfactory cortex (▶ Fig. 12.2).[49,50]

Several animal studies led to the development of clinical trials and a putative mechanism of action for hippocampal stimulation. Wyckhuys et al showed that high-frequency hippocampal stimulation decreases seizures in a kindled rat model of TLE.[106] Stimulation in seven kindled rats was compared to five control rats and a decrease in after-discharges in the kindled hippocampus was observed. The mechanism behind the effect of high-frequency stimulation on hippocampal discharges was evaluated by Lian et al using hippocampal slice culture. They suppressed picrotoxin- and high-potassium-induced epileptiform activity with high-frequency stimulation *in vitro*. This model not only supported high-frequency stimulation as the preferred parameter but also suggested that increased extracellular potassium and neuronal depolarization blockade are potential mechanisms for seizure control.[107]

The first major human trial for hippocampal stimulation in epilepsy was by Velasco et al in 13 patients with temporal lobe seizures.[108] Ten patients underwent high-frequency stimulation for 2 to 3 weeks prior to anterior temporal lobectomy. After several days of stimulation these patients had decreased interictal spikes and seizure frequency. Three remaining patients were tested chronically after permanent implantation of stimulation electrodes. Stimulation stopped temporal lobe seizures for 3 to 4 months.[108] In a long-term follow-up study, Velasco et al evaluated nine patients for 18 months. These patients were initially implanted with bilateral hippocampal electrodes for monitoring, but were not found to be good candidates for surgical resection. The electrodes were then replaced with permanent stimulating leads in order to examine whether long-term stimulation could attenuate seizure activity. Four of nine patients were seizure free. Interestingly, these patients did not have hippocampal sclerosis on MRI. The four patients who did have hippocampal sclerosis on preoperative imaging had an improvement in seizure frequency by 50 to 70%.[109]

The same year, Boon et al described 11 patients with chronic high-frequency hippocampal stimulation over 33 months. One patient achieved seizure freedom, one patient had more than 90% seizure reduction, and five patients had more than 50% seizure reduction. The remaining patients had less than 50% reduction.[110] This patient group was followed for another 8.5 years. Patients who did not respond to unilateral stimulation were switched to bilateral stimulation. Upon long-term follow-up, 6 of the 11 patients had more than 90% seizure reduction (3 with seizure freedom), 3 patients had 40 to 70% seizure reduction, and the rest had less than 30% reduction.[111] Interestingly, half of these patients did not have a mesial onset, thus confounding the broader implications of these results.

A study by Boex et al in 2011 described their experience in eight patients who were implanted with unilateral electrodes placed in the hippocampus on the more epileptogenic hemisphere, as determined by invasive monitoring. Interestingly, in this study, the DBS electrode was placed along the long axis of the hippocampus, as opposed to orthogonally. Two patients achieved seizure freedom, four patients had seizure reduction by 50 to 90%, and the other two had no changes in seizure frequency. Finally, a more recent study examined nine patients with unilateral (in MRI-positive lesions) and bilateral hippocampal stimulation (in MRI-negative patients). On average, they had 66 to 100% seizure reduction after 30 months.[112]

Given the results of these small trials, two large-scale clinical trials opened for enrollment: Controlled Randomized Stimulation Versus Resection trial (CoRaStiR), and the Medical versus Electrical Therapy for Temporal Lobe Epilepsy (METTLE) study. Unfortunately, neither study has published their results. METTLE was terminated for lack of enrollment and CoRaStiR completed enrollment in 2015 but their status is currently undetermined.

A parallel body of literature has recently emerged using forniceal stimulation to treat TLE with low-frequency stimulation.[113] This idea emerged from animal studies that showed decreased seizures from low-frequency amygdala stimulation in kindled rats.[114,115,116] A theoretical benefit to this approach is that it may minimize the impact surgical resection of the hippocampus may have on memory. In 2013, Koubeissi et al stimulated the fornix in 11 patients with mesial temporal lobe epilepsy (MTLE) during intracranial monitoring. They showed a reduction in hippocampal interictal spikes as well as a reduced propensity to seize for 2 days following stimulation. Interestingly, stimulation improved memory and recall.[113] These studies were the basis of a clinical trial that opened in 2015 investigating low-frequency electrical stimulation of the fornix in intractable MTLE (MTLE-DBS).

12.6 Responsive Neurostimulation

The above DBS stimulation protocols are derived from the movement disorders literature and are thus "open-loop." Most of these protocols provide continuous stimulation to the target of interest. Continuous protocols limit battery life and, in some cases, have been shown to exacerbate seizures. This was seen in a study with ANT and SNpr stimulation.[64] For this reason, a body of literature evaluating closed-loop stimulation has emerged. In a closed-loop system, or adaptive (responsive) neurostimulation (RNS), stimulation is delivered only when a seizure is detected.[117] As such, this technique depends on constant signal recording, real-time seizure identification, and subsequent stimulation, leaving room for a significant research effort.

To date, there are few studies evaluating this initial role of RNS. Fanselow et al reported seizure reduction with trigeminal nerve stimulation in response to seizure identification in the ventral posteromedial nucleus (VPM) thalamus and somatosensory cortex of PTZ mice.[118] Saillet et al presented seizure abatement in Genetic Absence Epilepsy Rat from Strasbourg (GAER) rats using closed-loop stimulation to SNpr while recording from cortex, striatum, and thalamus.[119] The safety of RNS in humans was first tested by Kossoff et al in 2004 in four patients with either subdural or depth electrodes tested externally. The procedure was tolerated well, seizures were altered, and seizure frequency was decreased.[120] Subsequently, a separate group showed 41% seizure reduction with RNS to ANT.[121] Because of these encouraging results, a randomized multicenter trial was performed in 191 blinded patients with focal seizures, with or without generalization.[122] After 1 month, seizure frequency was decreased by 37.9% in the stimulation group as opposed to 17.3% reduction in the no-stimulation group.[122] With interim follow-up, the authors reported 44% seizure reduction at 1 year and 53% seizure reduction at 2 years. Twenty percent of the patients achieved seizure freedom by 6 months.[123,124] Long-term follow-up in this same group showed a median seizure reduction of 51% at 3 years and 72% at 7 years. Twenty-nine percent of patients had more than 6 months of seizure freedom and 16% had seizure freedom for more than 1 year. The RNS device was granted FDA approval in 2013 and further trials are currently underway.

Data from two recent trials demonstrated the efficacy of RNS for seizures arising in the temporal lobe and eloquent neocortical areas.[125,126] Geller et al reported on 111 patients with refractory nonsurgical mesial TLE followed for 6.1 years. Compared to preoperative baseline, mean seizure reduction was 70%. Twenty-nine and fifteen percent of patients had a 6-month and 1-year seizure-free period, respectively. Interestingly, there was no correlation with seizure reduction and location of electrodes relative to the hippocampus, reflecting a complex mechanism underlying RNS efficacy.[125] Jobst et al described RNS in 126 patients with nonsurgical neocortical seizures, also with 6.1 years of follow-up. They showed a seizure reduction rate of 70% in patients with frontal and parietal seizure, 58% reduction in patients with temporal neocortical seizures, and 51% reduction in patients with multifocal seizures. Twenty-six percent of patients had a 6-month seizure-free period and 14% enjoyed 1 year of seizure freedom. Patients with MR-positive lesions benefited from improved outcomes and stimulation of eloquent areas did not cause neurological deficits.[126] Both studies showed the relative safety of RNS stimulation with implant-site infection being the most common adverse event at rates similar to other neurostimulation procedures.[125,126]

12.7 Conclusion

Despite encouraging results from the surgical management of patients with mesial temporal sclerosis, a significant proportion of medically and surgically refractory patients still remain untreated. For these patients, DBS has become a promising treatment. The literature, however, is unclear about the optimal location for each seizure type, stimulation parameters, or the mechanisms underlying efficacy. Each potential target is fraught with inconsistencies and problems, allowing room for large-scale multicenter trials.

By reviewing the literature, several conclusions can be drawn from each target. The cerebellum was the first structure to be stimulated. However, mounting evidence has suggested that cerebellar cortical stimulation is ineffective, and has raised questions regarding the Purkinje cell theory. Deep cerebellar nuclei are closer to the thalamus and thus are better targets. However, the circuitry of cerebellar outflow may prove to be too complex for the deep nuclei stimulation to be clinically effective. The thalamus became an obvious target due to its widespread cortical connections. The SANTE trial was encouraging for patients with focal seizures with or without generalization. Future large-scale trials should be performed to understand the role of ANT stimulation in treating generalized and TLE. CMT stimulation was effective in LG patients and suggested that further explorations in this patient cohort would be beneficial. Given CMT's connections to the reticular activating system, this would also be a potential target for generalized epilepsy patients. The nigral control of epilepsy theory provides a compelling mechanistic approach to treating seizures. Drawing from experience in movement disorders, the basal ganglia have become a very safe target for DBS. The clinical data for STN or

CN stimulation, however, comes from few studies and heterogeneous patients. Most animal studies looking at STN or CN stimulation are in models of focal seizures. It would be prudent to continue clinical studies of basal ganglia stimulation in patients with focal cortical seizures. Finally, direct stimulation of the hippocampus and surrounding structures has emerged as a new target for TLE. This could be an encouraging target for TLE patients who are not amenable to surgical resection.

References

[1] Ngugi AK, Bottomley C, Kleinschmidt I, Sander JW, Newton CR. Estimation of the burden of active and life-time epilepsy: a meta-analytic approach. Epilepsia. 2010; 51(5):883–890

[2] Jetté N, Sander JW, Keezer MR. Surgical treatment for epilepsy: the potential gap between evidence and practice. Lancet Neurol. 2016; 15(9):982–994

[3] Wiebe S, Blume WT, Girvin JP, Eliasziw M, Effectiveness and Efficiency of Surgery for Temporal Lobe Epilepsy Study Group. A randomized, controlled trial of surgery for temporal-lobe epilepsy. N Engl J Med. 2001; 345(5):311–318

[4] Nagel SJ, Najm IM. Deep brain stimulation for epilepsy. Neuromodulation. 2009; 12(4):270–280

[5] Saillet S, Langlois M, Feddersen B, et al. Manipulating the epileptic brain using stimulation: a review of experimental and clinical studies. Epileptic Disord. 2009; 11(2):100–112

[6] Morris GL, III, Gloss D, Buchhalter J, Mack KJ, Nickels K, Harden C. Evidence-based guideline update: vagus nerve stimulation for the treatment of epilepsy: report of the Guideline Development Subcommittee of the American Academy of Neurology. Neurology. 2013; 81(16):1453–1459

[7] Fisher RS, Velasco AL. Electrical brain stimulation for epilepsy. Nat Rev Neurol. 2014; 10(5):261–270

[8] Pahwa R, Factor SA, Lyons KE, et al. Quality Standards Subcommittee of the American Academy of Neurology. Practice parameter: treatment of Parkinson disease with motor fluctuations and dyskinesia (an evidence-based review): report of the Quality Standards Subcommittee of the American Academy of Neurology. Neurology. 2006; 66(7):983–995

[9] Fountas KN, Kapsalaki E, Hadjigeorgiou G. Cerebellar stimulation in the management of medically intractable epilepsy: a systematic and critical review. Neurosurg Focus. 2010; 29(2):E8

[10] Lega BC, Halpern CH, Jaggi JL, Baltuch GH. Deep brain stimulation in the treatment of refractory epilepsy: update on current data and future directions. Neurobiol Dis. 2010; 38(3):354–360

[11] Kandel A, Buzsáki G. Cerebellar neuronal activity correlates with spike and wave EEG patterns in the rat. Epilepsy Res. 1993; 16(1):1–9

[12] Krook-Magnuson E, Szabo GG, Armstrong C, Oijala M, Soltesz I. Cerebellar directed optogenetic intervention inhibits spontaneous hippocampal seizures in a Mouse model of temporal lobe epilepsy. eNeuro. 2014; 1(1):1

[13] Kros L, Eelkman Rooda OH, Spanke JK, et al. Cerebellar output controls generalized spike-and-wave discharge occurrence. Ann Neurol. 2015; 77(6): 1027–1049

[14] Kros L, Eelkman Rooda OHJ, De Zeeuw CI, Hoebeek FE. Controlling cerebellar output to treat refractory epilepsy. Trends Neurosci. 2015; 38(12):787–799

[15] Cooke PM, Snider RS. Some cerebellar influences on electrically-induced cerebral seizures. Epilepsia. 1955; 4:19–28

[16] Hablitz JJ, McSherry JW, Kellaway P. Cortical seizures following cerebellar stimulation in primates. Electroencephalogr Clin Neurophysiol. 1975; 38(4): 423–426

[17] Ebner TJ, Bantli H, Bloedel JR. Effects of cerebellar stimulation on unitary activity within a chronic epileptic focus in a primate. Electroencephalogr Clin Neurophysiol. 1980; 49(5–6):585–599

[18] Myers RR, Burchiel KJ, Stockard JJ, Bickford RG. Effects of acute and chronic paleocerebellar stimulation on experimental models of epilepsy in the cat: studies with enflurane, pentylenetetrazol, penicillin, and chloralose. Epilepsia. 1975; 16(2):257–267

[19] Cooper IS, Amin I, Gilman S. The effect of chronic cerebellar stimulation upon epilepsy in man. Trans Am Neurol Assoc. 1973; 98:192–196

[20] Cooper IS, Amin I, Upton A, Riklan M, Watkins S, McLellan L. Safety and efficacy of chronic stimulation. Neurosurgery. 1977; 1(2):203–205

[21] Cooper IS, Upton AR, Rappaport ZH, Amin I. Correlation of clinical and physiological effects of cerebellar stimulation. Acta Neurochir Suppl (Wien). 1980; 30:339–344

[22] Gilman S DG, Tennyson VM, Kremzner LT, Defendini, R CJ. Clinical, morphological, biochemical, and physiological effects of cerebellar stimulation. In Hambrecht FT. Functional Electrical Stimulation: Applications in Neural Prosthesis 1977:191–226

[23] Levy LF, Auchterlonie WC. Chronic cerebellar stimulation in the treatment of epilepsy. Epilepsia. 1979; 20(3):235–245

[24] Krauss GL, Koubeissi MZ. Cerebellar and thalamic stimulation treatment for epilepsy. Acta Neurochir Suppl (Wien). 2007; 97(Pt 2):347–356

[25] Velasco F, Carrillo-Ruiz JD, Brito F, et al. Double-blind, randomized controlled pilot study of bilateral cerebellar stimulation for treatment of intractable motor seizures. Epilepsia. 2005; 46(7):1071–1081

[26] Krauss GL, Fisher RS. Cerebellar and thalamic stimulation for epilepsy. Adv Neurol. 1993; 63:231–245

[27] Van Buren JM, Wood JH, Oakley J, Hambrecht F. Preliminary evaluation of cerebellar stimulation by double-blind stimulation and biological criteria in the treatment of epilepsy. J Neurosurg. 1978; 48(3):407–416

[28] Wright GD, McLellan DL, Brice JG. A double-blind trial of chronic cerebellar stimulation in twelve patients with severe epilepsy. J Neurol Neurosurg Psychiatry. 1984; 47(8):769–774

[29] Dow RS, Fernandez-Guardiola A, Manni E. The influence of the cerebellum on experimental epilepsy. Electroencephalogr Clin Neurophysiol. 1962; 14:383–398

[30] Hutton JT, Frost JD, Jr, Foster J. The influence of the cerebellum in cat penicillin epilepsy. Epilepsia. 1972; 13(3):401–408

[31] Babb TL, Mitchell AG, Jr, Crandall PH. Fastigiobulbar and dentatothalamic influences on hippocampal cobalt epilepsy in the cat. Electroencephalogr Clin Neurophysiol. 1974; 36(2):141–154

[32] Rubio C, Custodio V, Juárez F, Paz C. Stimulation of the superior cerebellar peduncle during the development of amygdaloid kindling in rats. Brain Res. 2004; 1010(1–2):151–155

[33] Sramka M, Fritz G, Galanda M, Nádvornik P. Some observations in treatment stimulation of epilepsy. Acta Neurochir (Wien). 1976(23) Suppl:257–262

[34] Jasper H. Diffuse projection systems: the integrative action of the thalamic reticular system. Electroencephalogr Clin Neurophysiol. 1949; 1(4):405–419, discussion 419–420

[35] Velasco M, Velasco F, Velasco AL, et al. Electrocortical and behavioral responses produced by acute electrical stimulation of the human centromedian thalamic nucleus. Electroencephalogr Clin Neurophysiol. 1997; 102(6):461–471

[36] Velasco M, Velasco F, Velasco AL, Jiménez F, Brito F, Márquez I. Acute and chronic electrical stimulation of the centromedian thalamic nucleus: modulation of reticulo-cortical systems and predictor factors for generalized seizure control. Arch Med Res. 2000; 31(3):304–315

[37] Velasco F, Velasco AL, Velasco M, Jiménez F, Carrillo-Ruiz JD, Castro G. Deep brain stimulation for treatment of the epilepsies: the centromedian thalamic target. Acta Neurochir Suppl (Wien). 2007; 97(Pt 2):337–342

[38] Starzl TE, Taylor CW, Magoun HW. Ascending conduction in reticular activating system, with special reference to the diencephalon. J Neurophysiol. 1951; 14(6):461–477

[39] Pantoja-Jiménez CR, Magdaleno-Madrigal VM, Almazán-Alvarado S, Fernández-Mas R. Anti-epileptogenic effect of high-frequency stimulation in the thalamic reticular nucleus on PTZ-induced seizures. Brain Stimul. 2014; 7(4):587–594

[40] Pinault D. The thalamic reticular nucleus: structure, function and concept. Brain Res Brain Res Rev. 2004; 46(1):1–31

[41] Zikopoulos B, Barbas H. Prefrontal projections to the thalamic reticular nucleus form a unique circuit for attentional mechanisms. J Neurosci. 2006; 26 (28):7348–7361

[42] Huguenard JR, McCormick DA. Thalamic synchrony and dynamic regulation of global forebrain oscillations. Trends Neurosci. 2007; 30(7):350–356

[43] Jones BE. From waking to sleeping: neuronal and chemical substrates. Trends Pharmacol Sci. 2005; 26(11):578–586

[44] Velasco F, Velasco M, Ogarrio C, Fanghanel G. Electrical stimulation of the centromedian thalamic nucleus in the treatment of convulsive seizures: a preliminary report. Epilepsia. 1987; 28(4):421–430

[45] Fisher RS, Uematsu S, Krauss GL, et al. Placebo-controlled pilot study of centromedian thalamic stimulation in treatment of intractable seizures. Epilepsia. 1992; 33(5):841–851

[46] Velasco F, Velasco M, Jiménez F, et al. Predictors in the treatment of difficult-to-control seizures by electrical stimulation of the centromedian thalamic nucleus. Neurosurgery. 2000; 47(2):295–304, discussion 304–305

[47] Velasco AL, Velasco F, Jiménez F, et al. Neuromodulation of the centromedian thalamic nuclei in the treatment of generalized seizures and the

[48] Valentín A, García Navarrete E, Chelvarajah R, et al. Deep brain stimulation of the centromedian thalamic nucleus for the treatment of generalized and frontal epilepsies. Epilepsia. 2013; 54(10):1823–1833

[49] MacLEAN PD. Psychosomatic disease and the visceral brain; recent developments bearing on the Papez theory of emotion. Psychosom Med. 1949; 11(6):338–353

[50] Papez JW. A proposed mechanism of emotion. 1937. J Neuropsychiatry Clin Neurosci. 1995; 7(1):103–112

[51] Oikawa H, Sasaki M, Tamakawa Y, Kamei A. The circuit of Papez in mesial temporal sclerosis: MRI. Neuroradiology. 2001; 43(3):205–210

[52] Mirski MA, Ferrendelli JA. Selective metabolic activation of the mammillary bodies and their connections during ethosuximide-induced suppression of pentylenetetrazol seizures. Epilepsia. 1986; 27(3):194–203

[53] Hamani C, Ewerton FI, Bonilha SM, Ballester G, Mello LE, Lozano AM. Bilateral anterior thalamic nucleus lesions and high-frequency stimulation are protective against pilocarpine-induced seizures and status epilepticus. Neurosurgery. 2004; 54(1):191–195, discussion 195–197

[54] Hamani C, Hodaie M, Chiang J, et al. Deep brain stimulation of the anterior nucleus of the thalamus: effects of electrical stimulation on pilocarpine-induced seizures and status epilepticus. Epilepsy Res. 2008; 78(2–3):117–123

[55] Mirski MA, Rossell LA, Terry JB, Fisher RS. Anticonvulsant effect of anterior thalamic high frequency electrical stimulation in the rat. Epilepsy Res. 1997; 28(2):89–100

[56] Covolan L, de Almeida AC, Amorim B, et al. Effects of anterior thalamic nucleus deep brain stimulation in chronic epileptic rats. PLoS One. 2014; 9(6):e97618

[57] Hodaie M, Wennberg RA, Dostrovsky JO, Lozano AM. Chronic anterior thalamus stimulation for intractable epilepsy. Epilepsia. 2002; 43(6):603–608

[58] Andrade DM, Zumsteg D, Hamani C, et al. Long-term follow-up of patients with thalamic deep brain stimulation for epilepsy. Neurology. 2006; 66(10):1571–1573

[59] Lim SN, Lee ST, Tsai YT, et al. Electrical stimulation of the anterior nucleus of the thalamus for intractable epilepsy: a long-term follow-up study. Epilepsia. 2007; 48(2):342–347

[60] Zhong XL, Lv KR, Zhang Q, et al. Low-frequency stimulation of bilateral anterior nucleus of thalamus inhibits amygdale-kindled seizures in rats. Brain Res Bull. 2011; 86(5–6):422–427

[61] Stypulkowski PH, Giftakis JE, Billstrom TM. Development of a large animal model for investigation of deep brain stimulation for epilepsy. Stereotact Funct Neurosurg. 2011; 89(2):111–122

[62] Osorio I, Overman J, Giftakis J, Wilkinson SB. High frequency thalamic stimulation for inoperable mesial temporal epilepsy. Epilepsia. 2007; 48(8):1561–1571

[63] Takebayashi S, Hashizume K, Tanaka T, Hodozuka A. Anti-convulsant effect of electrical stimulation and lesioning of the anterior thalamic nucleus on kainic acid-induced focal limbic seizure in rats. Epilepsy Res. 2007; 74(2–3):163–170

[64] Lado FA. Chronic bilateral stimulation of the anterior thalamus of kainate-treated rats increases seizure frequency. Epilepsia. 2006; 47(1):27–32

[65] Upton AR, Amin I, Garnett S, Springman M, Nahmias C, Cooper IS. Evoked metabolic responses in the limbic-striate system produced by stimulation of anterior thalamic nucleus in man. Pacing Clin Electrophysiol. 1987; 10(1 Pt 2):217–225

[66] Kerrigan JF, Litt B, Fisher RS, et al. Electrical stimulation of the anterior nucleus of the thalamus for the treatment of intractable epilepsy. Epilepsia. 2004; 45(4):346–354

[67] Fisher R, Salanova V, Witt T, et al. SANTE Study Group. Electrical stimulation of the anterior nucleus of thalamus for treatment of refractory epilepsy. Epilepsia. 2010; 51(5):899–908

[68] Salanova V, Witt T, Worth R, et al. SANTE Study Group. Long-term efficacy and safety of thalamic stimulation for drug-resistant partial epilepsy. Neurology. 2015; 84(10):1017–1025

[69] Tekriwal A, Baltuch G. Deep brain stimulation: expanding applications. Neurol Med Chir (Tokyo). 2015; 55(12):861–877

[70] Lawrence S. Medtronic prepares to head back to FDA with deep brain stimulation for epilepsy. https://www.fiercebiotech.com/medical-devices/medtronic-prepares-to-head-back-to-fda-deep-brain-stimulation-for-epilepsy. Published Feb 20, 2015. Accessed Feb 20, 2015

[71] Loddenkemper T, Pan A, Neme S, et al. Deep brain stimulation in epilepsy. J Clin Neurophysiol. 2001; 18(6):514–532

[72] Gale K, Iadarola MJ. GABAergic denervation of rat substantia nigra: functional and pharmacological properties. Brain Res. 1980; 183(1):217–223

[73] Iadarola MJ, Gale K. Substantia nigra: site of anticonvulsant activity mediated by gamma-aminobutyric acid. Science. 1982; 218(4578):1237–1240

[74] Xu SG, Garant DS, Sperber EF, Moshé SL. Effects of substantia nigra gamma-vinyl-GABA infusions on flurothyl seizures in adult rats. Brain Res. 1991; 566(1–2):108–114

[75] Redgrave P, Simkins M, overton P, Dean P. Anticonvulsant role of nigrotectal projection in the maximal electroshock model of epilepsy–I. Mapping of dorsal midbrain with bicuculline. Neuroscience. 1992; 46(2):379–390

[76] Parent A, Hazrati LN. Functional anatomy of the basal ganglia. II. The place of subthalamic nucleus and external pallidum in basal ganglia circuitry. Brain Res Brain Res Rev. 1995; 20(1):128–154

[77] Garant DS, Iadarola MJ, Gale K. Substance P antagonists in substantia nigra are anticonvulsant. Brain Res. 1986; 382(2):372–378

[78] Garant DS, Gale K. Infusion of opiates into substantia nigra protects against maximal electroshock seizures in rats. J Pharmacol Exp Ther. 1985; 234(1): 45–48

[79] Depaulis A, Snead OC, III, Marescaux C, Vergnes M. Suppressive effects of intranigral injection of muscimol in three models of generalized non-convulsive epilepsy induced by chemical agents. Brain Res. 1989; 498(1):64–72

[80] De Sarro G, De Sarro A, Meldrum BS. Anticonvulsant action of 2-chloroadenosine injected focally into the inferior colliculus and substantia nigra. Eur J Pharmacol. 1991; 194(2–3):145–152

[81] Chevalier G, Vacher S, Deniau JM, Desban M. Disinhibition as a basic process in the expression of striatal functions. I. The striato-nigral influence on tecto-spinal/tecto-diencephalic neurons. Brain Res. 1985; 334(2):215–226

[82] Velísková J, Velsek L, Moshé SL. Subthalamic nucleus: a new anticonvulsant site in the brain. Neuroreport. 1996; 7(11):1786–1788

[83] Smith Y, Bevan MD, Shink E, Bolam JP. Microcircuitry of the direct and indirect pathways of the basal ganglia. Neuroscience. 1998; 86(2):353–387

[84] Browning RA, Wang C, Nelson DK, Jobe PC. Effect of precollicular transection on audiogenic seizures in genetically epilepsy-prone rats. Exp Neurol. 1999; 155(2):295–301

[85] Depaulis A, Vergnes M, Marescaux C. Endogenous control of epilepsy: the nigral inhibitory system. Prog Neurobiol. 1994; 42(1):33–52

[86] Deransart C, Lê BT, Marescaux C, Depaulis A. Role of the subthalamo-nigral input in the control of amygdala-kindled seizures in the rat. Brain Res. 1998; 807(1–2):78–83

[87] Dybdal D, Gale K. Postural and anticonvulsant effects of inhibition of the rat subthalamic nucleus. J Neurosci. 2000; 20(17):6728–6733

[88] Ryan LJ, Sanders DJ. Subthalamic nucleus and globus pallidus lesions alter activity in nigrothalamic neurons in rats. Brain Res Bull. 1994; 34(1):19–26

[89] Vercueil L, Benazzouz A, Deransart C, et al. High-frequency stimulation of the subthalamic nucleus suppresses absence seizures in the rat: comparison with neurotoxic lesions. Epilepsy Res. 1998; 31(1):39–46

[90] Prabhu S, Chabardès S, Sherdil A, et al. Effect of subthalamic nucleus stimulation on penicillin induced focal motor seizures in primate. Brain Stimul. 2015; 8(2):177–184

[91] Benabid AL, Minotti L, Koudsié A, de Saint Martin A, Hirsch E. Antiepileptic effect of high-frequency stimulation of the subthalamic nucleus (corpus luysi) in a case of medically intractable epilepsy caused by focal dysplasia: a 30-month follow-up: technical case report. Neurosurgery. 2002; 50(6): 1385–1391, discussion 1391–1392

[92] Chabardès S, Kahane P, Minotti L, Koudsie A, Hirsch E, Benabid AL. Deep brain stimulation in epilepsy with particular reference to the subthalamic nucleus. Epileptic Disord. 2002; 4 Suppl 3:S83–S93

[93] Handforth A, DeSalles AA, Krahl SE. Deep brain stimulation of the subthalamic nucleus as adjunct treatment for refractory epilepsy. Epilepsia. 2006; 47 (7):1239–1241

[94] Wille C, Steinhoff BJ, Altenmüller DM, et al. Chronic high-frequency deep-brain stimulation in progressive myoclonic epilepsy in adulthood–report of five cases. Epilepsia. 2011; 52(3):489–496

[95] Meyer M. A study of efferent connexions of the frontal lobe in the human brain after leucotomy. Brain. 1949; 72(3):265–296, 3 pl

[96] Magill PJ, Bolam JP, Bevan MD. Relationship of activity in the subthalamic nucleus-globus pallidus network to cortical electroencephalogram. J Neurosci. 2000; 20(2):820–833

[97] Canteras NS, Shammah-Lagnado SJ, Silva BA, Ricardo JA. Afferent connections of the subthalamic nucleus: a combined retrograde and anterograde horseradish peroxidase study in the rat. Brain Res. 1990; 513(1):43–59

[98] Carpenter MB, Carleton SC, Keller JT, Conte P. Connections of the subthalamic nucleus in the monkey. Brain Res. 1981; 224(1):1–29

[99] Baker KB, Montgomery EB. Cortical evoked potentials from STN stimulation (Abstract). Soc Neurosci Abstr. 2000; 26:1226

[100] Mutani R, Fariello R. Effect of low frequency caudate stimulation on the EEG of epileptic neocortex. Brain Res. 1969; 14(3):749–753

[101] La Grutta V, Sabatino M, Gravante G, Morici G, Ferraro G, La Grutta G. A study of caudate inhibition on an epileptic focus in the cat hippocampus. Arch Int Physiol Biochim. 1988; 96(2):113–120

[102] Oakley JC, Ojemann GA. Effects of chronic stimulation of the caudate nucleus on a preexisting alumina seizure focus. Exp Neurol. 1982; 75(2):360–367

[103] Chkhenkeli SA. The inhibitory influence of the nucleus caudatus electrostimulation on the human amygdala and hippocampal activity at temporal lobe epilepsy. Bull Georgian Acad Sci. 1978; 4/6:406–411

[104] Chkhenkeli SA, Chkhenkeli IS. Effects of therapeutic stimulation of nucleus caudatus on epileptic electrical activity of brain in patients with intractable epilepsy. Stereotact Funct Neurosurg. 1997; 69(1–4 Pt 2):221–224

[105] Chkhenkeli SA, Sramka M, Lortkipanidze GS, et al. Electrophysiological effects and clinical results of direct brain stimulation for intractable epilepsy. Clin Neurol Neurosurg. 2004; 106(4):318–329

[106] Wyckhuys T, De Smedt T, Claeys P, et al. High frequency deep brain stimulation in the hippocampus modifies seizure characteristics in kindled rats. Epilepsia. 2007; 48(8):1543–1550

[107] Lian J, Bikson M, Sciortino C, Stacey WC, Durand DM. Local suppression of epileptiform activity by electrical stimulation in rat hippocampus in vitro. J Physiol. 2003; 547(Pt 2):427–434

[108] Velasco AL, Velasco M, Velasco F, et al. Subacute and chronic electrical stimulation of the hippocampus on intractable temporal lobe seizures: preliminary report. Arch Med Res. 2000; 31(3):316–328

[109] Velasco AL, Velasco F, Velasco M, Trejo D, Castro G, Carrillo-Ruiz JD. Electrical stimulation of the hippocampal epileptic foci for seizure control: a double-blind, long-term follow-up study. Epilepsia. 2007; 48(10):1895–1903

[110] Boon P, Vonck K, De Herdt V, et al. Deep brain stimulation in patients with refractory temporal lobe epilepsy. Epilepsia. 2007; 48(8):1551–1560

[111] Hauptmann C, Roulet JC, Niederhauser JJ, et al. External trial deep brain stimulation device for the application of desynchronizing stimulation techniques. J Neural Eng. 2009; 6(6):066003

[112] Boëx C, Seeck M, Vulliémoz S, et al. Chronic deep brain stimulation in mesial temporal lobe epilepsy. Seizure. 2011; 20(6):485–490

[113] Koubeissi MZ, Kahriman E, Syed TU, Miller J, Durand DM. Low-frequency electrical stimulation of a fiber tract in temporal lobe epilepsy. Ann Neurol. 2013; 74(2):223–231

[114] Weiss SR, Eidsath A, Li XL, Heynen T, Post RM. Quenching revisited: low level direct current inhibits amygdala-kindled seizures. Exp Neurol. 1998; 154 (1):185–192

[115] Weiss SR, Li XL, Rosen JB, Li H, Heynen T, Post RM. Quenching: inhibition of development and expression of amygdala kindled seizures with low frequency stimulation. Neuroreport. 1995; 6(16):2171–2176

[116] Zhong K, Wu DC, Jin MM, et al. Wide therapeutic time-window of low-frequency stimulation at the subiculum for temporal lobe epilepsy treatment in rats. Neurobiol Dis. 2012; 48(1):20–26

[117] Kahane P, Depaulis A. Deep brain stimulation in epilepsy: what is next? Curr Opin Neurol. 2010; 23(2):177–182

[118] Fanselow EE, Reid AP, Nicolelis MA. Reduction of pentylenetetrazole-induced seizure activity in awake rats by seizure-triggered trigeminal nerve stimulation. J Neurosci. 2000; 20(21):8160–8168

[119] Saillet SCG, Gharbi S, et al. Closed-loop control of seizures in a rat model of absence epilepsy using the BioMEA 14 system. Proceedings of Neural Engineering 4th International IEEE/EMBS Conference 2009;29 April to 2 May 2009; Antalya, Turkey. pp. 693–696

[120] Kossoff EH, Ritzl EK, Politsky JM, et al. Effect of an external responsive neurostimulator on seizures and electrographic discharges during subdural electrode monitoring. Epilepsia. 2004; 45(12):1560–1567

[121] Osorio I, Frei MG, Sunderam S, et al. Automated seizure abatement in humans using electrical stimulation. Ann Neurol. 2005; 57(2):258–268

[122] Morrell MJ, RNS System in Epilepsy Study Group. Responsive cortical stimulation for the treatment of medically intractable partial epilepsy. Neurology. 2011; 77(13):1295–1304

[123] Morrell M, Nair D. Long-term safety and efficacy of responsive brain stimulation in adults with medically intractable partial onset seizures. Neurology. 2017

[124] Bergey GK, Morrell MJ, Mizrahi EM, et al. Long-term treatment with responsive brain stimulation in adults with refractory partial seizures. Neurology. 2015; 84(8):810–817

[125] Geller EB, Skarpaas TL, Gross RE, et al. Brain-responsive neurostimulation in patients with medically intractable mesial temporal lobe epilepsy. Epilepsia. 2017; 58(6):994–1004

[126] Jobst BC, Kapur R, Barkley GL, et al. Brain-responsive neurostimulation in patients with medically intractable seizures arising from eloquent and other neocortical areas. Epilepsia. 2017; 58(6):1005–1014

13 Deep Brain Stimulation in Major Depression

Ian H. Kratter, R. Mark Richardson, Jordan F. Karp

Abstract

Deep brain stimulation (DBS) has emerged as a potential treatment for severe and treatment-refractory major depression. Significant advancements have been made over the past decades in the scientific understanding of the neural circuitry that regulates mood. DBS may provide an opportunity to therapeutically perturb specific pathways to produce an antidepressant effect. Since the initial trial reported in 2005, ongoing trials have sought to assess the efficacy and safety of the stimulation of one of several distinct brain targets. In this chapter, we review the history of DBS for depression, the rationale for the most studied targets, and the results to date that suggest that DBS might be an effective treatment for at least a subset of patients. We discuss current limitations and suggest future directions based on conceptual and technological progress in our understanding of depression and its treatment. Finally, we consider the safety and ethical implications of this investigative and invasive treatment.

Keywords: depression, antidepressant, DBS, bipolar, neuromodulation, circuit, response, remission, tractography, treatment-resistant

13.1 Introduction

Major depressive disorder, herein referred to simply as depression, is a clinical syndrome defined in the most recent edition of the Diagnostic and Statistical Manual of Mental Disorders as clinically significant distress or dysfunction lasting at least 2 weeks due to depressed mood or anhedonia combined with additional symptoms that may include feelings of worthlessness, impaired concentration, recurrent thoughts of death or suicide, or changes in baseline appetite, sleep, and motoric activity.[1] Depression represents a considerable public health concern: the World Health Organization's landmark 2010 Global Burden of Disease Study[2] as well as its 2013 update[3] both reported depression to be the second leading cause of years lived with disability in the world. This is at least partially due to the epidemiology of depression, which is notable for a high lifetime prevalence (related to it chronicity), high recurrence rates, and a substantial lack of access to effective treatments worldwide.[4]

Standard first- and second-line treatments for depression include psychotherapy and/or a variety of antidepressant medications. While these treatments are effective for many, the therapeutic effect from pharmacotherapy is delayed and often requires the trial of multiple medications before achieving satisfactory response. Indeed, the National Institute of Mental Health (NIMH)-funded Sequenced Treatment Alternatives to Relieve Depression (STAR*D) study found that remission did not occur in 63% of patients treated with a first-line antidepressant,[5] and only about half who received an adequate trial of two antidepressants remitted.[6] While the terminology is not standardized,[7,8] treatment-resistant depression (TRD) is generally defined as a lack of clinically meaningful response with two antidepressant treatment trials of adequate dose and duration.[6,9] TRD has been reported to range from 10 to 40% of all depressed patients, translating into a prevalence of 1 to 3% in the United States.[10,11,12] TRD is consistently associated with worse clinical outcomes[13] and exorbitant costs to society.[14]

This relatively high rate of TRD represents a major unmet clinical need and has motivated the ongoing use and trial of various interventional therapeutic approaches[15] including electroconvulsive therapy (ECT), transcranial magnetic stimulation, transcranial direct current stimulation, magnetic seizure therapy, vagus nerve stimulation, and epidural cortical stimulation. Of these, ECT has been the most extensively studied approach that continues to offer a relatively fast therapeutic response and remains the most effective antidepressant treatment available.[16] Limits to its use include adverse effects, particularly cognitive,[17,18] relapse of depression after ECT is stopped (even when medications are restarted),[19] and ongoing societal stigma.

Treatment for severe depression also has included ablative neurosurgical procedures.[20] Deep brain stimulation (DBS) emerged as a modern reversible descendant of these ablative interventions, and given the urgent need for more effective antidepressant therapies, DBS is actively being explored as an experimental treatment for TRD. In this chapter, we review the history leading to DBS as a potential treatment for depression, the brain regions that have been targeted based on an emerging understanding of depression as a disorder of neural circuitry, and the results of the associated clinical trials. We then discuss current limitations and elaborate on some of the issues and advances that are likely to play a crucial role in improving therapeutic outcomes of DBS for TRD. We conclude with a consideration of the ethical issues and risks inherent to this invasive and currently investigational intervention.

13.2 The Current State of DBS for Major Depression

In the 19th century, physicians began to describe closely the correlations between distinct brain lesions and behavioral changes, leading to the hypothesis that pathological mental states might be treated with the removal of a particular locus.[20] The first therapeutic surgery for patients suffering from schizophrenia was described by Buckhardt in 1888.[21] As a biological understanding of brain function grew, the putative importance of brain circuitry rather than distinct loci became increasingly hypothesized to be responsible for behavior, and neurosurgical treatments consequently began to shift toward disruption of white matter tracts.[22] In 1936, Moniz described the first clinical trial of the now-infamous prefrontal leucotomy for psychiatric illness, including depression.[23] The popularity of this procedure soared over the next two decades, only to recede with the discovery of chlorpromazine and other psychotropic medications in tandem with growing ethical concerns over psychiatric neurosurgery.[24] Still, the development of more advanced stereotactic techniques for neurosurgery led to the trial of focal ablations for intractable conditions, as exemplified by the anterior cingulotomy for both depression and obsessive-compulsive disorder (OCD).[25,26]

Concurrent with this refinement in neurosurgical procedures was the advent of techniques for repetitive intracranial stimulation, which ultimately developed into modern DBS. Although the efficacy and safety of DBS were established by its systematic use in movement disorders,[20] the concept has been applied to psychiatric problems since its inception.[27] Nevertheless, the 1991 report that chronic stimulation could function as a "reversible lesion" and safely mimic the effect of thalamotomy in the treatment of tremor[28] marked the major turning point in the widespread emergence of DBS. Eight years later Nuttin and colleagues reported chronic stimulation of the anterior limb of the internal capsule (ALIC) led to symptomatic improvement in three out of four patients with intractable OCD,[29] setting the stage for the application of DBS to TRD.

We now will review the major results of this application by target. Please see ▶ Table 13.1 for a listing of all DBS trials described in this chapter and additional case reports of one or two subjects that are not discussed in the main text.

13.2.1 Initial DBS Application to Depression: Targeting the Subcallosal Cingulate

The first modern studies of DBS for depression

Utilizing results obtained from the rapidly advancing field of neuroimaging, especially positron emission tomography (PET), Mayberg in 1997 proposed a hypothesis linking depression to cortical, subcortical, and limbic dysregulation.[30] Her hypothesis synthesized imaging results from patients with depression after a traumatic brain injury, induction of transient sadness in healthy subjects, and changes in brain metabolism following successful pharmacological antidepressant treatment. Specifically, the subcallosal cingulate (SCC) (also known as the subgenual cingulate or Brodmann area 25) is metabolically hyperactive in depression, and decreased metabolism in the same region correlates with clinical response to a variety of antidepressant treatments. Based on this hypothesis, Mayberg and colleagues first initiated a trial of high-frequency DBS of the SCC white matter in six subjects with severe TRD, using the standard approach for DBS used in movement disorders.[31] In this initial cohort described in 2005, acute postimplantation antidepressant effects were reported by all subjects in conjunction with stimulation. Examples included decreased feelings of emptiness, heightened sense of awareness, and brightening of the room with sharpened visual details.[31] After 6 months of chronic stimulation, four of the subjects met criteria for treatment response, with three demonstrating full or near full remission.

Subsequent open-label and small controlled studies

Given the success in this small open-label trial and the absence of major adverse effects linked to acute or chronic DBS, the study was expanded to a total of 20 subjects in 2008. Clinical benefits were observed in the first few months and were progressive until reaching a stable plateau after 6 months. After 1 year of stimulation, 55% of subjects were responders and 35% achieved full remission or near full remission.[32] PET scans of eight responders demonstrated widespread changes in limbic and cortical metabolism providing plausible biological correlates to the treatment response. Specific metabolic changes included decreased activity in orbital cortex, medial frontal cortex, and insula as well as increased activity in lateral prefrontal and parietal cortex, anterior midcingulate, and posterior cingulate areas.[32] Longer-term follow-up of the same subjects in 2011 revealed average response and remission rates of 55% and 35%, respectively at the final follow-up visit 3 to 6 years after the procedure.[33] Serious adverse events included two suicides that occurred after some degree of response had been achieved, although analysis suggested both cases were secondary to an acute relapse of a depressive episode and not an adverse effect of any stimulation parameter change or chronic DBS itself.

To expand beyond the open-label design, in 2012 the next trial of DBS of the SCC white matter included an initial 4-week, single-blind, sham stimulation phase. This was followed by 24 weeks of open-label active stimulation and then a single-blind discontinuation phase before resuming active treatment for 2 years. Notably, this study also included subjects with bipolar II disorder.[34] The first three subjects who underwent the discontinuation phase experienced complete relapse within 2 weeks with significant distress and suicidal ideation. Out of concern for subject safety, this phase was removed for remainder of the subjects. Results were notable for a significant but mild antidepressant effect of initial sham treatment, followed by a progressively more robust effect of chronic DBS over the course of multiple months. After 2 years, the clinical remission rate was 58% without distinction between subjects with unipolar or bipolar depression, and no episodes of hypomania or mania emerged.[34]

With this continued success, investigators sought, in 2012, to replicate these results across three different medical centers in Canada with a prospective, open-label trial of 21 subjects for 12 months.[35] Improvement was again progressive over the first few months, with clinical gains observed at 3 months generally maintained at 1 year. However, outcomes were less impressive with a response rate of 29%, though if the definition of treatment response had been liberalized from a 50% reduction in symptom burden to a 40% improvement, then the response rate would have increased to 62%. While all prior studies had delivered stimulation using voltage-controlled pulse generators, this study utilized a constant-current mode of delivery based on the theory that such stimulation would be independent of the variable impedance of the electrode–tissue interface. As such, less adjustment of stimulation parameters might be required, though it was unclear if that was indeed the case.

The promise of DBS targeting the SCC for TRD as reported by the initial studies described above led additional investigators to pursue their own trials. In 2012, a group in Spain first reported clinically meaningful improvement after 3 to 6 months of stimulation with a 12-month remission rate of 50% in an open-label study of eight subjects.[36] This group reported that using bipolar stimulation (two contacts on the electrode are activated—one as the cathode and one as the anode)

Table 13.1 Summary of all Published Reports of DBS for Depression on MEDLINE (as of 11/29/2017)

Author	Target	Laterality	Patients	Stimulation mode	Mean (or range of) stimulation parameters			Follow-up (months)	Response/remission at final time point	Comments
					Amplitude or current	Frequency (Hz)	Pulse width (µs)			
Mayberg et al.[31]	SCC	Bilateral	6	Monopolar	4 V	130	60	6	66%/33%	One responder also achieved near remission
Lozano et al.[32]	SCC	Bilateral	20	Monopolar	3.5–5 V	130	90	12	55%/15%	Includes 6 patients from Mayberg et al.[31]; 1 patient with bipolar II disorder; 35% achieved near remission
Neimat et al.[37]	SCC	Bilateral	1	Monopolar	4.5 V	130	60	30	100%/100%	Case report of patient treated with DBS ~ 1 year after therapeutic ablative cingulotomy
Guinjoan et al.[38]	SCC	Unilateral and bilateral	1	Monopolar	4.5 V	120	90	18	100%/100%	Case report
Kennedy et al.[33]	SCC	Unilateral and bilateral	20	Monopolar	4.3 V	124.7	70.6	36–72 (mean 42.1)	55%/35%	Same 20 patients as Lozano et al.[32] only 14 completed follow-ups; response/remission rates based on intent-to-treat analysis; 2 probable suicides
Holtzheimer et al.[15]	SCC	Bilateral	17	Monopolar	5–10 mA	130	91	24	92%/58%	Seven patients with bipolar II disorder
Lozano et al.[35]	SCC	Bilateral	21	Not reported	5.2 mA	128.1	93.9	12	29%/NR	Sixty-two percent of patients showed response if defined as a 40% reduction in symptoms; 1 suicide
Puigdemont et al.[36]	SCC	Bilateral	8	Bipolar	4.2 V	135	90	12	63%/50%	
Merkl et al.[39]	SCC	Bilateral	6	Monopolar	5 V	130	90	6–8	33%/33%	Follow-up imaging of one patient that achieved remission revealed stimulating contacts located in posterior gyrus rectus bilaterally (see Accolla et al.[40])
Ramasubbu et al.[41]	SCC	Bilateral	4	Monopolar	0–10.5 V	2 – 185	60–450	6	50% / 0%	6-month follow-up does not include initial 3 months of randomized testing of stimulation parameters
Torres et al.[42]	SCC	Bilateral	1	NR	6 mA	130	91	9	100%/100%	Bipolar I disorder with psychotic features
Puigdemont et al.[43]	SCC	Bilateral	5	Bipolar	3.5–5 V	130–135	120–240	6	N/A	Double-blind, randomized, sham-controlled crossover study of a subset of patients from Puigdemont et al.[36]
Accolla et al.[40]	SCC	Bilateral	2	Monopolar	5 V	130	90	6	0%/0%	Results from 2 of 5 patients (#1 and #5) as other 3 included patients already reported in Merkl et al.[39]
Torres et al.[44]	SCC	Bilateral	2		6–8 mA	130	90–91	25–46	100%/100%	Extended follow-up of patient from Torres et al.[42] in addition to 1 patient with rapid cycling bipolar II

Table 13.1 (*Continued*) Summary of all Published Reports of DBS for Depression on MEDLINE (as of 11/29/2017)

Author	Target	Laterality	Patients	Stimulation mode	Amplitude or current	Frequency (Hz)	Pulse width (μs)	Follow-up (months)	Response/remission at final time point	Comments
Riva-Posse et al.[45]	SCC	Bilateral	11	Monopolar	6–8 mA	130	90	12	82%/55%	Testing of prospective targeting of specific axon bundles using tractography
Holtzheimer et al.[46]	SCC	Bilateral	90	Monopolar	4–8 mA	130	91	6	N/A	Double-blind, randomized, sham-controlled trial with subsequent open-label phase that was terminated early; 2 suicides
Schlaepfer et al.[47]	NAcc	Bilateral	3	Monopolar	0–5 V	145	90	1.4–5.1	33%/0%	Forty-two percent improvement in HDRS after 1 week of stimulation reported
Bewernick et al.[48]	NAcc	Bilateral	10	Both	1.5–10 V	100–150	60–210	12	50%/30%	1 suicide
Bewernick et al.[49]	NAcc	Bilateral	11	Both	1.5–10 V	100–150	60–210	12–48	46%/9%	Includes 10 patents from Bewernick et al.[48]; 1 suicide
Sousa et al.[50]	NAcc	Bilateral	1	Bipolar	4.2 V	150	150	5	100%/100%	Patient with comorbid bipolar I and OCD actually implanted to target refractory OCD and saw remission of depression; developed panic attacks with subsequent stimulation parameter adjustments
Malone et al.[51]	VC/VS	Bilateral	15	Both	6.7 V	127	113	6–51 (mean 23.5)	53%/40%	One patient with bipolar I disorder included and experienced two episodes of hypomania that resolved with stimulation and medication adjustments
Dougherty et al.[52]	VC/VS	Bilateral	30	Both	0–8 V	NR	90–210	24	23%/20%	Data from the open-label continuation phase after initial blinded phase of RCT was completed; 1 completed suicide
Bergfeld et al.[53]	vALIC	Bilateral	25	Monopolar	2.5–6 V	30–190	60–150	12	40%/20%	Results represent end of open-label phase; mean improvement of 9.5 points on HAM-D-17 scale between active and sham conditions in crossover phase
Schlaepfer et al.[54]	slMFB	Bilateral	7	Bipolar	2–3 V	130	60	2.8–7.6	86%/57%	One patient with bipolar disorder; response and remission rates based on MADRS instead of HDRS and would be lower if HDRS had been used
Fenoy et al.[55]	slMFB	Bilateral	4	Bipolar	3 V	130	60	6	75%/25%	One patient lost early in treatment and final rating score carried forward
Bewernick et al.[56]	slMFB	Bilateral	8	Bipolar	2–3 V	130	60	12	75%/50%	Includes 7 patients from Schlaepfer et al[62]; response and remission rates based on MADRS instead of HDRS and would be lower if HDRS had been used

Table 13.1 (*Continued*) Summary of all Published Reports of DBS for Depression on MEDLINE (as of 11/29/2017)

| Author | Target | Laterality | Patients | Mean (or range of) stimulation parameters | | | | Follow-up (months) | Response/ remission at final time point | Comments |
				Stimulation mode	Amplitude or current	Frequency (Hz)	Pulse width (μs)			
Blomstedt et al.[57]	slMFB	Bilateral	1	Bipolar	2.8–3 V	130	60	24	0%/0%	Comorbid anorexia nervosa; trial aborted due to intolerable visual side effects and patient underwent second DBS procedure at BNST (see same reference below)
Jiménez et al.[58]	ITP	Bilateral	1	Bipolar	2.5 V	130	450	24	100%/100%	Comorbid borderline personality disorder and bulimia; explanted after 3 years for unclear reasons without relapse per Jiménez et al.[60]
Sartorius et al.[59]	LHb	Bilateral	1	Monopolar	10.5 V	165	60	12	100%/100%	Target was stria medullaris thalami, the major afferent bundle of the LHb; a second patient implanted at this site is referenced in Kiening and Sartorius,[61] but insufficient information is provided to list here
Blomstedt et al.[57]	BNST	Bilateral	1	Monopolar	4.3 V	130	120	12	100%/100%	Comorbid anorexia nervosa; second DBS procedure after aborted trial at MFB (see same reference above)

Abbreviations: BNST, bed nucleus of stria terminalis; HDRS, Hamilton Depression Rating Scale; ITP, inferior thalamic peduncle; LHb, lateral habenula; N/A, not applicable; NAcc, nucleus accumbens; NR, not reported; SCC, subcallosal cingulate; slMFB, superolateral medial forebrain bundle; vALIC, ventral anterior limb of the internal capsule; VC/VS, ventral capsule/ventral striatum.

improved clinical efficacy, whereas previous studies of DBS at this target had utilized monopolar stimulation (one of the contacts on the electrode is programmed to be cathode to the implanted pulse generator case). Monopolar stimulation leads to radial current diffusion out from the stimulating electrode in a spherical manner, whereas bipolar stimulation creates a narrower and more focused field with maximal effect near the cathode.[62]

To further their analysis, the Barcelona group followed these initial results with a double-blind, randomized, sham-controlled crossover study in 2015 to confirm efficacy and measure the effects of discontinuation in a subset of the same subjects.[43] Subjects who had been implanted and had achieved at least 3 months of sustained clinical remission were randomized to receive either 3 months of sham stimulation followed by 3 months of active stimulation or vice versa. During active stimulation, four out of five subjects maintained response scores and none relapsed. During sham stimulation, only two subjects remained in remission, and one subject was withdrawn from the trial due to a serious relapse during the sham phase. Statistical analysis revealed a statistically significant effect of active stimulation. Limitations of this important step forward included small sample size and the sampling bias inherent to the study design.

A German group published their initial results in 2013, soon after the first report from the Spanish group. They studied both acute and chronic stimulation in a group of six subjects with TRD. High-intensity stimulation for 24 hours with rotating homologous contact pairs over 5 consecutive days after surgery was found to have modest antidepressant effects at best, but chronic stimulation over approximately 6 months did lead to remission in two subjects.[39] Of note, subsequent imaging revealed that the stimulating contacts in one of the responders were actually located in the posterior gyrus rectus bilaterally.[40]

Contemporaneously, a Canadian group sought to address ongoing questions regarding optimal stimulation parameters by adjusting the frequency and pulse width in four subjects in a double-blind, random manner over the first 3 months following electrode implantation and then monitoring symptoms for another 6 months.[41] In 2013, they reported that after stimulation with the optimized parameters, two subjects met criteria for treatment response. The authors also noted that increased pulse width seemed to be associated with clinical improvement.

Multisite-controlled study powered for efficacy testing

These relatively consistent reports of clinical efficacy in a significant number of subjects led to the initiation of a multicenter, prospective, randomized controlled trial (RCT) for TRD. Known as the BROdmann Area 25 DEep brain Neuromodulation (BROADEN) study and sponsored by industry (St. Jude Medical), the randomized phase of the trial lasted 6 months and compared active versus sham conditions in a double-blind paradigm. The trial was halted early in 2013 by the study sponsor because it failed a short-term futility analysis.[63] The complete results were published in 2017.[46] Ninety subjects were implanted across 13 investigational sites, with 60 subjects randomized to active treatment and the remaining 30 received sham stimulation. Both groups demonstrated a statistically significant and mild improvement in depressive symptoms after 6 months, but there was no statistical difference between treatment groups in response or remission rates (20 and 5% for stimulation versus 17 and 7% in sham, respectively).

After 6 months, all subjects eligible and willing to continue entered an open-label phase of stimulation lasting 6 more months. Subjects and investigators remained blinded as to whether each participant had received active or sham stimulation during the randomized phase, and blinding was successful based on subjects' inability to correctly guess their treatment condition beyond random chance. At the end of this additional period, in comparison to symptom burden at the end of the randomized phase, both groups demonstrated a mild and progressive improvement that did not reach statistical significance. Seventy-seven subjects continued in an ongoing follow-up study for up to 4 years. Data from up to 30 months was reported because not all subjects reached the final time point prior to study termination. With longer-term treatment, response/remission rates at 12, 18, and 24 months were 29%/14%, 53%/18%, and 49%/26%, respectively. Overall, chronic DBS was well tolerated and most serious adverse events were attributed to the primary mood disorder. Two deaths by suicide occurred, both during the 6-month open-label phase in subjects who had received sham stimulation during the randomized phase. The 18 and 24-month follow-up response rates of approximately 50% support the cumulative clinical effect of chronic stimulation and suggest that confirmatory efficacy testing be delayed until after at least 1 year of DBS for TRD.

13.2.2 Targeting the Nucleus Accumbens

The nucleus accumbens (NAcc) plays a critical role in reward-seeking, motivation, and addiction.[64,65] Schlaeffer and others hypothesized that DBS of this region might be efficacious in TRD via modulation of the apathy and anhedonia that is frequently part of the depression syndrome. Their brief first report in 2008 included three subjects (two were monozygotic twins), who were alternated between bilateral stimulation or no stimulation in a double-blind manner over the course of several weeks.[47] A mean improvement of 42% in depressive ratings was noted after the first week, and improvement in depressive symptoms correlated with stimulation but not control. In fact, symptomatic worsening during the control phase was severe enough to require resumption of stimulation prior to the end of the 4-week blinded placebo period in two of the subjects. Although improvement was rapid—noted on a scale of days to weeks—the study lasted only a few months and accordingly was unable to assess for stability of response.

Based on this preliminary success, in 2010, the authors expanded the study to an open-label trial of 10 subjects who were followed for 1 year.[48] The study had initially been planned to be sham-controlled, but this design was abandoned after enrolling the first three subjects due to acute worsening of symptoms during the sham phase. Responses were seen at 1 month and were progressive throughout the trial. At 1 year, 50% of subjects were responders and 30% met criteria for remission. A secondary measure of anxiety also demonstrated significant improvement and subjects engaged in increased levels of activity (e.g., returning to work part-time, starting a new hobby, establishing a daily structure, making new acquaintances). Interestingly, PET after 6 months of stimulation demonstrated significantly decreased metabolism in the amygdala of responders as compared to that of nonresponders, similar to successful antidepressant medication treatment studies of amygdala activity.[66] Notable adverse events following parameter adjustment included one subject with psychosis and two subjects with hypomania. One subject committed suicide, though this did not appear to be attributable to DBS itself. A subsequent report in 2012 followed up some of these subjects for upto 4 years and found that the antidepressant effect (or lack of treatment response) remained stable.[49]

13.2.3 Targeting the Ventral Capsule/Ventral Striatum

The rationale for extending the NAcc target (ventral striatum) for TRD to include the adjacent white matter (ventral anterior limb of internal capsule), a region collectively referred to as the ventral capsule/ventral striatum (VC/VS), came from trials of DBS for refractory OCD that reported concomitant improvement in depressive symptoms.[67,68] Accordingly, Malone and colleagues proceeded with an initial open-label trial spread across three clinical sites targeting the VC/VS in 15 subjects with TRD (1 with bipolar depression) in 2009. Maximal response was seen after 3 months of stimulation, and a 40% response rate was recorded after 6 months. By the end of the study (mean of 23.5 months), the response rate was 53% and the remission rate was 40%.[51] In a non-peer-reviewed article the next year, the lead author reported that addition of two more subjects and extended follow-up to 67 months (mean 37.4 months) had improved the results to 71% response rate and 35% remission rate.[69]

Multi-site, randomized double-blind sham-controlled trial

These promising results led to the first RCT of DBS of the VC/VS for TRD in 2015. In what was to be a study adequately powered to test efficacy (n = 208), the RECLAIM RCT was designed as a randomized, double-blind sham-controlled study for 16 weeks followed by an open-label continuation phase for at least 2 years. The trial was halted early due to disappointing results from the first 30 subjects.[52] During the controlled phase, only 3 out of 15 subjects receiving active stimulation responded, compared to 2 out of 14 control subjects. The continuation phase resulted in only a meager improvement in the response rate (23%). One subject committed suicide during the study. Importantly, since monopolar stimulation is more likely to lead to noticeable physical effects (i.e., paresthesia at the pulse generator site) which could break the blind, bipolar stimulation was used exclusively during the blinded phase. Interestingly, only subjects undergoing active treatment experienced an increased frequency of mood-related adverse events, including three subjects who experienced hypomanic or manic episodes despite no prior history of bipolar disorder.

Randomized sham-controlled trial after open-label optimization

Despite this setback, a Dutch group that had previously described significant antidepressant response during their experiences with VC/VS DBS for treatment-refractory OCD proceeded with a separate trial of this target for TRD in 2016. Referring to the DBS target as ventral ALIC (vALIC), they studied 25 subjects with an open-label design for 1 year during which setting optimization was attempted, followed by a double-blind, randomized crossover phase for two blocks of 6 weeks.[53] First responses were noted after approximately 2 months, and at the end of the open-label phase 40% of subjects were responders and 20% were in clinical remission. Sixteen subjects remained in the study and proceeded to the crossover phase. Tellingly, all responders from the open-label phase had to be prematurely crossed over to active from sham phase due to an increase in depressive symptoms. Active DBS led to a statistically significant improvement in depression severity with a mean improvement of 9.5 points on the Hamilton Depression Rating Scale (HDRS).[70] Significance was not lost with post-hoc inclusion of the nine subjects who did not proceed to the crossover phase, arguing against the result being attributable to potential bias. Notable adverse events included five suicide attempts (none clearly linked to stimulation itself), mania in two subjects, and hypomania in one subject. Two subjects who withdrew from the study and whose DBS accordingly had been stopped died shortly afterward, one via suicide and one via legal euthanasia in the Netherlands.

13.2.4 Targeting the Medial Forebrain Bundle

Building on prior results suggesting that stimulation of NAcc could modulate the brain's intrinsic reward circuit and thereby produce antidepressant effects, other components of functionally connected reward circuitry have also been studied clinically as targets for DBS. The superolateral branch of the medial forebrain bundle (slMFB) is a central component of the mesolimbic dopaminergic reward circuit and connects multiple brain regions involved in reward processing such as the ventral tegmental area (VTA), lateral and medial hypothalamus, VS, NAcc, and limbic prefrontal cortex.[71] In 2013, the Bonn group published an initial open-label trial of DBS targeting the slMFB in a group of seven subjects with TRD.[54] Notably, the slMFB cannot be identified with conventional magnetic resonance imaging (MRI), and each subject underwent diffusion tensor imaging to identify the implantation target. Treatment response was noted quite quickly as compared to prior DBS trials: six subjects experienced improvement of symptoms within 2 days, and four met the criterion for treatment response after 1 week. Subjects were followed for up to 33 weeks (minimum of 12), and at the last observation 86% and 57% were responders and remitters, respectively. Secondary measures of anxiety and functioning also improved. All subjects experienced oculomotor adverse events with certain stimulation settings consistent with the target being located near oculomotor nerve fibers.

With these initial encouraging results, the group updated their experience in a 2017 publication, including one more subject and describing longer follow-up.[56] At 1 year follow-up, six of eight subjects were responders, four of whom were in remission also. Some subjects were followed for up to 4 years, and the response appeared stable and durable. Oculomotor effects continued to be a ubiquitous adverse event. Curiously, one subject who had experienced stable remission requested device explantation against medical advice without explanation after

27 months, but he remained stable in his remission for the next year.

To further examine the slMFB target, a group in Texas began a clinical trial to replicate the prior findings and in 2016 published a preliminary report with data from their first four subjects.[55] One week following implantation, the subjects entered a single-blind sham stimulation phase lasting 4 weeks, after which they were unblinded for the subsequent 12 months of stimulation. Mean depression ratings improved considerably during the sham period but did not reach the level of statistical significance ($p = 0.101$). Within 1 week of active stimulation, however, the difference became statistically significant, and three of four subjects met criterion for response. Unfortunately, one of the responders was then lost to follow-up, but after 6 months the two responders had maintained the response and even continued to improve. All subjects experienced vertical diplopia, but such oculomotor adverse events were mostly transient. A potentially important additional finding was that structural connectivity between the stimulation sites and the medial prefrontal cortex was much stronger in the three responders than in the nonresponder.[55]

Of note, all slMFB trials utilized the Montgomery–Åsberg Depression Rating Scale (MADRS)[72] to calculate response and remission rates, whereas all the previous studies described in this review used the HDRS to assess the primary depression outcome. Comparison of MADRS with HDRS results in these studies indicates that use of the MADRS led to a higher proportion of subjects meeting criteria for treatment efficacy, raising several questions including: (1) whether the MADRS may be a more sensitive depression measure for use in future studies, and (2) whether the use of the MADRS in the slMFB studies artificially inflated the response rates compared to studies of other targets which used the HDRS.

13.2.5 DBS for Bipolar Depression

The depressive episodes encountered in bipolar disorder represent another treatment challenge for modern psychiatry with only a few medications available with the Food and Drug Administration (FDA) approval for this condition. TRD in bipolar disorder is a common clinical dilemma.[73] Although modern neuroscience has revealed clear differences in the pathophysiology of unipolar depression and bipolar disorder, there is also evidence for involvement of similar neural networks during depressive episodes, and mania and hypomania have been rare reported side effects of DBS for TRD and movement disorders.[73] Accordingly, DBS has been considered in severe cases of bipolar TRD.[74] Indeed, several of the trials already described in this chapter targeting the SCC,[32,34] VC/VS,[51] and slMFB[54] have included individuals experiencing bipolar depression, and overall efficacy and tolerability have been indistinguishable from subjects with unipolar TRD in this small sample size. Additional successful treatment of bipolar TRD with DBS is also described in several case reports (see ▶ Table 13.1), but overall this area of study remains very much in its infancy.

13.2.6 Ongoing DBS trials

Various trials of DBS for TRD are in planning, ongoing, or awaiting reporting of results. A search of clinicaltrials.gov on October 18, 2017, was performed using the query terms "deep brain stimulation" and "depression" without filtering by country. Results were then sorted to reflect only studies testing for treatment efficacy in a primary mood disorder (unipolar or bipolar depression). Finally, studies that were classified as withdrawn or completed with results available were also excluded. Targeted brain regions include SCC, VC/VS, NAcc, and slMFB as discussed above in addition to the inferior thalamic peduncle and the capsula interna/bed nucleus of the stria terminalis; see ▶ Table 13.2 for results of this search. Of note, some trials identified had not updated their status in some time and may reflect studies that have already been completed and reported or were never launched.

13.3 The Future of DBS for Major Depression

A careful review of the published evidence demonstrates that DBS may be an effective treatment for TRD. While there has been considerable variability, response rates in the 30 to 50% range (sometimes higher, see ▶ Table 13.1), along with cases of sustained remission and cases of re-emergence of severe symptoms when crossing from active to sham stimulation, are quite impressive results, particularly in the context of a severely ill patient population that has already been failed by scores of pharmacological, psychotherapeutic, and noninvasive stimulation interventions. Although mania, hypomania, psychosis, motor effects, and suicides have been reported during these trials, in general DBS for TRD is well tolerated, and there are at least five distinct but promising brain targets currently in study. Like treatment with antidepressant medications, meaningful and sustained antidepressant effects of DBS appear to be delayed in onset by weeks to months. However, unlike antidepressant medications, relapse when DBS is abruptly ceased (i.e., consequent to battery depletion or crossover from active stimulation to sham stimulation) is much swifter.

Despite the promise, many limitations and questions remain. Although some subjects plainly respond to DBS, the factors that underlie response remain obscure, and expectation bias must always be considered as a source of response variability. Clinical presentation does not predict response, and currently there is no validated rational means to link a unique patient with the most promising DBS target for that patient. Further, the most appropriate measurements of treatment response remain debatable, and ongoing diagnostic challenges and ethical concerns remain at the collective forefront of the field. These limitations are underscored by the early termination of two of the three RCTs that have occurred to date (the BROADEN and the RECLAIM trials).

While the challenges are great, the need for effective treatments for TRD is greater. Results thus far strongly suggest that DBS has the potential not only to help meet that need, but also to contribute to the understanding of affective neural networks such that highly effective but less invasive antidepressant treatments might be developed. In the remainder of this chapter, we elaborate on some of these challenges, discuss putative explanations for discordant results obtained, and suggest guidance for future trials with an emphasis on confirming target engagement.

Table 13.2 Ongoing Trials of DBS for Treatment-Resistant Depression Indexed on clinicaltrials.gov (as of 10/18/2017)

NCT number	Title	Recruitment	Target	Enrollment	Study design	Primary depression outcome measure(s)	Sponsor/collaborators	Completion date
NCT00296920	Deep Brain Stimulation for Refractory Major Depression	Completed	SGC	10	Open-label	HDRS	University Health Network, Toronto/National Alliance for Research on Schizophrenia and Depression	Not listed
NCT01435148	Deep Brain Stimulation in Treatment Resistant Depression	Not listed	SGC or VACNAC	8	Double-blind, randomized, crossover	MADRS	North Bristol NHS Trust/ University of Bristol	December 2012
NCT02889250	Deep Brain Stimulation to Relieve Depression	Not yet recruiting	SCCWM	6	Open-label	MADRS, suicidality	University of Pittsburgh	March 2020
NCT00367003	Deep Brain Stimulation for Treatment Resistant Depression	Recruiting	SCCWM	20	Open-label	HDRS	Emory University/The Dana Foundation	September 2018
NCT00122031	Deep Brain Stimulation for Treatment-Refractory Major Depression	Completed	VC/VS	13	Open-label	HDRS	University Hospital, Bonn/ Medtronic	January 2011
NCT03254017	Remotely Programmed Deep Brain Stimulation of the Bilateral Habenula for Treatment-Resistant Major Depression: An Open Label Pilot Trial	Recruiting	Habenula	6	Open-label	MADRS, HDRS	Ruijin Hospital	August 2019
NCT00555698	Feasibility, Safety and Efficacy of Deep Brain Stimulation for Depression	Completed	ALIC	8	Open-label	MADRS, HDRS	Medtronic/The Cleveland Clinic/ Ohio State University	February 2011
NCT01973478	Deep Brain Stimulation in Patients with Chronic Treatment-Resistant Depression	Active, not recruiting	NAcc	40	Double-blind, randomized, sham-controlled	HDRS	Rennes University Hospital	February 2020

Table 13.2 (*Continued*) Ongoing Trials of DBS for Treatment-Resistant Depression Indexed on clinicaltrials.gov (as of 10/18/2017)

NCT number	Title	Recruitment	Target	Enrollment	Study design	Primary depression outcome measure(s)	Sponsor/collaborators	Completion date
NCT01801319	A Clinical Evaluation of Subcallosal Cingulate Gyrus Deep Brain Stimulation for Treatment-Resistant Depression	Active, not recruiting	SCG	40	Double-blind, randomized, placebo-controlled, crossover	HDRS	St. Jude Medical	December 2017
NCT01898429	Deep Brain Stimulation (DBS) for Treatment-Resistant Depression (TRD)	Completed	SCCWM	5	Double-blind, randomized, cross-over	HDRS	Dartmouth-Hitchcock Medical Center	December 2016
NCT01569711	Deep Brain Stimulation of Nucleus Accumbens for Chronic and Resistant Major Depressive Disorder	Completed	NAcc	6	Open-label	HDRS	Rennes University Hospital	May 2013
NCT01778790	Deep Brain Stimulation of the Superolateral Branch of the Medial Forebrain Bundle (slMFB) for the Treatment of Refractory Major Depression	Not listed	slMFB	12	Randomized, sham-controlled	MADRS	University Hospital, Bonn	August 2015
NCT01095263	Effects of Deep Brain Stimulation in Treatment-Resistant Major Depression	Not listed	slMFB	7	Double-blind, randomized, sham-controlled	MADRS	University Hospital, Bonn	June 2015
NCT00531726	Berlin Deep Brain Stimulation Depression Study	Not listed	SCCWM	20	Multicenter, double-blind, randomized, sham-controlled	MADRS, HDRS	Charite University, Berlin, Germany/University Hospital Carl Gustav Carus/Ludwig-Maximilians - University of Munich/Hannover Medical School	September 2013
NCT02046330	Deep Brain Stimulation (DBS) Therapy for Treatment-Resistant Depression	Recruiting	slMFB	10	Open-label	MADRS	The University of Texas Health Science Center, Houston/Medtronic	November 2019

Table 13.2 (Continued) Ongoing Trials of DBS for Treatment-Resistant Depression Indexed on clinicaltrials.gov (as of 10/18/2017)

NCT number	Title	Recruitment	Target	Enrollment	Study design	Primary depression outcome measure(s)	Sponsor/collaborators	Completion date
NCT01331330	European Deep Brain Stimulation (DBS) Depression Study	Completed	SCCWM	9	Multicenter, double-blind, randomized, two treatment settings	MADRS	St. Jude Medical	January 2015
NCT01834560	SubGenual CG25 Deep Brain Stimulation in Severe Resistant Depression	Active, not recruiting	SCCWM	5	Open-label	HDRS	University Hospital, Grenoble	December 2017
NCT01921543	Deep Brain Stimulation in Treatment Refractory Depression	Terminated	ITP & CI/BNST	7	Double-blind, randomized, crossover	HDRS	Universitaire Ziekenhuizen Leuven/Medtronic	October 2013
NCT01984710	DBS for TRD Medtronic Activa PC + S	Recruiting	SCCWM	20	Open-label	HDRS	Emory University/Hope for Depression Research Foundation/The Dana Foundation	September 2023
NCT01798407	DBS of the Lateral Habenula in Treatment-Resistant Depression	Recruiting	Habenula	6	Open-label for 1 year, responders then enter double-blind discontinuation phase	HDRS	Baylor College of Medicine	February 2020
NCT01268137	DBS in Treatment Resistant Major Depression	Not listed	SCCWM	8	Open-label for 6–9 months, then randomized, crossover phase	HDRS	Fundació Institut de Recerca de l'Hospital de la Santa Creu i Sant Pau/Fondo de Investigacion Sanitaria	June 2011
NCT01476527	Deep Brain Stimulation for the Treatment of Refractory Bipolar Disorder	Not listed	Not reported	6	Open-label	MADRS, HDRS	University Health Network, Toronto	Not listed
NCT01372722	Deep Brain Stimulation (DBS) for Treatment Resistant Bipolar Disorder	Not listed	NAcc	12	Double-blind, randomized, crossover	MADRS	University Hospital, Bonn	July 2015
NCT01069952	Electrical Stimulation of the Internal Capsule for Intractable Depression	Completed	VC/VS	5	Not reported	HDRS	Butler Hospital/Medtronic	Not listed

Abbreviations: CI/BNST, capsula interna/bed nucleus of the stria terminalis; ITP, inferior thalamic peduncle; SCCWM, subcallosal cingulate white matter; SCG, subcallosal cingulate gyrus; slMFB, superolateral branch from the main medial forebrain bundle; SGC, subgenual cingulate cortex; VACNAC, ventral anterior capsule nucleus accumbens.

13.3.1 Depression is Heterogeneous and its Treatment is Susceptible to Placebo Response

Depression is a clinical syndrome defined by a combination of reported and observed symptoms and signs. It is inherently heterogeneous, and diagnostic criteria can be met by numerous combinations of symptoms[1] that occur in concert with unique social and environmental stressors that synergize in a dysfunctional manner. While historically clinicians have divided depression into various phenomenological subtypes, such as melancholic or atypical, these have been predictive neither of treatment response nor underlying biology. Attempts to improve the validity of the diagnosis and treatment response remain hindered by the lack of validated biomarkers, although promising recent results suggest the potential for breakthroughs in this regard.[75,76,77,78] Finally, comorbidity with other psychiatric illnesses—or frank misdiagnosis—presents grave challenges to the execution of valid and generalizable clinical trials.

Most trials reported thus far have been open-label in design. While this reflects the experimental nature of the intervention and the proof-of-concept aims of many of these trials, it also is attributable to the belief that the subjects selected for these trials, having been severely ill and already having been failed by dozens of medication combinations and interventional treatment modalities, are minimally susceptible to a placebo response.[79] Results from the RCT of VC/VS[52] and sham stimulation phases of otherwise unblinded trials[34,43,55] call this presumption into question. In fact, the desperation of these patients, who have exhausted almost all other treatment options and who may lose all hope if "brain surgery can't even fix me," combined with the intensity of the surgical intervention and study requirements, may create a scenario where a placebo effect might be anticipated rather than dismissed. This underscores the importance of future studies attempting to include a control condition of sufficient duration to allow more definitive conclusions regarding treatment efficacy.

13.3.2 Lessons from Randomized Controlled Trial Design

To date there have been three double-blind, sham-controlled RCTs, and each is worthy of closer scrutiny. In the RECLAIM trial, Doughtery et al. reported a double-blind, sham-controlled, multicenter RCT targeting VC/VS that was halted after 30 subjects due to minimal clinical response.[52] Subjects in the active treatment arm experienced a higher rate of mood-related adverse events, such as mania even in the absence of a bipolar disorder history, arguing for the engagement in at least some subjects of mood-relevant neural circuitry.

Why, then, were statistically significant therapeutic clinical effects lacking? While a variety of explanations have been offered—including inadequate duration of treatment, variability across treatment sites, and insufficiently sensitive measures of treatment response[80]—another possible explanation may be the lack of optimized stimulation parameters. All DBS trials include close attention to the selection of which contacts to use for chronic stimulation and the choice of stimulation parameters

(i.e., amplitude, frequency, and pulse width) to promote an antidepressant response. This iterative process of surveying contacts and adjusting parameters may promote or instead delay onset of clinical benefit given the lack of immediate indicators of sustained response (which in contrast usually are observed with acute DBS for movement disorders). This approach may also result in higher stimulation settings than actually needed for an antidepressant effect. The RECLAIM project, however, chose settings for the blinded phase based on two overnight trials. Further, only bipolar stimulation was allowed during the blinded phase as it was believed to reduce risk of breaking the blind. Finally, the eventual blinded phase lasted only 16 weeks. Afterwards, subjects continued in an open treatment phase and stimulation parameters were again allowed to be modified. Improvement, while still less in magnitude than that noted in prior studies, was more significant after 24 months of ongoing stimulation, again consistent with other observations of delayed onset of therapeutic effect and the crucial role of progressive and systematic optimization of stimulation parameters over this longer time scale.

In the case of the BROADEN trial, Holtzheimer and others reported the largest RCT of DBS to date, with 90 subjects receiving implantation targeting the SCC white matter. Although symptomatic improvement was noted, active treatment was not statistically different from sham, and a futility analysis indicated that the study had a 17% chance of success if continued. The industry sponsor of the trial accordingly elected to end enrollment, though it is worth noting that this result did not actually meet the prespecified definition of futility agreed upon by the FDA when approving the trial (10%)[46] and likely reflects some degree of financial considerations.

While clearly representing another disappointing result, BROADEN also offers lessons for future trials. In particular, the experimental design and stimulation selection procedure are again worthy of closer inspection. The surgical target was chosen on a purely anatomical basis, and there was no intraoperative testing for acute effects of stimulation. In fact, the contact chosen for chronic stimulation was selected by a subgroup of the authors based on apparent proximity to the predefined target. After 2 weeks of postoperative recovery, monopolar stimulation was initiated at the chosen contact and at predefined stimulation settings. If at least 10% improvement was not noted 2 weeks later, then the amplitude was increased. After another 4 weeks, this process was repeated. Another 4 weeks later (now 10 weeks after onset of stimulation), a second contact was activated if response remained insufficient. Modification of other parameters was not allowed, nor were any further stimulation changes permitted beyond 10 weeks. The 26-week trial period was not extended even if optimization had continued for the first 10 weeks, meaning some participants may have received only 16 weeks of partially-optimized stimulation prior to primary outcome assessment. Given that the subject population in this study had a mean duration of their current depressive episode of 12 years, which is considerably longer than that seen in previous studies targeting the SCC,[46] the treatment duration may simply have been too short to capture a more robust therapeutic response capable of separating from placebo, especially in the possible setting of inadequate stimulation optimization. The significantly improved results achieved after further stimulation parameter adjustments and an additional 18 to 24 months of stimulation support this notion.

These study designs contrast notably with the paradigm employed by Bergfeld and colleagues in their trial of vALIC DBS.[53] They enrolled 25 subjects who underwent an open-label optimization phase after implantation. Stimulation parameters were serially adjusted based on assessment of response and any adverse events only after maintaining the settings for a minimum of 1 week, and this optimization strategy continued until a stable response was maintained for 4 consecutive weeks or after a maximum of 52 weeks. (This phase initially was to last a maximum of 6 months but was eventually extended during the trial, and six subjects still exceeded the new maximum for logistical reasons.) Only then was a subject randomized in a double-blinded manner into blocks of sham or active treatment for 6 weeks each. Notably, the mean duration of the optimization phase was nearly 1 year even though mean time to earliest detectable response in the subset of subjects who responded was only 53.6 days. Given the relative success of this trial, a longer and more sustained period of stimulation optimization combined with increased treatment duration may be necessary for improved efficacy. Further, some degree of flexibility in trial design may be imperative to capturing this.

Critics will point out, however, that this study design tends to lead to increased relative drop out of nonresponders, a selection bias that may result in falsely inflated efficacy despite the authors' attempts to account for it statistically. There is also a concern that the rapid worsening of symptoms after transition to sham stimulation could represent a rebound or discontinuation effect directly attributable to the abrupt stopping of the stimulation (i.e., similar to discontinuation syndromes experienced after stopping antidepressant medications that may include depressed mood and irritability but do not represent recurrence of syndromic depression), rather than the cessation of a direct therapeutic effect, a confound not well addressed by this study design.[81,82] Finally, this abrupt worsening could represent a "nocebo effect"[83]; although subjects were blinded, they could accurately predict the stimulation setting.[53]

13.3.3 Confirming Functional Target Engagement—A Necessary Next Step?

Although many of the studies have been uncontrolled, evidence to date suggests that DBS can lead to improvement and sometimes even complete remission in a subset of patients with severe TRD. This is perhaps best illustrated by the number of studies and reports that noted symptomatic worsening in treatment responders when stimulation was intentionally or unintentionally discontinued.[34,43,47,48,53,59,58] Unfortunately, many patients do not respond; even after 1 year's worth of stimulation optimization in the vALIC trial, only about 40% of subjects responded to treatment.[53] What might explain why some subjects respond robustly while others not at all?

The engagement of specific axon fibers, and by extension the specific neural circuits they serve, may be crucial to the answer. DBS implantation has been based mostly on anatomical coordinates rather than prospective modeling of the activation of particular fiber tracts by a range of electrical field doses. While modern neurosurgical techniques are quite precise, the acceptable ranges for implantation of electrodes still have been sufficiently large such that the desired target may not be consistently engaged.[84] Conversely, the slMFB DBS target cannot be identified by standard structural imaging and requires the use of diffusion-based tractography to estimate the precise location of the axon bundle to be targeted. While early promising results with the targeting of slMFB may simply be attributable to this representing a superior target for TRD, another possibility is that the functional nature of its targeting may increase the probability that the intended brain circuitry is stimulated.

As others have pointed out,[85] studies of brain stimulation for other indications also support the concept of engaging a functionally connected circuit. Direct stimulation for intractable tinnitus, for example, is only effective if the stimulation target demonstrates functional connectivity with the desired auditory pathways.[86,87] More generally, resting state functional connectivity predicts the success of invasive and noninvasive brain stimulation of distinct anatomical targets for a variety of neuropsychiatric disorders.[88] In the case of DBS for TRD, preoperative tractography combined with retrospective analysis revealed that all 11 subjects that ultimately responded to stimulation of SCC had electrodes located such that they engaged a distinct set of converging white matter bundles (forceps minor, uncinate fasciculus, cingulate, and fronto-striatal fibers), whereas nonresponders did not consistently show these connections.[89] This connectomic approach has now been applied prospectively by using probabilistic tractography to plan surgical targeting and thereby increasing the likelihood of engagement of the desired fibers (▶ Fig. 13.1).[45] Considerably less stimulation parameter optimization was required with this approach, and out of a new cohort of 11 subjects, 8 and 9 were responders after 6 and 9 months of stimulation, respectively.

To what extent might target engagement be confirmed intraoperatively? DBS implantation surgery traditionally has relied on confirmation of lead placement in the desired anatomic site based on microelectrode recordings in awake patients that allow functional characterization of single neuron firing, in addition to test stimulation. More recently, interventional/intraoperative MRI-guided implantation under general anesthesia has been validated as an accurate technique for implanting leads in the desired anatomic target, producing expected functional outcomes in Parkinson's disease (See Chapter 4, Intraoperative Imaging-based Lead Implantation). The anatomic targets in TRD, however, are less well defined in terms of their electrophysiological signatures, suggesting that asleep MRI-guided surgery could be a reasonable approach for placing leads in a desired stimulation target. Such MRI-guided surgery would also facilitate prospective use of tractography or other imaging data for lead targeting by allowing real-time visualization of the implanted lead in relation to structures of interest. The obvious trade-off for asleep DBS surgery is the inability to test for undesirable side effects that may occur acutely with stimulation and may be of paramount importance in patients with TRD. Ultimately, the best method for lead implantation in TRD likely will be determined by a combination of understanding the underlying functional and structural physiology of the target network, need to test for clinical benefits and/or side effects, and a given patient's ability to undergo awake surgery.

**Evolution of surgical targeting
for SCC DBS for depression**

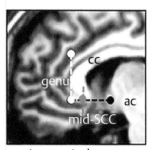

Anatomical target
stereotactic MRI

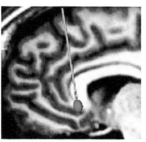

Volume of tissue
activated with
therapeutic DBS

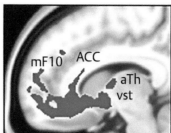

Common white matter
tracts impacted by
effective DBS

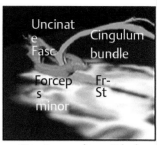

Tractography guided
surgical targeting
in a single patient

Fig. 13.1 The evolution of surgical targeting of the subcallosal cingulate region. Progression (*left* to *right*) from an anatomical "gray matter" target, to identification of the "white matter" tracts activated, to tractography allowing identification of the involved pathways. This approach allows individualized target refinement and produces improved therapeutic outcomes. Genu, genus of the corpus callosum; Mid-SCC, mid subcallosal cingulate; Ac, anterior commissure; mF10, medial frontal Brodmann Area 10; ACC, anterior cingulate cortex; aTh, anterior thalamus; vSt, ventral striatum; Fr-st, frontal striatal fibers. (Reused with permission from Deeb et al, Proceedings of the Fourth Annual Deep Brain Stimulation Think Tank: A Review of Emerging Issues and Technologies. Front Integr Neurosci. 2016 Nov. 22;10:38.)

13.3.4 Neuroethics of DBS for TRD

The philosophical and practical implications of implanting a device in the brain of a human who has treatment-resistant psychiatric illness must be considered in order for the field to proceed in a manner that assures beneficence, respect for persons, and justice.[90] Recognizing the necessity for neuroethics research to proceed in tandem with cutting edge neuroscience and brain-device investigation, the Neuroethics Division of the Brain Research through Advancing Innovative Neurotechnologies (BRAIN) Multi-Council Working group wrote in the report *BRAIN 2025: A Scientific Vision*, "Although brain research entails ethical issues that are common to other areas of biomedical science, it entails special ethical considerations as well. Because the brain gives rise to consciousness, our innermost thoughts and our most basic human needs, mechanistic studies of the brain have already resulted in new social and ethical questions."[91] To achieve this goal, National Institutes of Health recently announced grant support to explore neuroethics questions related to BRAIN initiative research.[92] While the field is rich for a variety of ethical inquiries related to DBS, we predict cutting edge areas of neuroethics research, which will develop over the coming decade, include: (1) minimizing therapeutic misconceptions of very ill participants in clinical trials,[93,94] (2) informed consent procedures with psychiatrically ill patients,[94,95] (3) digital security and ownership of big data generated from implanted devices that both stimulate and record neural activity and capture global positioning,[96] and (4) ethical obligations of clinical investigators, device manufacturers, and insurers in the ongoing provision of care to graduates of DBS clinical trials in the absence of an FDA-approved indication and associated reimbursement by insurance companies and Medicare.[95]

13.4 Conclusion

As TRD represents an enormous disease burden to the world, DBS has emerged as both a promising treatment modality and a unique opportunity to learn more about the brain circuitry that underlies depression and antidepressant response. Although many small studies have suggested treatment efficacy, the results of randomized trials have been less encouraging, and only a subset of patients seem to respond to the treatment. Fortunately, emerging technologies and approaches that identify objective biomarkers of depression and precisely target defined neural pathways provide reason for optimism. Ultimately, treatment optimization may require a combination of approaches. Patients might initially undergo functional MRI and electroencephalography (EEG) in combination with assessment of serum biomarkers to identify neurophysiological subtypes of depression that will more likely respond to stimulation of a specific brain target.[75,76,97] Then, tractography and advanced connectomics might be used to precisely identify the surgical target.[45] Finally, EEG, magnetoencephalography, further imaging, and/or serum biomarkers might be utilized as complementary measures of treatment response and to guide further optimization. Given the risks of adverse effects and the multiple ethical issues associated with employing an experimental neurosurgical procedure in a very ill and highly vulnerable patient population, ongoing study should proceed purposefully and methodically.

References

[1] American Psychiatric Association. Diagnostic and Statistical Manual of Mental Disorders. 5th ed. Arlington, VA: American Psychiatric Publishing; 2013

[2] Vos T, Flaxman AD, Naghavi M, et al. Years lived with disability (YLDs) for 1160 sequelae of 289 diseases and injuries 1990–2010: a systematic analysis for the Global Burden of Disease Study 2010. Lancet. 2012; 380(9859):2163–2196

[3]   Vos T, Barber RM, Bell B, et al. Global Burden of Disease Study 2013 Collaborators. Global, regional, and national incidence, prevalence, and years lived with disability for 301 acute and chronic diseases and injuries in 188 countries, 1990–2013: a systematic analysis for the Global Burden of Disease Study 2013. Lancet. 2015; 386(9995):743–800

[4]   Thornicroft G, Chatterji S, Evans-Lacko S, et al. Undertreatment of people with major depressive disorder in 21 countries. Br J Psychiatry. 2017; 210(2):119–124

[5]   Trivedi MH, Rush AJ, Wisniewski SR, et al. STAR*D Study Team. Evaluation of outcomes with citalopram for depression using measurement-based care in STAR*D: implications for clinical practice. Am J Psychiatry. 2006; 163(1):28–40

[6]   Fava M. Diagnosis and definition of treatment-resistant depression. Biol Psychiatry. 2003; 53(8):649–659

[7]   Berlim MT, Turecki G. What is the meaning of treatment resistant/refractory major depression (TRD)? A systematic review of current randomized trials. Eur Neuropsychopharmacol. 2007; 17(11):696–707

[8]   Conway CR, George MS, Sackeim HA. Toward an evidence-based, operational definition of treatment-resistant depression: when enough is enough. JAMA Psychiatry. 2017; 74(1):9–10

[9]   Souery D, Papakostas GI, Trivedi MH. Treatment-resistant depression. J Clin Psychiatry. 2006; 67 Suppl 6:16–22

[10] Holtzheimer PE, Mayberg HS. Stuck in a rut: rethinking depression and its treatment. Trends Neurosci. 2011; 34(1):1–9

[11] Kornstein SG, Schneider RK. Clinical features of treatment-resistant depression. J Clin Psychiatry. 2001; 62 Suppl 16:18–25

[12] Narang P, Retzlaff A, Brar K, Lippmann S. Deep brain stimulation for treatment-refractory depression. South Med J. 2016; 109(11):700–703

[13] Fekadu A, Wooderson SC, Markopoulo K, Donaldson C, Papadopoulos A, Cleare AJ. What happens to patients with treatment-resistant depression? A systematic review of medium to long term outcome studies. J Affect Disord. 2009; 116(1–2):4–11

[14] Mrazek DA, Hornberger JC, Altar CA, Degtiar I. A review of the clinical, economic, and societal burden of treatment-resistant depression: 1996–2013. Psychiatr Serv. 2014; 65(8):977–987

[15] Holtzheimer PE, Mayberg HS. Neuromodulation for treatment-resistant depression. F1000 Med Rep. 2012; 4(November):22

[16] Kellner CH, Greenberg RM, Murrough JW, Bryson EO, Briggs MC, Pasculli RM. ECT in treatment-resistant depression. Am J Psychiatry. 2012; 169(12):1238–1244

[17] Ingram A, Saling MM, Schweitzer I. Cognitive side effects of brief pulse electroconvulsive therapy: a review. J ECT. 2008; 24(1):3–9

[18] Tielkes CEM, Comijs HC, Verwijk E, Stek ML. The effects of ECT on cognitive functioning in the elderly: a review. Int J Geriatr Psychiatry. 2008; 23(8):789–795

[19] Flint AJ, Gagnon N. Effective use of electroconvulsive therapy in late-life depression. Can J Psychiatry. 2002; 47(8):734–741

[20] Cleary DR, Ozpinar A, Raslan AM, Ko AL. Deep brain stimulation for psychiatric disorders: where we are now. Neurosurg Focus. 2015; 38(6):1–24

[21] Manjila S, Rengachary S, Xavier AR, Parker B, Guthikonda M. Modern psychosurgery before Egas Moniz: a tribute to Gottlieb Burckhardt. Neurosurg Focus. 2008; 25(1):E9

[22] Holtzheimer PE, Mayberg HS. Deep brain stimulation for psychiatric disorders. Annu Rev Neurosci. 2011; 34:289–307

[23] Moniz E. Prefrontal leucotomy in the treatment of mental disorders. Am J Psychiatry. 1937; 93(6):1379–1385

[24] Wind JJ, Anderson DE. From prefrontal leukotomy to deep brain stimulation: the historical transformation of psychosurgery and the emergence of neuroethics. Neurosurg Focus. 2008; 25(1):E10

[25] Patel SR, Aronson JP, Sheth SA, Eskandar EN. Lesion procedures in psychiatric neurosurgery. World Neurosurg. 2013; 80(3–4):31.e9–31.e16

[26] Volpini M, Giacobbe P, Cosgrove GR, Levitt A, Lozano AM, Lipsman N. The history and future of ablative neurosurgery for major depressive disorder. Stereotact Funct Neurosurg. 2017; 95(4):216–228

[27] Hariz MI, Blomstedt P, Zrinzo L. Deep brain stimulation between 1947 and 1987: the untold story. Neurosurg Focus. 2010; 29(2):E1

[28] Benabid AL, Pollak P, Gervason C, et al. Long-term suppression of tremor by chronic stimulation of the ventral intermediate thalamic nucleus. Lancet. 1991; 337(8738):403–406

[29] Nuttin B, Cosyns P, Demeulemeester H, Gybels J, Meyerson B. Electrical stimulation in anterior limbs of internal capsules in patients with obsessive-compulsive disorder. Lancet. 1999; 354(9189):1526

[30] Mayberg HS. Limbic-cortical dysregulation: a proposed model of depression. J Neuropsychiatry Clin Neurosci. 1997; 9(3):471–481

[31] Mayberg HS, Lozano AM, Voon V, et al. Deep brain stimulation for treatment-resistant depression. Neuron. 2005; 45(5):651–660

[32] Lozano AM, Mayberg HS, Giacobbe P, Hamani C, Craddock RC, Kennedy SH. Subcallosal cingulate gyrus deep brain stimulation for treatment-resistant depression. Biol Psychiatry. 2008; 64(6):461–467

[33] Kennedy SH, Giacobbe P, Rizvi SJ, et al. Deep brain stimulation for treatment-resistant depression: follow-up after 3 to 6 years. Am J Psychiatry. 2011; 168(5):502–510

[34] Holtzheimer PE, Kelley ME, Gross RE, et al. Subcallosal cingulate deep brain stimulation for treatment-resistant unipolar and bipolar depression. Arch Gen Psychiatry. 2012; 69(2):150–158

[35] Lozano AM, Giacobbe P, Hamani C, et al. A multicenter pilot study of subcallosal cingulate area deep brain stimulation for treatment-resistant depression. J Neurosurg. 2012; 116(2):315–322

[36] Puigdemont D, Pérez-Egea R, Portella MJ, et al. Deep brain stimulation of the subcallosal cingulate gyrus: further evidence in treatment-resistant major depression. Int J Neuropsychopharmacol. 2012; 15(1):121–133

[37] Neimat JS, Hamani C, Giacobbe P, et al. Neural stimulation successfully treats depression in patients with prior ablative cingulotomy. Am J Psychiatry. 2008; 165(6):687-693

[38] Guinjoan SM, Mayberg HS, Costanzo EY, et al. Asymmetrical contribution of brain structures to treatment-resistant depression as illustrated by effects of right subgenual cingulum stimulation. J Neuropsychiatry Clin Neurosci. 2010; 22(3):265–277

[39] Merkl A, Schneider GH, Schönecker T, et al. Antidepressant effects after short-term and chronic stimulation of the subgenual cingulate gyrus in treatment-resistant depression. Exp Neurol. 2013; 249:160–168

[40] Accolla EA, Aust S, Merkl A, et al. Deep brain stimulation of the posterior gyrus rectus region for treatment resistant depression. J Affect Disord. 2016; 194:33–37

[41] Ramasubbu R, Anderson S, Haffenden A, Chavda S, Kiss ZHT. Double-blind optimization of subcallosal cingulate deep brain stimulation for treatment-resistant depression: a pilot study. J Psychiatry Neurosci. 2013; 38(5):325–332

[42] Torres CV, Ezquiaga E, Navas M, de Sola RG. Deep brain stimulation of the subcallosal cingulate for medication-resistant type I bipolar depression: case report. Bipolar Disord. 2013; 15(6):719-721

[43] Puigdemont D, Portella M, Pérez-Egea R, et al. A randomized double-blind crossover trial of deep brain stimulation of the subcallosal cingulate gyrus in patients with treatment-resistant depression: a pilot study of relapse prevention. J Psychiatry Neurosci. 2015; 40(4):224–231

[44] Torres CV, Ezquiaga E, Navas M, García Pallero MA, Sola RG. Long-term Results of Deep Brain Stimulation of the Subcallosal Cingulate for Medication-Resistant Bipolar I Depression and Rapid Cycling Bipolar II Depression. Biol Psychiatry. 2017; 81(4):e33-e34

[45] Riva-Posse P, Choi KS, Holtzheimer PE, et al. A connectomic approach for subcallosal cingulate deep brain stimulation surgery: prospective targeting in treatment-resistant depression. Mol Psychiatry. 201 8; 23:843–849

[46] Holtzheimer PE, Husain MM, Lisanby SH, et al. Subcallosal cingulate deep brain stimulation for treatment-resistant depression: a multisite, randomised, sham-controlled trial. Lancet Psychiatry. 2017; 4(11):839–849

[47] Schlaepfer TE, Cohen MX, Frick C, et al. Deep brain stimulation to reward circuitry alleviates anhedonia in refractory major depression. Neuropsychopharmacology. 2008; 33(2):368–377

[48] Bewernick BH, Hurlemann R, Matusch A, et al. Nucleus accumbens deep brain stimulation decreases ratings of depression and anxiety in treatment-resistant depression. Biol Psychiatry. 2010; 67(2):110–116

[49] Bewernick BH, Kayser S, Sturm V, Schlaepfer TE. Long-term effects of nucleus accumbens deep brain stimulation in treatment-resistant depression: evidence for sustained efficacy. Neuropsychopharmacology. 2012; 37(9):1975–1985

[50] Sousa MB, Reis T, Reis A, Belmonte-De-Abreu P. New-onset panic attacks after deep brain stimulation of the nucleus accumbens in a patient with refractory obsessive-compulsive and bipolar disorders: A case report. Rev Bras Psiquiatr. 2015; 37(2):182-183

[51] Malone DA, Jr, Dougherty DD, Rezai AR, et al. Deep brain stimulation of the ventral capsule/ventral striatum for treatment-resistant depression. Biol Psychiatry. 2009; 65(4):267–275

[52] Dougherty DD, Rezai AR, Carpenter LL, et al. A randomized sham-controlled trial of deep brain stimulation of the ventral capsule/ventral striatum for chronic treatment-resistant depression. Biol Psychiatry. 2015; 78(4):240–248

[53] Bergfeld IO, Mantione M, Hoogendoorn MLC, et al. Deep brain stimulation of the ventral anterior limb of the internal capsule for treatment-re-

sistant depression: a randomized clinical trial. JAMA Psychiatry. 2016; 73 (5):456–464

[54] Schlaepfer TE, Bewernick BH, Kayser S, Mädler B, Coenen VA. Rapid effects of deep brain stimulation for treatment-resistant major depression. Biol Psychiatry. 2013; 73(12):1204–1212

[55] Fenoy AJ, Schulz P, Selvaraj S, et al. Deep brain stimulation of the medial forebrain bundle: distinctive responses in resistant depression. J Affect Disord. 2016; 203:143–151

[56] Bewernick BH, Kayser S, Gippert SM, Switala C, Coenen VA, Schlaepfer TE. Deep brain stimulation to the medial forebrain bundle for depression- long-term outcomes and a novel data analysis strategy. Brain Stimul. 2017; 10(3): 664–671

[57] Blomstedt P, Naesström M, Bodlund O. Deep brain stimulation in the bed nucleus of the stria terminalis and medial forebrain bundle in a patient with major depressive disorder and anorexia nervosa. Clin case reports. 2017; 5 (5):679-684

[58] Jiménez F, Velasco F, Salin-Pascual R, et al. A patient with a resistant major depression disorder treated with deep brain stimulation in the inferior thalamic peduncle. Neurosurgery. 2005; 57(3):585–593, discussion 585–593

[59] Sartorius A, Kiening KL, Kirsch P, et al. Remission of major depression under deep brain stimulation of the lateral habenula in a therapy-refractory patient. Biol Psychiatry. 2010; 67(2):e9–e11

[60] Jiménez F, Nicolini H, Lozano AM, Piedimonte F, Salín R, Velasco F. Electrical Stimulation of the Inferior Thalamic Peduncle in the Treatment of Major Depression and Obsessive Compulsive Disorders. World Neurosurg. 2013; 80(3-4):S30.e17-S30.e25

[61] Kiening K, Sartorius A. A new translational target for deep brain stimulation to treat depression. EMBO Mol Med. 2013; 5(8):1151-1153

[62] Deli G, Balas I, Nagy F, et al. Comparison of the efficacy of unipolar and bipolar electrode configuration during subthalamic deep brain stimulation. Parkinsonism Relat Disord. 2011; 17(1):50–54

[63] Morishita T, Fayad SM, Higuchi M-A, Nestor KA, Foote KD. Deep brain stimulation for treatment-resistant depression: systematic review of clinical outcomes. Neurotherapeutics. 2014; 11(3):475–484

[64] Han MH, Nestler EJ. Neural substrates of depression and resilience. Neurotherapeutics. 2017; 14(3):677–686

[65] Cooper S, Robison AJ, Mazei-Robison MS. Reward circuitry in addiction. Neurotherapeutics. 2017; 14(3):687–697

[66] Drevets WC. Neuroimaging abnormalities in the amygdala in mood disorders. Ann N Y Acad Sci. 2003; 985(1):420–444

[67] Greenberg BD, Malone DA, Friehs GM, et al. Three-year outcomes in deep brain stimulation for highly resistant obsessive-compulsive disorder. Neuropsychopharmacology. 2006; 31(11):2384–2393

[68] Nuttin BJ, Gabriëls LA, Cosyns PR, et al. Long-term electrical capsular stimulation in patients with obsessive-compulsive disorder. Neurosurgery. 2003; 52 (6):1263–1272, discussion 1272–1274

[69] Malone DA, Jr. Use of deep brain stimulation in treatment-resistant depression. Cleve Clin J Med. 2010; 77 Suppl 3:S77–S80

[70] Hamilton M. A rating scale for depression. J Neurol Neurosurg Psychiatry. 1960; 23(23):56–62

[71] Gálvez JF, Keser Z, Mwangi B, et al. The medial forebrain bundle as a deep brain stimulation target for treatment resistant depression: A review of published data. Prog Neuropsychopharmacol Biol Psychiatry. 2015; 58:59–70

[72] Montgomery SA, Åsberg M. A new depression scale designed to be sensitive to change. Br J Psychiatry. 1979; 134(4):382–389

[73] Lipsman N, McIntyre RS, Giacobbe P, Torres C, Kennedy SH, Lozano AM. Neurosurgical treatment of bipolar depression: defining treatment resistance and identifying surgical targets. Bipolar Disord. 2010; 12(7):691–701

[74] Gippert SM, Switala C, Bewernick BH, et al. Deep brain stimulation for bipolar disorder-review and outlook. CNS Spectr. 2017; 22(3):254–257

[75] Drysdale AT, Grosenick L, Downar J, et al. Resting-state connectivity biomarkers define neurophysiological subtypes of depression. Nat Med. 2017; 23(1): 28–38

[76] Gadad BS, Jha MK, Czysz A, et al. Peripheral biomarkers of major depression and antidepressant treatment response: current knowledge and future outlooks. J Affect Disord. 201 8; 233:3–14

[77] Downar J, Geraci J, Salomons TV, et al. Anhedonia and reward-circuit connectivity distinguish nonresponders from responders to dorsomedial prefrontal repetitive transcranial magnetic stimulation in major depression. Biol Psychiatry. 2014; 76(3):176–185

[78] Yuan H, Mischoulon D, Fava M, Otto MW. Circulating microRNAs as biomarkers for depression: many candidates, few finalists. J Affect Disord. 201 8; 233

[79] Schatzberg AF, Kraemer HC. Use of placebo control groups in evaluating efficacy of treatment of unipolar major depression. Biol Psychiatry. 2000; 47(8): 736–744

[80] Schlaepfer TE. Deep brain stimulation for major depression—steps on a long and winding road. Biol Psychiatry. 2015; 78(4):218–219

[81] Etkin A. A glimmer of hope for depression. Sci Transl Med. 2016; 8(335): 335ec62

[82] Bentzley BS, Pannu J, Badran BW, Halpern CH, Williams NR. It takes time to tune. Ann Transl Med. 2017; 5(7):171–174

[83] Youngerman BE, Sheth SA. Deep brain stimulation for treatment-resistant depression: optimizing interventions while preserving valid trial design. Ann Transl Med. 2017; 5 Suppl 1:S1

[84] Richardson RM, Ghuman AS, Karp JF. Results of the first randomized controlled trial of deep brain stimulation in treatment-resistant depression. Neurosurgery. 2015; 77(2):N23–N24

[85] De Ridder D, Vanneste S, Langguth B. Deep brain stimulation of the ventral anterior limb of the internal capsule for treatment-resistant depression: possibilities, limits and future perspectives. Ann Transl Med. 2017; 5(7):167

[86] De Ridder D, Vanneste S. Targeting the parahippocampal area by auditory cortex stimulation in tinnitus. Brain Stimul. 2014; 7(5):709–717

[87] De Ridder D, Joos K, Vanneste S. Anterior cingulate implants for tinnitus: report of 2 cases. J Neurosurg. 2016; 124(4):893–901

[88] Fox MD, Buckner RL, Liu H, Chakravarty MM, Lozano AM, Pascual-Leone A. Resting-state networks link invasive and noninvasive brain stimulation across diverse psychiatric and neurological diseases. Proc Natl Acad Sci U S A. 2014; 111(41):E4367–E4375

[89] Riva-Posse P, Choi KS, Holtzheimer PE, et al. Defining critical white matter pathways mediating successful subcallosal cingulate deep brain stimulation for treatment-resistant depression. Biol Psychiatry. 2014; 76 (12):963–969

[90] National Commission for the Protection of Human Subjects of Biomedical and Behavioral Research. The Belmont Report: Ethical Principles and Guidelines for the Protection of Human Subjects of Research. Bethesda, MD; 1978. http://ohsr.od.nih.gov/guidelines/belmont.html

[91] Brain Research through Advancing Innovative Neurotechnologies (BRAIN) Working Group. BRAIN 2025: A Scientific Vision.; 2014. https://www.braininitiative.nih.gov/2025/index.htm

[92] National Institutes of Health. RFA-MH-18-500. BRAIN Initiative: Research on the Ethical Implications of Advancements in Neurotechnology and Brain Science (R01). 2017. https://grants.nih.gov/grants/guide/rfa-files/RFA-MH-18-500.html

[93] Leykin Y, Christopher PP, Holtzheimer PE, et al. Participants' perceptions of deep brain stimulation research for treatment-resistant depression: risks, benefits, and therapeutic misconception. AJOB Prim Res. 2011; 2(4):33–41

[94] Fisher CE, Dunn LB, Christopher PP, et al. The ethics of research on deep brain stimulation for depression: decisional capacity and therapeutic misconception. Ann N Y Acad Sci. 2012; 1265:69–79

[95] Rabins P, Appleby BS, Brandt J, et al. Scientific and ethical issues related to deep brain stimulation for disorders of mood, behavior, and thought. Arch Gen Psychiatry. 2009; 66(9):931–937

[96] Pycroft L, Boccard SG, Owen SLF, et al. Brainjacking: implant security issues in invasive neuromodulation. World Neurosurg. 2016; 92:454–462

[97] Broadway JM, Holtzheimer PE, Hilimire MR, et al. Frontal theta cordance predicts 6-month antidepressant response to subcallosal cingulate deep brain stimulation for treatment-resistant depression: a pilot study. Neuropsychopharmacology. 2012; 37(7):1764–1772

14 Deep Brain Stimulation in Tourette Syndrome

Fatu S. Conteh, Ankur Butala, Kelly Mills, Christina Jackson, William S. Anderson, Shenandoah Robinson

Abstract

Tourette Syndrome (TS) is a neuropsychiatric disorder characterized by repetitive, stereotyped motor and vocal tics; it is often accompanied by obsessive-compulsive disorder or attention deficit hyperactive disorder symptoms. Symptoms severity varies considerably with many patients having tics refractory to several pharmacologic or psychotherapeutic trials. For these patients, deep brain stimulation (DBS) has emerged as a viable treatment option. In this chapter, we review the diagnosis, management, and pathophysiology of TS relevant to neuromodulation. Current delivery by DBS electrodes allows alteration of dysfunctional corticostriatothalamic circuits implicated in DBS. We review the safety profile, relative reversibility, and titratability of DBS. Numerous reports and studies of DBS in TS support efficacy, ranging from 30% to more than 90% for TS symptoms assessed via standardized rating scales. We consider patient selection and surgical consideration, and analyze the published electrode targets: thalamic nuclei, subthalamic nucleus, globus pallidum, ventral internal capsule, nucleus accumbens, and substantia nigra. Finally, we review limitations including the Food and Drug Administration's investigational device exemption status, incomplete understanding of pathophysiology, or established biomarkers to inform postimplantation DBS programming. However, as more well-designed research in these areas emerge, DBS will likely prove to be an indispensable option for TS treatment.

Keywords: Tourette syndrome, tics, deep brain stimulation, neuromodulation

14.1 Introduction

Gilles de la Tourette syndrome (TS) is a complex neuropsychiatric and neurodevelopmental disorder whose treatment has been a challenge since Dr. Gilles de la Tourette first described it in 1885.[1,2,3,4] Its evolving epidemiology, elusive etiology, and heterogeneous character are driving changes in its diagnosis and treatment. Deep brain stimulation (DBS) is emerging as a promising treatment for patients with severe, refractory TS, and research into its application and safety continues to unfold.

14.2 Epidemiology of Tourette Syndrome

Once considered a rare disorder, TS has now been shown to be prevalent in all cultures[5,6,7] with wide range of reported incidence worldwide. Prevalence rates between 0.03 and 5.26%[5,7,8] have been reported in various population prevalence studies, but an international TS prevalence of 1% is safe to assume.[6,8] For the United States, at least, a more reliable estimate is that of The Diagnostic and Statistical Manual of Mental Disorders-5 (DSM-5), which gives prevalence ranges of 3 to 8 per 1,000 school-aged children and 3 per 1,000 in the U.S. population, with the male to female ratio ranging from 2:1 to 4:1, with a lower frequency in the African American and Hispanic populations.[9] Such wide variations in prevalence reflect the wide differences in study methodologies, diagnostic criteria, and variations in cultural awareness of TS. However, as more studied factors gain in precision, the need for and impact of novel treatments like DBS will be better quantified.

14.3 Characteristics of Tourette Syndrome

The initial description of TS included, among other symptoms, motor tics and vocal tics of varying complexity, intensity, duration, and frequency.[2,4] Tics are defined as sudden, rapid, recurrent, stereotyped, and nonrhythmic motor movements or vocalizations of varying intensity, frequency, and duration.[9] The criteria for diagnosing TS according to the DSM-5 is that an individual should have multiple motor and one or more vocal tics not due to a substance or a medical condition, starting before age of 18 years, and lasting for at least 1 year.[9] The presence of both motor and vocal tics is important in distinguishing TS from other tic disorders that are characterized by either motor or vocal tics. There are other diagnostic criteria for TS, as in the ICD-10 Classification of Mental and Behavioral Disorders, and the Chinese Classification of Mental Disorders-3 (CCMD-3), both of which are comparable to the DSM-5, although there's a higher prevalence of TS with CCMD-3.[10,11]

Tics usually begin between the ages of 4 and 6 years, peak in frequency around 10 years, and decrease during the adolescent and adult years. Most individuals never achieve complete remission.[7] According to DSM-5 description, tics may be either simple or complex, with a waxing and waning frequency.[9] Simple motor tics include eye blinking, shoulder shrugging, extremity extension, or head turning.[9] Simple vocal tics range from throat clearing to grunting or sniffing. Complex tics involve a combination of motor and/or vocal tics and include copropraxia (an obscene or sexual movement), echopraxia (an imitation of someone's movements), palilalia (repetition of sounds), echolalia (repeating the last heard word or phrase), or coprolalia (an obscene, ethnic, religious, or socially unacceptable utterance).[9] Coprolalia is an uncommon vocal tic with 10 to 15% prevalence in TS patients and usually occurs at a later age.[5] Among other features of tics are their suppressibility—individuals can voluntarily suppress a tic, although the tic usually rebounds with a greater intensity. Tics are also characterized by premonitory urges that are somatic sensations preceding the tic and can be suppressed. Because many tics occur in response to pathological urges where some degree of suppressibility is possible, the term "unvoluntary" has been applied to emphasize their location on a spectrum between voluntary and involuntary behavior.[12]

14.3.1 Comorbidities

The diagnostic challenge and complexity of TS lies not only in the varied character of tics that can present in a patient, but also in the various psychiatric, mood, and personality disorders that are usually comorbid with the tics. The most common are DSM-5 autism spectrum disorder (ASD), obsessive-compulsive disorder (OCD) or behavior (OCB), attention deficit hyperactive disorder (ADHD), oppositional defiant disorder (ODD), conduct disorder (CD), anxiety and depression. Migraines are also common in TS patients and are reported to occur in 25% cases.[13,14] Comorbid self-injurious behaviors (SIB), although rare, can be life-threatening and warrant intervention.[15,16] In one cross-sectional study,[17] diagnostic interviews of TS participants and their family members were conducted to find out the lifetime prevalence, heritability, ages of maximal risk, age at onset, and associations with symptom severity of comorbid disorders with TS. It was found that 85.7% of TS patients have one or more comorbid psychiatric disorder, with 57.7% patients having at least two.[17] A majority of their study population (72.1%) met the criteria for OCD or ADHD, and other mood disorders such as anxiety and disruptive behavior, each can be diagnosed in 30% of their interviewees.[17] The greatest risk for onset of these comorbidities was between 4 and 10 years, with ADHD and disruptive behaviors preceding tic onset and OCD, and anxiety beginning within a year before or after tic onset.[17] Furthermore, it was found, through genetic factors, that OCD further predisposes TS individuals to mood disorders and ADHD to disruptive behaviors. OCD was more common in females, adults and adolescents, and ADHD was more prevalent in males and children.[17] However, the study did not specifically isolate the prevalence of SIB which is one of the comorbidities that has a significant impact in selecting TS patients for DBS.[17,18,19]

14.3.2 Tic Measurement Scales

Various measurement and screening tools have been developed to aid in the diagnosis and management of TS and other tic disorders. One of the most widely used scale is the Yale Global Tic Severity Scale (YGTSS), which is a 15- to 20-minute clinician-rated scale covering multiple aspects of the patient's tics, including number, frequency, intensity, complexity, interference, and overall impairment.[2,20] The advantage of the YGTSS lies in its internal consistency, interrater reliability, and convergent and divergent validity.[20] In addition, the total tic severity subscore of the YGTSS can identify clinically significant changes of tics,[20] which is useful in evaluating responses to treatment in the clinical or research setting. However, the training requirement and the length of time to administer YGTSS can limit its use, especially in a fast-paced outpatient setting. Other measurement scales such as the Premonitory Urges for Tics Scale (PUTS) and the Rush Video-Based Tic Rating Scale (RVBTRS) are different in the dimensions they address and the methodology of tic evaluation, respectively, and are recommended as complements to the YGTSS.[21] The PUTS is the only scale that evaluates premonitory urges that are a defining characteristic of tics.[20] An important drawback of this scale is that its metric has a low yield in patients less than 10 years of age.[20] Similar to the YGTSS, the RVBTRS assesses tics along a list of dimensions, albeit a less exhaustive list.[20] It is, however, the only validated scale that uses video recordings to allow clinicians to get an objective measure of tics and also measure the ability of the patient to actively inhibit tics.[20] Specific scales, such as Tourette Disorder Scale, Motor tic, Obsessions and compulsions, Vocal tic Evaluation Survey (MOVES), and Autism-Tics, AD/HD and Other Comorbidities Inventory (A-TAC) are also available to assess for tics and their comorbid conditions.

14.4 Pathophysiology of Tourette Syndrome

The etiology of TS is still unknown, but several studies have suggested a strong genetic influence.[22,23] Twins studies have reported concordance as high as 86% in monozygotic twins, and family studies have shown that first-degree relatives of TS individuals are at greater risk of developing TS.[2,24] Further, genetic studies of TS argue for a multigenetic etiology, which might explain the co-occurrence of some psychiatric disorders with tics. Genome-wide association studies (GWAS) have identified several genes that might be related to TS, but only one gene on chromosome 2p, *NRXN1* (Neurexin 1) has reached genome-wide significance.[25,26] Many of the genes that have been implicated in TS are connected to neurotransmitters like dopamine and serotonin which have been shown to play key roles in various movement disorders.[21,23,25] For example, dopamine receptor D2 (DRD2), monoamine oxidase-A (MAO-A), and dopamine transporter-1 (DAT1) have all been suspects that are supported clinically by the efficacy of dopamine antagonists in suppressing tics.[24,25,27]

Surgery to manage TS symptoms lies in the theory that disruptions in the cortico-striato-thalamo-cortical network (CSTC) underlie the pathophysiology of TS.[2,27] The CSTC pathway includes circuits connecting the frontal cortex with deep subcortical structures such as the thalamus and the basal ganglia (BG), where parallel circuits are segregated based on cortical regions and functions. Notably, the BG is a crucial modulatory station for the CSTC loop circuitry, disinhibiting and inhibiting thalamus via the direct (striatum → GPi and SNr → thalamus) and indirect (STN → GPi and SNr → thalamus) pathway, respectively (▶ Fig. 14.1).[2,27] The striatum is thought to participate in the formation of complex preservative behaviors and facial movements, and stereotyped behaviors that are characteristics of TS and OCD.[27] Neuropathological and neuroanatomical evidence suggest that TS is the result of an aberrant focus of striatal neurons inhibiting globus pallidus pars interna (GPi) and substantia nigra pars reticulata (SNr) neurons, resulting in disinhibition of competing motor patterns and execution of adventitious behaviors (tics) (▶ Fig. 14.1).[27]

14.5 Treatment for Tourette Syndrome

As the frequency of tics waxes and wanes, some individuals with TS can tolerate their tics with moderate discomfort. However, for those in whom tics become a psychosocial impairment, create functional problems, or cause physical discomfort, treatment is indicated.[24,28] In many instances, the treatment approach also has to be targeted at comorbidities that are often more debilitating than the tics and may confound treatment results.[24,29,30] Behavioral modification methods and pharmacological treatment are first line and can be used exclusively or in combination.[24,28]

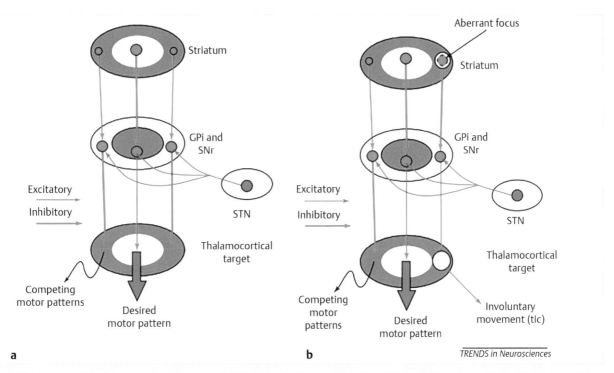

Fig. 14.1 The basal ganglia in a **(a)** normal patient versus **(b)** TS patient. In the normal circuitry, striatal inhibition of the globus pallidus interna (GPi) and substantia nigra pars reticulata (SNr) is less and subthalamic nucleus predominantly excites inhibitory GPi and SNr neurons, which inhibits thalamocortical targets and prevents involuntary movements (i.e., a tic). However, in the TS circuitry, an aberrant focus of striatal inhibitory neurons causes striatal inhibition of the GPi to predominate causing disinhibition of the thalamocortical target, allowing involuntary movements (tics) to occur. (Used with permission from Albin RL, Mink JW. Recent advances in Tourette syndrome research. Trends in Neurosciences. Elsevier; 2006.)

Behavioral modification methods include various refinements of cognitive behavioral therapy (CBT), which have been shown to be effective for tic reduction, with and without medication.[24] Examples of CBT include contingency management, relaxation training, habit reversal training (HRT), and comprehensive behavioral interventions (CBIT). Contingency management aims to control tics through the contingencies surrounding the tics (praise, rewords, and punishment).[24] Relaxation training reduces factors that exacerbate tics, such as stress and anxiety, and has been shown to be effective, although its effects are short-lived.[24] CBIT combines various aspects of other behavioral methods with the primary component being HRT. There have also been reports of possible benefits with acupuncture and alternative dieting therapies.[24]

The pharmacological management of TS involves several medications that alter neurotransmitters such as dopamine, norepinephrine, serotonin, and gamma-aminobutyric acid (GABA). These medications allow 30 to 65% improvement in tics, although the evidence for their effectiveness has been minimal to fair.[24,28] It must be noted that prior to starting any pharmacological treatment, it is important to identify the primary driver of disability as comorbid conditions such as OCD or ADHD respond well to specific medications.

A two-tiered approach to medication selection is recommended.[24] The first-tier medications are usually for mild TS symptoms and include the non-neuroleptics, like clonidine, guanfacine, topiramate, baclofen, and the benzodiazepines (▶ Table 14.1).[24] These drugs act primarily by decreasing noradrenergic or GABAergic neurotransmission. Their tic suppression effect is less than the neuroleptics, but these drugs are especially useful in TS patients with concomitant ADHD (clonidine, guanfacine) or anxiety (benzodiazepines).[24,28,29] Sedation is a common side effect with clonidine, guanfacine, and the benzodiazepines.[29] Blood pressure variability is especially a concern with clonidine and guanfacine may cause mania in patients with a high risk for bipolar disorder.[29]

Tier 2 medications are the typical neuroleptics such as haloperidol and pimozide and the atypical neuroleptics such as risperidone and olanzapine. These medications are classic D2 antagonists that decrease dopaminergic input to the BG. They have been shown to be 70 to 80% successful in suppressing tics.[24] However, it must be noted that tier 2 medications are usually used only after failure of tier 1 medications or for severe tics. The typical neuroleptics, especially haloperidol, have been shown to be very effective at suppressing severe tics, however, their side effects, including sedation, weight gain, metabolic derangements, and extrapyramidal symptoms like parkinsonism and tardive dyskinesia, limit their use.[24,28,29] Consequently, the atypical neuroleptics are supplanting the typical neuroleptics for treatment of severe tics, and some of these like risperidone have been shown to be equally effective.[31,32] Unlike typical neuroleptics, such as haloperidol, with a predominantly D2 antagonistic activity, the atypical neuroleptics, such as risperidone, are antagonists at D2, 5-HT2-A, and 5-HT2-C receptors.[28] However, metabolic derangements, especially weight gain, are a major concern and patients should have regular liver function tests, lipids, prolactin, and glucose labs while on atypical neuroleptics.[28,29]

Table 14.1 Treatment approaches for Tourette Syndrome

Nonpharmacological therapy	Pharmacological therapy	Surgical approaches
Behavioral modification methods	**Tier 1**	DBS
Contingency management	Clonidine	
Relaxation training	Guanfacine	
Cognitive behavioral therapy	Topiramate	
HRT	Baclofen	
CBIT	Levetiracetam	
	Clonazepam	
Alternative dietary therapies	**Tier 2**	Lesioning
Vitamin B6	Pimozide	
Magnesium	Fluphenazine	
Qufeng Zhidong Recipe	Risperidone	
Clerodendrum inerme plant	Aripiprazole	
	Haloperidol	
	Ziprasidone	
	Olanzapine	
	Quetiapine	
Acupuncture	**Other medications (tier 3)**	
Repetitive TMS	Tetrabenazine	
	Dopamine agonists	
	Pergolide	
	Pramipexole	
	Δ-9-THC	
	Donepezil	
	Botulinum toxin	
	Sulpiride and tiapride	
Treatment approach		
First line	**Second line**	**Third line**
Behavioral modification methods and/or tier 1	Initiate tier 2 medication and/or tier 1 or tier 3 medication	Tier 3
		DBS

Abbreviations: CBIT, comprehensive behavioral intervention for tics; DBS, deep brain stimulation; HRT, habit reversal training; TMS, transcranial magnetic stimulation.
Source: Adapted from Singer[24].

More recently, valbenazine vesicular monoamine transporter-2 (VMAT2) inhibitor has been considered in clinical trials and has shown promising results with significant improvement in symptoms as measured by the Clinical Global Impression scale.[33] However clinical trials for other VMAT2 inhibitors such as tetrabenazine and deutetrabenazine, have not been convincing.[34,35] Other trial data for therapies like cannabinoids for TS, specifically delta 9-tetrahydrocannabinol (Δ-9-THC), remain inconclusive with positive, yet small improvements in tic frequency and severity.[36,37,38]

Most TS patients have tics that are benign and do not cause any functional impairment;[16] however, about 5% of TS patients develop malignant TS, which is defined in one study as requiring two or more emergency room visits, or one or more hospitalizations due to TS symptoms or its comorbidities.[15,16] In some cases, TS individuals can have violent motor tics that result in severe neurological injuries like cervical myelopathy, stroke, spinal cord injury (especially with violent head jerking), and arterial dissection.[3,16] For these patients, neurosurgery may be a strong consideration. (▶ Table 14.1)

14.5.1 History of Lesioning

Neurosurgery to treat TS started with various ablative interventions at locations ranging from the frontal lobe to various subcortical structures to the cerebellum.[39,40] Many of these surgeries were reported to decrease tic frequency with minimal side effects, but some were ineffective, lacked accurate tic measurement scales and follow-up, and resulted in major complications such as quadriplegia.[39] Hassler and Dieckmann's thalamotomies, performed in the 1970s, were notable for their location, i.e., the intralaminar and medial thalamic nuclei, and ventro-oralis internus (Voi).[1,39] They reported 70 to 100% tic reduction when these sites were lesioned in each of the three patients.[39] Later thalamic DBS studies would report electrode placement at the centromedian nucleus–substantia periventricularis–Voi (CM–Spv–Voi) complex, stimulation of which would encompass the nuclei lesioned by Hassler and Dieckmann.[39]

14.5.2 Deep Brain Stimulation for Tourette Syndrome

The transition from lesioning to DBS began with Vandewalle's 1999 report in which they performed high-frequency DBS on a 42-year-old man with intractable TS, placing the electrodes at the CM–Spv–Voi complex to target the thalamic nuclei lesioned by Hassler.[39,41] They followed this case with two more similar ones and reported 70 to 90% tic reduction in all three patients.[39,41,42] Vandewalle and colleagues chose DBS because of its safety, reversibility, and adjustability, and since then the number of DBS cases and targets have been steadily rising.[39,43]

In their review of DBS for TS, Schrock et al identified at least seven different targets among the 120 cases reported, including: thalamus, GPi (postrema and anteromedial), GPe, the ventral anterior internal capsule, nucleus accumbens, and the substantia nigra.[19] Among these, the CM–Spv–Voi complex of the thalamus and the GPi are the most frequently targeted.

A 2016 systematic review and meta-analysis of DBS showed a significant symptom reduction in 80% of patients with an absolute YGTSS score reduction of 43.5 points.[44] Furthermore, their analysis of randomized, double-blinded controlled studies showed that DBS was effective in treating both vocal and motor tics in GTS, with a significantly greater reduction of vocal tics than motor tics.[44]

Thalamus

The thalamus is a major DBS target for TS treatment. Many studies target the motor thalamus, but despite the use of a common nomenclature to report targeted territories, the specific area that was stimulated varies across studies. Two widely used nomenclatures for the human motor thalamus are that of Hassler and Hirai and Jones.[45] In Hassler's classification, the motor thalamus is divided into lateral-polar (*lateropolaris, Lpo*), oral (*ventral-oralis anterior, Voa; ventral-oralis posterior, Vop*; and *ventral-oralis intermediate, Voi*), intermediate (*ventrointermedius, Vim*), and caudal (*ventrocaudalis, Vc*) segments.[45] In contrast, Hirai and Jones divided the motor thalamus into ventral anterior (VA), ventral medial (VM), ventral lateral (VL), and ventral posterior (lateral, VPL).[45] However, there is some level of overlap between the two systems. Hassler's Lpo, Voa, and Vop correspond to Jones's VA and VL (anterior) which receive pallidal afferents and project to the premotor cortex. Jones's VL (posterior) corresponds to Hassler's Vim and Voi, which receive deep cerebellar afferents and projects to the motor cortex.[45] The caudal segment of Hassler system corresponds to the posterior segment of Jones, receives medial lemniscus afferents, and sends efferents to the somatosensory cortex (▶ Fig. 14.2 and ▶ Table 14.2).

The intralaminar nuclei (the CM, and the parafasicular nucleus, Pf) and the Spv are also frequently used in DBS for TS. These nuclei form connections that are believed to regulate cortical, limbic, and striatal circuits whose dysfunction is implicated in the pathophysiology of TS.[43,47,48,49] The Spv has connections with the prefrontal cortex, nucleus accumbens, and amygdala, and it participates in awareness of vicerosensory stimuli and response to stress.[47] The CM–Pf complex is notable for its prevalent connections to the motor and limbic areas of the BG and is implicated in sensorimotor learning.[47,49] Despite their distinct projections, these nuclear regions are essentially similar in their morphology, electrophysiology, and connections to the cerebral cortex, striatum, and specific limbic nuclei.[43,47,49] They contain matrix cells, which are different from the typical thalamic relay cells in their diffuse projections to layer I of the cerebral cortex, and they receive major input from the reticular activating system, which might explain resulting side effects in arousal and energy levels when these nuclei are stimulated.[19,41,42,47,49]

Studies that report stimulation of only thalamic nuclei demonstrate 19 to 100% improvement on the YGTSS score.[19] For example, DBS of the Vop–Voa–Voi complex in two patients resulted in 75 to 100% improvement of the YGTSS score.[19] However, this is one of the few studies that target the Vop–Voa–Voi complex. Many thalamic DBS studies target the Voi, the midline periventricular nuclei, and the intralaminar CM–Pf complex. In their initial 1993 and 2003 publications, Visser-Vandewalle and

Table 14.2 Thalamic nuclei and their cortical projections

Input	Hassler	Hirai and Jones	Cortical projection
Pallidum	Voa, Vop	VLa	Premotor
Deep cerebellar	Vim, Voi	VLp	Motor
Medial lemniscus	Vci, Vce	VPM, VPL	Somatosensory

Abbreviations: Voa, ventral-oralis anterior; Vop, ventral-oralis posterior; Vim, ventrointermedius; Voi, ventral-oralis internus, VPL, ventral lateral posterior; VLa, Ventral lateral anterior nucleus; VLp, Ventral lateral posterior nucleus; VPM, Ventral posterior medial nucleus.

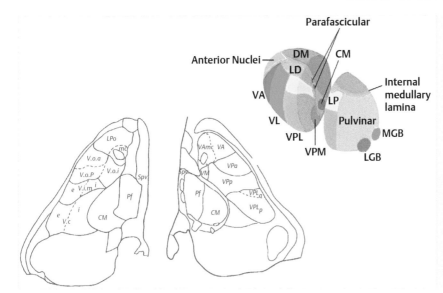

Fig. 14.2 Classification of thalamic nuclei according to Hassler (*left*) and Hirai and Jones (*right*).[45,46] (Reused with permission from Oxford Journals and University of Texas Health Science Center at Houston.)

colleague reported stimulation of the CM–Spv–Voi complex and achieving almost complete elimination of tics as measured by the RVBTRS.[19,41,42] Side effects from DBS of these targets included reduced energy levels and sexual dysfunction. The first randomized control trial (RCT) targeting the CM–Pf complex in five patients reported a 43.6% mean improvement in tics by the YGTSS.[50] Two patients, however, had a 4.3 to 260.9% increase in tic exacerbation, and one patient had an adverse effect of acute psychosis.

Other combinations of thalamic nuclei have also been used as targets. In his study of DBS therapy for 18 patients with severe TS, the largest prospective trial of DBS in TS to date, Servello targeted the CM–Pf complex along with the Voa and achieved 64.7% mean tic improvement on the YGTSS.[19,51] All of the 18 cases of TS were resistant to standard medical management and psycho-behavioral interventions for 6 months. Reported adverse events include transient vertigo and visual deficits.

Globus pallidus pars interna (GPi)

The GPi is frequently stimulated in Parkinson's disease (PD) and dystonia with good results.[52,53,54] Several case reports of DBS targeting the posterior-ventral-lateral GPi for TS have shown as high as 88% improvements in tics on the YGTSS.[19,55] A controlled, double-blind, randomized crossover study with electrodes both in the GPi and in the CM–Pf complex reported a 65 to 96% improvement of tics by the YGTSS when the GPi was stimulated, and a 30 to 64% improvement when the CM–Pf complex was stimulated, and a 43 to 76% improvement when both nuclei were stimulated.[56] Adverse effects of stimulating the GPi include hemorrhage and bradykinesia.

Globus pallidus pars externa (GPe)

Case reports of stimulating the GPe for TS demonstrated an 81 to 71% reduction in tics at 6 months, but with significant worsening at 2 years due to battery failure.[19,57,58] Interestingly, these reports show significant reductions in comorbid conditions as measured by their respective measurement scales. There were no reported adverse events.[19,57,58]

Ventral internal capsule/ventral striatum (VC/VS)

DBS of the VC/VS is approved for the treatment of refractory OCD in the United States under a Humanitarian Device Exemption (HDE) from the Food and Drug Administration (FDA). When applied to the treatment of TS, the reports are conflicting in terms of efficacy. Flaherty et al performed DBS targeting the VC/VS in a 37-year-old woman with severe TS and reported a 25% reduction in tics after 18 months.[19,59] Shields et al reported similar results with VC stimulation in a 40-year-old woman with head-snapping tics.[60] However, one lead extension in this patient fractured due to residual head snapping, so the electrodes were removed and reimplanted in the CM, after which the patient saw a significant reduction in tics.[60] Servello demonstrated improved tics when the VC/VS was simulated concurrently with the thalamus.[19,61] Other studies have reported a 41 to 56% improvement in YGTSS score with stimulation of the internal capsule/nucleus accumbens.[19]

Subthalamic nucleus (STN)

To date, there has been only one report of stimulation of the STN in a 38-year-old man with TS and PD.[62] The patient experienced a 97% reduction in his tics by the RVTRS, with no reported complications, but only with short-term follow-up (i.e., 1 year).

14.5.3 Selection Criteria

The heterogeneous nature of TS presentation and course makes patient selection for this procedure very difficult. Recognizing the growing interest in using DBS to treat tics in TS patients, the Tourette Syndrome Association (TSA) gathered a group of TS and DBS experts to develop the 2006 TSA guidelines to guide the selection of DBS for TS. These guidelines included exclusion and inclusion criteria for clinical trials and recommendations for reliable outcome measures and monitoring. In 2014, another panel of experts was constituted to revise the 2006 guidelines based on the growing evidence for DBS in TS.

The basic guidelines

In the 2006 guidelines, a DSM-IV diagnosis of TS was recommended which was then revised to a DSM-5 diagnosis in the more recent guidelines.[19,43] The age limit of 25 years in the previous guidelines was also removed, and an ethics committee consultation was also suggested for cases less than 18 years.[19,43] The recommendations for assessing tic severity remained unchanged—the tic disorder must be with functional impairment, with YGTSS score greater than 35/50, and must be documented with standardized video assessment.[19] The criteria regarding the accompanying neuropsychiatric comorbidities remained unchanged as well—tics should be the major symptom causing disability, and comorbid conditions should be stably treated and assessed using valid rating scales.[19] Criteria for failed conventional therapy were modified to include offering a trial of CBT rather than the old recommendation of evaluating the patient for suitability of behavioral interventions.[19] For psychosocial factors, a recommendation was added that a caregiver be available to accompany the patient for frequent follow-up, and that psychogenic tics, embellishment, factitious symptoms, personality disorders, and malingering be recognized and addressed.[19] Lastly, a recommendation for documentation of no active suicidal or homicidal ideation (SI/HI) was included.[19]

Inclusion and exclusion criteria

The most recent inclusion criteria are similar to those mentioned in the basic guidelines with added stipulations that individuals should demonstrate the ability to adhere to recommended treatments, and that the neuropsychological profile of the candidates should show that he or she could tolerate the demands of surgery, postoperative follow-up, and a possible poor outcome (see list below).[19] TS patients should be excluded from having DBS if there is a history of active SI/HI within 6 months of surgery, or active or recent substance abuse.[19] The subject should also be excluded if there is any structural lesion on brain magnetic resonance imaging (MRI), malingering, factitious disorder, or psychogenic tics, and if they have any medical, neurological, or psychiatric disorder that can increase the risk of failed DBS or interference with postop management.[19] Studies like the 2014 FDA-approved clinical trial of DBS for TS at Johns Hopkins (NCT 01817517) has adopted most of the TSA guidelines, including the inclusion and exclusion criteria, with few modifications.

TSA Inclusion and Exclusion Criteria for TS DBS

Inclusion Criteria

- DSM-V diagnosis of TS by expert clinician.
- Age is not a strict criterion. Local ethics committee involvement for cases involving persons < 18 years, and for cases considered "urgent" (e.g., impending paralysis from head-snapping tics).
- Tic severity: YGTSS score > 35/50.
- Tics are primary cause of disability.
- Tics are refractory to conservative therapy (failed trials of medications from 3 classes, CBIT offered).
- Comorbid medical, neurological, and psychiatric disorders are treated and stable x 6 months.
- Psychosocial environment is stable.
- Demonstrated ability to adhere to recommended treatments.
- Neuropsychological profile indicates candidate can tolerate demands of surgery, postoperative follow-up, and possibility of poor outcome.

Exclusion Criteria

- Active suicidal or homicidal ideation within 6 months.
- Active or recent substance abuse.
- Structural lesions on brain MRI.
- Medical, neurological, or psychiatric disorders that increase the risk of a failed procedure or interference with postoperative management.
- Malingering, factitious disorder, or psychogenic tics.

Source: Adapted from Schrock et al.[19]

Pre- and postoperative outcome measures

Successful application of DBS for TS not only requires careful selection of patients but also gathering the relevant pre- and postoperative information that is crucial to the surgery and subsequent management. The important preoperative information needed includes measurement of tic type and severity, evaluation of comorbidities using validated measurement and rating scales (YGTSS, RVTRS, etc.), documentation of TS medications including failed trials with start and stop dates, and measurement of quality of life or function.[19] In addition, the locations of the target(s) and leads, postop MRI or computed tomography (CT) for lead verification, and geometry of stimulation (bipolar versus monopolar, lead contact spacing, and location relative to target) are important.[19] Postoperatively, programming of the implanted pulse generator (IPG) and recording of outcome and adverse events should be noted. Common side effects to look for include exacerbation of tics, psychiatric comorbidities, dyskinesias, and immediate surgical complications such as hemorrhage and stroke.[63,64,65]

14.6 Surgical Flow and DBS Lead Placement

The surgery for DBS lead placement in TS has not been standardized, but it is typically performed with the patient intubated with or without microelectrode recordings (MER) to assist with localization and macrostimulation to look for stimulation-induced effects such as tetany. Despite the variation in nuclear targets for TS, there are key steps that are common across surgical approaches. These include defining the target location, refining the target location with an MER system, and confirming proper lead placement with imaging.

Defining the target location can be performed indirectly through the use of stereotactic coordinates or directly through visualization of the target nucleus on MRI. In indirect target localization, MRI or CT images are used to allow for high-resolution determination of stereotactic coordinates relative to a common reference point, such as the AC-PC line.[66] Using direct or indirect target localization often depends on the targeted nucleus. For example, many cases of subthalamic nucleus (STN) DBS lead placement have used direct MRI visualization, and some studies have shown direct visualization to be more superior to indirect localization for STN lead placement.[67]

Furthermore, frame-based, frameless, or intraoperative MRI techniques may all be used for lead placement.[66,68] In frame-based procedures, proper frame fixation is important for matching anatomical structures with MER signals in refining the target location for final DBS lead placement.

MER identifies action potential (or "spikes") from single neurons or local field potential (LFPs) from a group of neurons. Although MERs of various nuclei may differ between disease states,[69] specific subcortical brain structures can still be precisely localized on the basis of the characteristic amplitude, frequency, and pattern of their neuronal action potential or LFP. Recordings from the thalamic nuclei (Vo/CM-Pf) in TS patients typically exhibit a low-frequency (2.5–8 Hz) burst firing pattern from thalamic relay cells with alpha (8–13 Hz) LFPs,[70,71] and the frequency of action potentials in the VC, Vim, and Vop has been previously described in tremor and Parkinson's patients.[72] Furthermore, the GPe is characterized by irregular, higher frequency (50 ± 21 Hz) patterns from pause cells with intermittent lower frequency (18 ± 12 Hz) patterns from burst cells,[72] and the GPi shows a constant pattern of high-frequency (82 ± 24 Hz) action potentials.[72] Recordings in the nucleus accumbens show higher beta LFPs,[71] and the STN can be identified by its high background noise and frequent spontaneous discharges.[69] This step in refining the target location based on MER can be important after MRI stereotactic localization, as MRI images may demonstrate distortion. However, the use of MER usually increases the surgery time and may increase the risk of

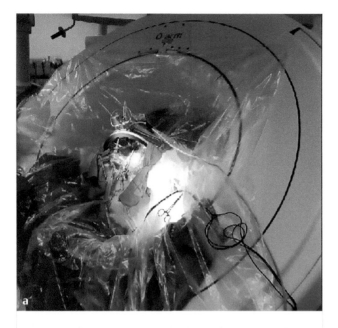

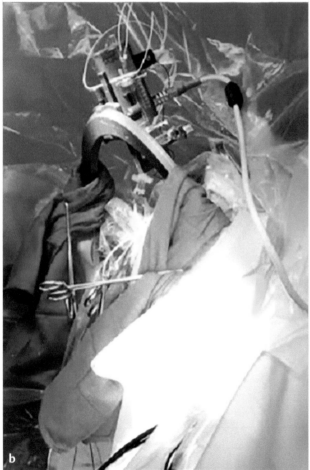

Fig. 14.3 (a, b) Standard frame-based deep brain stimulation setup used for lead placement. The operative field has been positioned inside an O-Arm intraoperative CT scanner, with the frame and microelectrode recording hardware attached to the frame.

complications such as hemorrhage of subcortical vessels due to multiple passes of the electrode[73] (▶ Fig. 14.3).

After the target has been refined and the DBS lead has been positioned at the desired target, prior to lead anchoring, the final lead location is tested intraoperatively with test stimulation. During the test stimulation, the voltage is increased, and the patient's extremities are examined for any tetanic responses or paresthesias in the case of thalamic targeting. The specific adverse effects elicited inform the neurosurgeon of the proximity of the DBS lead relative to certain structures and can also help guide postoperative programming of the IPG.

14.7 Postoperative Programming of the Pulse Generator for the DBS System

Postoperative programming of the IPG is performed transcutaneously and is aimed at finding the optimal stimulation parameters that will produce maximal tic suppression with minimal side effects and prolonged battery life (see ▶ Table 14.3 for one illustrative example from the clinical trial at Johns Hopkins). The typical DBS system consists of a quadripolar electrode attached to a lead that is connected to the neurostimulator/IPG via a lead extension. Each generator setting is a combination of a few parameters: the electrode polarity, pulse width, amplitude, and frequency.

Electrode polarity can be set as monopolar, which usually involves programming an electrode contact as the cathode with the IPG case as anode to produce a diffuse current stimulating a volume around the contact. Bipolar settings treat two electrode contacts as either anodal or cathodal to create a narrower and more focused stimulation volume.[74] The amplitude of stimulation determines the diameter or length of the stimulation volume. Also, tissue inhomogeneity and anisotropy has been shown to influence the shape of the stimulation volume.[75] The pulse width sets the duration of the current, and the frequency determines the rate at which the current is delivered. Stimulation frequency of the thalamus, GPi, and IC/Nac range from 60 to 200 Hz, amplitudes range between 1.5 and 6 V with constant voltage stimulation, and the pulse width can range from 60 to 210 μsecond.[43,74,76,77,78,79]

At present, there is no consensus on optimal postoperative DBS parameters in TS, and general ranges utilized are analogous to observations from other disorders. In practice, premonitory urge or subjective discomfort or frequency of motoric/vocal tics in office is utilized as a proxy for stimulation adjustments. For example, certain side effects such as vertigo and sedation often may respond to changes in amplitude and changes in frequency.[43] In the absence of a clear clinical correlate, basic principles of programming include reshaping or moving the volume of tissue activation to avoid stimulation of structures causing side effects, and increasing the amplitude and modifying the pulse width if symptoms persists.[77]

DBS programming in TS, in particular, highlights the limitations of existing open-loop systems. In open-loop systems,

Table 14.3 DBS settings and outcome of a patient from the TS DBS clinical trial at Johns Hopkins

Evaluation	Highest prior to surgery	At initial settings	2 weeks after initial settings
DBS settings		L - 4.0 V 130 Hz 60 µsec 1- Case + | R - 4.0 V 130 Hz 60 µsec 10- Case +	L - 5.0 V 130 Hz 60 µsec 1- Case + | R - 5.0 V 130 Hz 60 µsec 10- Case +
Total motor tic score	11	7	4
Total phonic tic score	18	11	7
Total tic score	28	18	11

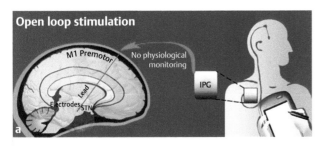
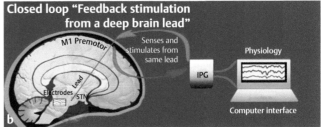
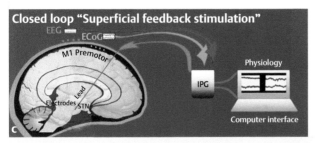
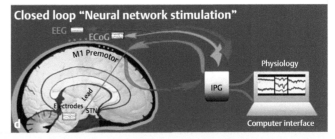

Fig. 14.4 Different modes of DBS. **(a)** Current DBS systems are mainly open-loops systems. **(b–d)** Possible modes of closed-loop systems. ECoG: electrocorticography, EEG: electroencephalogram, LFP: local field potential.[80]

stimulation parameters are preprogrammed by the physician and stimulation is delivered in a continuous and chronic fashion, regardless of the local neural environment (▶ Fig. 14.4a).[80] Given the intermittent and variable nature of tic expression and that TS patients often suffer from stimulation-induced complication, open-loop systems in DBS programming for TS may not be ideal. Closed-loop systems such as responsive or adaptive DBS (aDBS) are now being developed as an alternative.[80] These systems allow for real-time neural activity recordings to inform generator "on" or "off" settings, turning "on" only when symptoms appear, further preventing side effects and prolonging battery life.[43] One of the challenges to this paradigm, however, lies in identifying neural activity indicative of the pathologic or treated state. Early work has demonstrated consistent electrophysiological correlates detected via electrocorticography strips placed on the precentral gyrus for more complex or longer tics treated by triggered post-event depth electrode stimulation activation.[81] Other works have shown that LFPs, electrically evoked compound action potentials (ECAP), or the neurochemical environment may be used as feedbacks (▶ Fig. 14.4b).[80] For instance, increased thalamic gamma band activity has been shown to correlate with symptom relief following DBS in TS patients.[82] Cases of intermittent stimulation showing efficacy support the concept that continuous stimulation may not be required for tic reduction and at least one case of closed-loop ("responsive") DBS has been reported.[83,84]

14.8 Future Directions

DBS in TS has been a steadily growing field, but it is still a small field with broad reported ranges in its therapeutic efficacy, improvement in YGTSS ranging from 7 to 100%.[19] The lack of a coherent pathophysiology, the variable symptomatology of TS, and nonspecific pharmacotherapies have led neurosurgeons to stimulate numerous targets. In future, well-designed research and emerging close-loop systems such as adaptive DBS may provide more insight into the pathophysiology of TS, elucidate the clinical effect of different TS DBS targets, and enhance our understanding of the mechanism of DBS in TS. All this will help to fine-tune programming parameters to maximize tic reduction, prevent side effects, and guide the selection and application of DBS in TS.

References

[1] Rickards H, Wood C, Cavanna AE. Hassler and Dieckmann's seminal paper on stereotactic thalamotomy for Gilles de la Tourette syndrome: translation and critical reappraisal. Mov Disord. 2008; 23(14):1966–1972

[2] Gunduz A, Okun MS. A Review and Update on Tourette Syndrome: Where Is the Field Headed? Curr Neurol Neurosci Rep. 2016; 16(4):37

[3] Kumar A, Trescher W, Byler D. Tourette Syndrome and Comorbid Neuropsychiatric Conditions. Curr Dev Disord Rep. 2016; 3(4):217–221

[4] Lajonchere C, Nortz M, Finger S. Gilles de la Tourette and the discovery of Tourette syndrome. Includes a translation of his 1884 article. Arch Neurol. 1996; 53(6):567–574

[5] Robertson MM. The prevalence and epidemiology of Gilles de la Tourette syndrome Part 2: Tentative explanations for differing prevalence figures in GTS, including the possible effects of psychopathology, aetiology, cultural differences, and differing phenotypes. J Psychosom Res.

[6] Robertson MM, Eapen V, Cavanna AE. The international prevalence, epidemiology, and clinical phenomenology of Tourette syndrome: a cross-cultural perspective. J Psychosom Res. 2009; 67(6):475–483

[7] Robertson MM. The prevalence and epidemiology of Gilles de la Tourette syndrome Part 1: The epidemiological and prevalence studies. J Psychosom Res.

[8] Scharf JM, Miller LL, Gauvin CA, Alabiso J, Mathews CA, Ben-Shlomo Y. Population prevalence of Tourette syndrome: a systematic review and meta-analysis. Mov Disord. 2015; 30(2):221–228

[9] American Psychiatric Association. Diagnostic and Statistical Manual of Mental Disorders. 2013.

[10] Yang C, Zhang L, Zhu P, Zhu C, Guo Q. The prevalence of tic disorders for children in China: A systematic review and meta-analysis. Medicine (Baltimore). 2016; 95(30):e4354

[11] World Health Organization. The ICD-10 Classification of Mental and Behavioural Disorders.

[12] The Tourette Syndrome Classification Study Group. Definitions and classification of tic disorders. Arch Neurol. 1993; 50(10):1013–1016

[13] Kwak C, Vuong KD, Jankovic J. Migraine headache in patients with Tourette syndrome. Arch Neurol. 2003; 60(11):1595–1598

[14] Singer HS. Tourette syndrome: from behaviour to biology. Lancet Neurol. 2005; 4(3):149–159

[15] Cheung M-YC, Shahed J, Jankovic J. Malignant Tourette syndrome. Mov Disord. 2007; 22(12):1743–1750

[16] Patterson AL, Choudhri AF, Igarashi M, McVicar K, Shah N, Morgan R. Severe Neurological Complications Associated With Tourette Syndrome. Pediatr Neurol. 2016; 61:99–106

[17] Hirschtritt ME, Lee PC, Pauls DL, et al. Tourette Syndrome Association International Consortium for Genetics. Lifetime prevalence, age of risk, and genetic relationships of comorbid psychiatric disorders in Tourette syndrome. JAMA Psychiatry. 2015; 72(4):325–333

[18] Ganos C. Tics and Tourette: update on pathophysiology and tic control. Curr Opin Neurol. 2016; 29(4):513–518

[19] Schrock LE, Mink JW, Woods DW, et al. Tourette Syndrome Association International Deep Brain Stimulation (DBS) Database and Registry Study Group. Tourette syndrome deep brain stimulation: a review and updated recommendations. Mov Disord. 2015; 30(4):448–471

[20] Martino D, Pringsheim TM, Cavanna AE, et al. Members of the MDS Committee on Rating Scales Development. Systematic review of severity scales and screening instruments for tics: Critique and recommendations. Mov Disord. 2017; 32(3):467–473

[21] Mink JW, Walkup J, Frey KA, et al. Tourette Syndrome Association, Inc. Patient selection and assessment recommendations for deep brain stimulation in Tourette syndrome. Mov Disord. 2006; 21(11):1831–1838

[22] Pauls DL, Fernandez TV, Mathews CA, State MW, Scharf JM. The Inheritance of Tourette Disorder: A review. J Obsessive Compuls Relat Disord. 2014; 3(4):380–385

[23] Georgitsi M, Willsey AJ, Mathews CA, State M, Scharf JM, Paschou P. The Genetic Etiology of Tourette Syndrome: Large-Scale Collaborative Efforts on the Precipice of Discovery. Front Neurosci. 2016; 10:351

[24] Singer HS. Treatment of tics and tourette syndrome. Curr Treat Options Neurol. 2010; 12(6):539–561

[25] Ünal D, Akdemir D. Neurobiology of Tourette Syndrome. [Article in Turkish]. Turk Psikiyatr Derg. 2016; 27(4):275–285

[26] Paschou P, Forde NJ, Rizzo R, Stern JS, Mathews CA. The First World Congress on Tourette Syndrome and Tic Disorders: Controversies and Hot Topics in Etiology and Treatment. 2016;10.

[27] Albin RL, Mink JW. Recent advances in Tourette syndrome research. Trends in Neurosciences. 2006; 29(3):175–182

[28] Hartmann A, Worbe Y. Pharmacological treatment of Gilles de la Tourette syndrome. Neurosci Biobehav Rev. 2013; 37(6):1157–1161

[29] Roessner V, Plessen KJ, Rothenberger A, et al. ESSTS Guidelines Group. European clinical guidelines for Tourette syndrome and other tic disorders. Part II: pharmacological treatment. Eur Child Adolesc Psychiatry. 2011; 20(4):173–196

[30] Hartmann A, Martino D, Murphy T. Gilles de la Tourette syndrome—a treatable condition? Rev Neurol (Paris). 2016; 172(8–9):446–454

[31] Bruun RD, Budman CL. Risperidone as a treatment for Tourette syndrome. J Clin Psychiatry. 1996; 57(1):29–31

[32] Lombroso PJ, Scahill L, King RA, et al. Risperidone treatment of children and adolescents with chronic tic disorders: a preliminary report. J Am Acad Child Adolesc Psychiatry. 1995; 34(9):1147–1152

[33] Kim ES. Valbenazine: First Global Approval. Drugs. 2017; 77(10):1123–1129

[34] Jankovic J, Jimenez-Shahed J, Budman C, et al. Deutetrabenazine in Tics Associated with Tourette Syndrome. Tremor Other Hyperkinet Mov (N Y). 2016; 6:422

[35] Jankovic J, Glaze DG, Frost JD, Jr. Effect of tetrabenazine on tics and sleep of Gilles de la Tourette syndrome. Neurology. 1984; 34(5):688–692

[36] Müller-Vahl KR, Schneider U, Koblenz A, et al. Treatment of Tourette syndrome with □9-tetrahydrocannabinol (THC): a randomized crossover trial. Pharmacopsychiatry. 2002; 35(2):57–61

[37] Müller-Vahl KR, Schneider U, Prevedel H, et al. Delta 9-tetrahydrocannabinol (THC) is effective in the treatment of tics in Tourette syndrome: a 6-week randomized trial. J Clin Psychiatry. 2003; 64(4):459–465

[38] Curtis A, Clarke CE, Rickards HE. Cannabinoids for Tourette Syndrome. Cochrane Database Syst Rev. 2009(4):CD006565

[39] Temel Y, Visser-Vandewalle V. Surgery in Tourette syndrome. Mov Disord. 2004; 19(1):3–14

[40] Anderson WS, Lenz FA. Lesioning and stimulation as surgical treatments for psychiatric disorders. Neurosurg Q. 2009; 19(2):132–143

[41] Vandewalle V, van der Linden C, Groenewegen HJ, Caemaert J. Stereotactic treatment of Gilles de la Tourette syndrome by high frequency stimulation of thalamus. Lancet. 1999; 353(9154):724

[42] Visser-Vandewalle V, Temel Y, Boon P, et al. Chronic bilateral thalamic stimulation: a new therapeutic approach in intractable Tourette syndrome. Report of three cases. J Neurosurg. 2003; 99(6):1094–1100

[43] Andrade P, Visser-Vandewalle V. DBS in Tourette syndrome: where are we standing now? J Neural Transm (Vienna). 2016; 123(7):791–796

[44] Baldermann JC, Schüller T, Huys D, et al. Deep Brain Stimulation for Tourette-Syndrome: A Systematic Review and Meta-Analysis. Brain Stimul. 2016; 9(2):296–304

[45] Hamani C, Dostrovsky JO, Lozano AM. The motor thalamus in neurosurgery. Neurosurgery. 2006; 58(1):146–158, discussion 146–158

[46] Neuroanatomy Online. Lab 8 - Higher Motor Function - Thalamic Nucleus. http://nba.uth.tmc.edu/neuroanatomy/L8/Lab08p10_index.html. Accessed October 28, 2017

[47] Benarroch EE. The midline and intralaminar thalamic nuclei: anatomic and functional specificity and implications in neurologic disease. Neurology. 2008; 71(12):944–949

[48] Bentivoglio M, Fiorella Contarino M, Lee KH, et al. Deep brain stimulation for Tourette syndrome: the case for targeting the thalamic centromedian–parafascicular complex. Mini Rev Front Neurol. 2016; 7:193

[49] Testini P, Zhao CZ, Stead M, Duffy PS, Klassen BT, Lee KH. centromedian-parafascicular complex deep brain stimulation for Tourette syndrome: a retrospective study. Mayo Clin Proc. 2016; 91(2):218–225

[50] Maciunas RJ, Maddux BN, Riley DE, et al. Prospective randomized double-blind trial of bilateral thalamic deep brain stimulation in adults with Tourette syndrome. J Neurosurg. 2007; 107(5):1004–1014

[51] Servello D, Porta M, Sassi M, Brambilla A, Robertson MM. Deep brain stimulation in 18 patients with severe Gilles de la Tourette syndrome refractory to treatment: the surgery and stimulation. J Neurol Neurosurg Psychiatry. 2008; 79(2):136–142

[52] Follett KA, Weaver FM, Stern M, et al. CSP 468 Study Group. Pallidal versus subthalamic deep-brain stimulation for Parkinson's disease. N Engl J Med. 2010; 362(22):2077–2091

[53] Zhang X-H, Li J-Y, Zhang Y-Q, Li Y-J. deep brain stimulation of the globus pallidus internus in patients with intractable Tourette syndrome: a 1-year follow-up study. Chin Med J (Engl). 2016; 129(9):1022–1027

[54] Perlmutter JS, Mink JW. Deep. Brain Stimul. 2006; 29:229–257

[55] Dehning S, Mehrkens J-H, Müller N, Bötzel K. Therapy-refractory Tourette syndrome: beneficial outcome with globus pallidus internus deep brain stimulation. Mov Disord. 2008; 23(9):1300–1302

[56] Welter M-L, Mallet L, Houeto J-L, et al. Internal pallidal and thalamic stimulation in patients with Tourette syndrome. Arch Neurol. 2008; 65(7):952–957

[57] Filho OV, Ragazzo PC, Silva DJ, Sousa JT, Ribeiro TMC, Oliveira PM. Bilateral globus pallidus externus deep brain stimulation (GPe-DBS) for the treatment of Tourette syndrome: An ongoing prospective controlled study. Stereotact Funct Neurosurg. 2007; 85(1):42–43

[58] Piedimonte F, Andreani JCM, Piedimonte L, et al. Behavioral and motor improvement after deep brain stimulation of the globus pallidus externus in a case of Tourette syndrome. Neuromodulation. 2013; 16(1):55–58, discussion 58

[59] Flaherty AW, Williams ZM, Amirnovin R, et al. Deep brain stimulation of the anterior internal capsule for the treatment of Tourette syndrome: technical case report. Neurosurgery. 2005; 57(4 Suppl):E403; discussion E403

[60] Shields DC, Cheng ML, Flaherty AW, Gale JT, Eskandar EN. Microelectrode-guided deep brain stimulation for Tourette syndrome: within-subject comparison of different stimulation sites. Stereotact Funct Neurosurg. 2008; 86(2):87–91

[61] Servello D, Sassi M, Brambilla A, et al. De novo and rescue DBS leads for refractory Tourette syndrome patients with severe comorbid OCD: a multiple case report. J Neurol. 2009; 256(9):1533–1539

[62] Martinez-Torres I, Hariz MI, Zrinzo L, Foltynie T, Limousin P. Improvement of tics after subthalamic nucleus deep brain stimulation. Neurology. 2009; 72 (20):1787–1789

[63] Lyons KE, Wilkinson SB, Overman J, Pahwa R. Surgical and hardware complications of subthalamic stimulation: a series of 160 procedures. Neurology. 2004; 63(4):612–616

[64] Seijo FJ, Alvarez-Vega MA, Gutierrez JC, Fdez-Glez F, Lozano B. Complications in subthalamic nucleus stimulation surgery for treatment of Parkinson's disease. Review of 272 procedures. Acta Neurochir (Wien). 2007; 149(9):867–875, discussion 876

[65] Vergani F, Landi A, Pirillo D, Cilia R, Antonini A, Sganzerla EP. Surgical, medical, and hardware adverse events in a series of 141 patients undergoing subthalamic deep brain stimulation for Parkinson disease. World Neurosurg. 2010; 73(4):338–344

[66] Dormont D, Seidenwurm D, Galanaud D, Cornu P, Yelnik J, Bardinet E. Neuroimaging and deep brain stimulation. Am J Neuroradiol. 2010; 31(1):15–23

[67] Schlaier J, Schoedel P, Lange M, et al. Reliability of atlas-derived coordinates in deep brain stimulation. Acta Neurochir (Wien). 2005; 147(11):1175–1180, discussion 1180

[68] Bjartmarz H, Rehncrona S. Comparison of accuracy and precision between frame-based and frameless stereotactic navigation for deep brain stimulation electrode implantation. Stereotact Funct Neurosurg. 2007; 85(5):235–242

[69] Kobayashi K, Katayama Y. Intraoperative microelectrode recording. In: Deep Brain Stimulation for Neurological Disorders. Cham: Springer International Publishing; 2015:39–48.

[70] Marceglia S, Servello D, Foffani G, et al. Thalamic single-unit and local field potential activity in Tourette syndrome. Mov Disord. 2010; 25(3):300–308

[71] Priori A, Giannicola G, Rosa M, et al. Deep brain electrophysiological recordings provide clues to the pathophysiology of Tourette syndrome. Neurosci Biobehav Rev. 2013; 37(6):1063–1068

[72] Israel Z, Burchiel KJ. Microelectrode Recording in Movement Disorder Surgery. (Liu S, ed.). New York: Thieme Medical Publishers, Inc; 2004

[73] Maiti TK, Konar S, Bir S, Kalakoti P, Nanda A. Intra-operative micro-electrode recording in functional neurosurgery: Past, present, future. J Clin Neurosci. 2016; 32:166–72 2016

[74] Volkmann J, Herzog J, Kopper F, Deuschl G. Introduction to the programming of deep brain stimulators. Mov Disord. 2002; 17 Suppl 3:S181–S187

[75] Mcintyre CC, Mori S, Sherman DL, Thakor N V, Vitek JL. Electric field and stimulating influence generated by deep brain stimulation of the subthalamic nucleus. Clin Neurophysiol. 2004; 115 3:589–595

[76] Motlagh MG, Smith ME, Landeros-Weisenberger A, et al. Lessons Learned from Open-label Deep Brain Stimulation for Tourette Syndrome: Eight Cases over 7 Years.

[77] Neuner I, Podoll K, Lenartz D, Sturm V, Schneider F. Deep brain stimulation in the nucleus accumbens for intractable Tourette syndrome: follow-up report of 36 months. Biol Psychiatry.; 65:e5–e6

[78] Viswanathan A, Jimenez-Shahed J, Baizabal Carvallo JF, Jankovic J. Deep brain stimulation for Tourette syndrome: target selection. Stereotact Funct Neurosurg. 2012; 90(4):213–224

[79] Ackermans L, Temel Y, Cath D, et al. Dutch Flemish Tourette Surgery Study Group. Deep brain stimulation in Tourette syndrome: two targets? Mov Disord. 2006; 21(5):709–713

[80] Almeida L, Martinez-Ramirez D, Rossi PJ, Peng Z, Gunduz A, Okun MS. Chasing tics in the human brain: development of open, scheduled and closed loop responsive approaches to deep brain stimulation for Tourette syndrome. J Clin Neurol. 2015; 11(2):122–131

[81] Deeb W, Giordano JJ, Rossi PJ, et al. Proceedings of the Fourth Annual Deep Brain Stimulation Think Tank: A Review of Emerging Issues and Technologies. Front Integr Neurosci. 2016; 10:38

[82] Maling N, Hashemiyoon R, Foote KD, Okun MS, Sanchez JC. Increased Thalamic Gamma Band Activity Correlates with Symptom Relief following Deep Brain Stimulation in Humans with Tourette Syndrome. PLoS One. 2012; 7(9): e44215

[83] Molina R, Okun MS, Shute JB, et al. Report of a patient undergoing chronic responsive deep brain stimulation for Tourette syndrome: proof of concept. J Neurosurg. 201 8; 129(2):308–314

[84] Rossi PJ, Opri E, Shute JB, et al. Scheduled, intermittent stimulation of the thalamus reduces tics in Tourette syndrome. Parkinsonism Relat Disord. 2016; 29:35–41

15 Deep Brain Stimulation for Emerging Psychiatric Indications

Brett E. Youngerman, Smit Shah, Sameer A. Sheth

Abstract

Deep brain stimulation (DBS) has become a mainstay treatment for some neurological conditions, including Parkinson's disease, essential tremor, and dystonia. It has also demonstrated promise for a few psychiatric indications, including obsessive-compulsive disorder and depression. Previous chapters of this text book provide detailed, up-to-date accounts of the state of the science for these disorders. The success of DBS for these indications has led groups around the world to use this surgical platform to treat a variety of other neuropsychiatric disorders. The implicit assumption is that these disorders are manifestations of network-level dysfunction; if we can understand the underlying network and identify accessible nodes within it, we can perhaps treat disorders resulting from its dysfunction with targeted therapy such as DBS. In this chapter, we review the current state of DBS for these emerging indications, including anorexia nervosa, addiction and substance use disorders, aggressive and self-injurious behavior, post-traumatic stress disorder, and schizophrenia.

Keywords: anorexia nervosa, post-traumatic stress disorder, addiction, self-injurious behavior, schizophrenia

15.1 Introduction

Inspired by the success of deep brain stimulation (DBS) for the treatment of movement disorders and advances in the understanding of neural circuit dysfunction underlying brain disease, the last decade has seen a tremendous renewal of interest in neurosurgical interventions for the treatment of psychiatric disorders.[1,2] DBS for movement disorders, including Parkinson's disease, essential tremor, and dystonia, has demonstrated robust efficacy and it has become standard practice for appropriately selected patients. In 2009, the Food and Drug Administration (FDA) awarded DBS a Humanitarian Device Exemption (HDE) for obsessive-compulsive disorder (OCD) and evidence has continued to accumulate in favor of its efficacy.[2,3] As covered elsewhere in this book, DBS is under investigation for the treatment of refractory epilepsy, Tourette syndrome, and major depression.

In this chapter, we review the literature investigating the use of DBS for other emerging psychiatric applications, including anorexia nervosa (AN), addiction and substance use disorders, aggressive and self-injurious behavior (SIB), post-traumatic stress disorder (PTSD), and schizophrenia. For each indication, we briefly review the epidemiology and burden of refractory disease. We discuss advances in neuroanatomical and functional understanding of the diseases, including select human imaging and animal model findings, and the theoretical basis for proposed targets. Finally, we summarize the reported clinical experience with DBS for each indication.

15.2 Anorexia Nervosa

Anorexia nervosa (AN) is a chronic eating disorder characterized by abnormal patterns of eating behavior and distorted body image.[4] Features include strict attitudes toward body weight and shape along with abnormal perception of body image. Individuals with AN demonstrate restricted food intake along with ritualized consumption of a low-calorie diet. AN is more common in women than men, with a lifetime prevalence as high as 2% in American women.[5] Acute interventions include nutrition and treating the medical sequelae of prolonged starvation. Mainstays of longer-term therapy aimed at behavior modification include medications (i.e., selective serotonin reuptake inhibitors and antipsychotics) and cognitive behavioral therapy. However, approximately 30% of patients do not significantly improve, and mortality rates approach 15%, inclusive of medical complications and suicide.[6] Family therapy has been relatively successful for the treatment of adolescents, who have the best prognosis,[7] but there has been minimal improvement in treatments for adults, who are often highly refractory to intervention.[4]

Imaging studies in patients with AN have suggested certain reproducible patterns of neural dysfunction. Studies have demonstrated general sequelae likely related to poor nutrition including cerebral atrophy of both gray and white matter and a secondary relative increase in cerebrospinal fluid volume. More specifically, anorexic patients have different responses to distorted body image from controls including hyperactivity in the prefrontal cortex and inferior parietal lobule, suggesting dysfunction in perceptual pathways.[8] They may also have different appetite regulation and dysfunction in the reward system, which is associated with comorbid mood disorders.[9] Exposure to food is associated with abnormal activity in the insula, orbitofrontal cortex, and multiple regions of the cingulate cortex. These patients may also experience anxiety provocation and amygdala activation upon eating or exposure to food.[10]

AN has high comorbidity with mood disorders and OCD and shares many of the behavioral phenotypes. There has been significant overlap in neurosurgical targets for both OCD and depression. In the past, lesioning procedures including anterior capsulotomy, thalamotomy, and limbic leucotomy demonstrated success for highly refractory cases of AN, but adoption has been limited, largely due to the risk of permanent side effects.[11,12] Success of DBS for OCD has led to interest in its use for AN treatment.

DBS for AN has been reported in the subcallosal cingulate sulcus (SCC), the nucleus accumbens (NAcc), and ventral capsule/ventral striatum (VC/VS), all of which have been targets for depression, OCD, or both. However, investigation of these targets in AN is at an earlier stage, with evidence limited to open-label case series and reports (▶ Table 15.1).

Lipsman et al initially demonstrated promising results of DBS of the SCC in six patients with AN at 9-months follow-up.[13] As

Table 15.1 Selected studies of DBS for anorexia nervosa

Author	Patients	Study type	Target	Follow-up	Outcome
Lipsman et al.[14]	16[a]	Prospective, open label	SCC	1 year	Increase in mean BMI from 13.83 (SD = 1.49) to 17.34 (SD = 3.40), p = 0.0009 Improvement in depression, anxiety, and affective regulation Changes in PET glucose metabolism
Lipsman et al.[13]	6	Prospective, open label	SCC	9 months	Three out of six patients had an increase in BMI Four out of six patients had improvement in depression, anxiety, affective regulation, and AN-related obsessions and compulsions Changes in PET glucose metabolism
Wu et al.[18]	2	Case series	NAcc	1 year	Increase in BMI from 13.3 and 12.9 at baseline to 18.0 and 20.8, respectively Improvement in anxiety, depression, and attitudes toward food
Wang et al.[17]	4	Case series	NAcc	Multiple years	Increase in mean BMI from 11.9 to 19.6 Remission after DBS explant
McClaughlin et al.[19]	1	Case report	VC/VS	NA	Improvement in eating habits and BMI

Abbreviations: AN, anorexia nervosa; BMI, body mass index; NA, not available; NAcc, nucleus accumbens; SCC, subcallosal cingulate sulcus; VC/VS, ventral capsule/ventral striatum.

[a]Includes six patients from Lipsman et al.[13]

of their most recent publication, 16 patients aged 20 to 60 years with chronic (average duration 18 years), treatment-resistant AN (restricting or binge-purging subtype) have undergone DBS of the SCC and open-label continuous stimulation.[14] At 1 year, mean body mass index (BMI; normal range 18.5–25) increased from 13.83 (SD = 1.49) to 17.34 (SD = 3.40) kg/m^2 (p = 0.0009). Patients also experienced significant improvements in depression, anxiety, and affective regulation. Given the precarious health of patients with chronic anorexia, the primary endpoint of the trial was safety. Serious adverse events were largely attributable to the underlying disorder with few major procedure-related complications.

Positron-emission tomography (PET) imaging at 6 and 12 months showed significant changes in glucose metabolism in multiple brain structures implicated in AN, suggesting that DBS can alter relevant brain circuitry. Activity in the SCC and the immediately adjacent anterior cingulate was reduced with chronic stimulation, and parietal areas including the supramarginal gryus and cuneus developed significant hyperactivity over time. The cingulate plays an important role in selective processing and the assignment of reward value to external stimuli, both of which are abnormal in patients with AN.[15] There are direct projections from the SCC to the affected parietal areas. Prior studies had shown hyperactivity in the anterior cingulate and hypometabolism in the parietal regions in both acutely ill and recovered AN patients.[16] The PET findings suggest a reversal of the functional imaging abnormalities seen in AN and thus a potential therapeutic mechanism for the intervention.

The primary limitation of the study was its open label nature, making it susceptible to placebo effect and other biases. However, the sustained clinical improvement at 1-year follow-up and objective imaging changes are promising. The authors plan continued long-term follow-up and favor a sham-controlled, randomized trial. They also favor inclusion of hormonal markers in future trials, as there are often significant hormonal disturbances in patients with AN, and such biomarkers offer an objective outcome metric not always available in studies of psychiatric disease.

Evidence for the NAcc and VC/VS is more limited. Wu et al reported on two patients who underwent DBS of the NAcc and experienced increases in BMI from 13.3 and 12.9 at baseline to 18.0 and 20.8, respectively, at 1-year follow-up.[17] They also had improvement in anxiety and depressive symptoms, and in attitudes toward food. Notably, they had normalization of core temperature and heart rate. In another report, four patients who underwent NAcc DBS experienced an increase in average BMI from 11.9 to 19.6 over varying multi-year time periods with persistent benefit after removal.[18] However, these patients were all adolescents with relatively short histories (less than 2.5 years) of AN. Given that this cohort is more likely to have resolution of symptoms with medication and therapy,[7] these findings may be influenced by natural history. Finally, in a single case report of VC/VS DBS primarily for OCD, the patient had improvement in comorbid AN including eating habits and BMI.[19]

15.3 Addiction and Substance Use Disorders

Addiction is a broad category of disorders characterized by compulsive, repetitive engagement in behaviors with negative physical, psychological, or social consequences.[20] Addiction includes substance use disorders, as well as other potentially compulsive behaviors such as gambling. The annual prevalence is over 30% for smoking, 7% for alcohol abuse, and 5% for other illicit drug use.[21] While there is often a component of increased tolerance and physical withdrawal in substance use disorders, preoccupation with the addictive behavior and relapse often occur in the absence of these effects or after they have subsided.[22] These clinical observations, along with numerous imaging and animal model studies, suggest that addiction involves underlying or longer-term brain dysfunction, most likely in the reward system.

Neural mechanisms of addiction are well studied and have led to a focus on the NAcc as a potential target for stimulation. Psychoactive substances lead to activation of the reward system. Dopaminergic neurons project from the ventral tegmental area (VTA) to the VS (including the NAcc), the amygdala and septal nuclei, and the prefrontal and cingulate cortices.[22,23,24] The connections between the VTA and NAcc modulate reward learning and repetitive behavior, making them particularly relevant in addiction.

Several targets have been studied for surgical lesions in patients with addiction. Lesions of the anterior cingulate, hypothalamus, and subcallosal white matter have all been attempted in open-label series, with varying measures of efficacy and adverse effects.[23] In 2003, Gao et al reported 28 patients who underwent bilateral NAcc ablation for addiction.[25] The study suffered from poor follow-up, but complete remission was reported in 7 patients (mean follow-up 15 months), and an additional 10 patients relapsed within 6 months but experienced alleviation of withdrawal symptoms. There was a 19.2% rate of serious complications including temporary memory loss and personality changes, which further limited adoption. However, the advent of DBS has offered the opportunity for a less destructive, titratable intervention.

Animal studies have demonstrated that stimulation of the NAcc attenuates behaviors learned in association with substances of abuse.[26,27,28] It is not clear if stimulation acts by reducing the rewarding value of the substance or by decreasing the association between behavior and reward.[29]

There are several small series and case reports describing DBS for primary or comorbid abuse of heroin, alcohol, or cigarette smoking (▶ Table 15.2). Two case reports describe patients treated with bilateral NAcc stimulation for heroin addiction. Zhou et al reported a patient who was explanted after 3 years but remained abstinent at last follow-up of 6 years.[30] The patient treated by Valencia-Alfonso et al remained abstinent at 6 months. Interestingly, in the latter report, different stimulation parameters reportedly correlated reliably with increases or decreases in drug use, cravings, and intracranial EEG responses to images of heroin.[31]

Kuhn and colleagues reported two successful cases of NAcc DBS for chronic alcoholism. In the first case, a patient treated for severe anxiety and depression did not see improvement in these symptoms but did have resolution of his comorbid alcoholism at 1 year.[32] A second patient later underwent implantation primarily for chronic alcoholism and achieved abstinence at 1-year follow-up.[33] Notably, this patient also had improvement in error-related negativity, an electrophysiological marker linked to the anterior cingulate cortex. In a small initial series of three patients from another institution, two of the three patients who underwent NAcc DBS for alcoholism were abstinent at 1 year.[34] In an expanded series of five patients, however, only two remained abstinent at 4 years, though all patients had significant reductions in alcohol consumption and cravings.[35]

Evidence for NAcc DBS for smoking comes exclusively from observed changes in patients treated for other primary indications. In a single case report, a patient who responded successfully to treatment of her OCD also experienced concurrent smoking cessation (and weight loss), which was sustained at 2-year follow-up.[36] In a series of 10 smokers who underwent DBS primarily for Tourette syndrome, OCD, or anxiety, only 3 patients had stopped smoking at 30 months.[37] The use of retrospective self-assessment of baseline nicotine dependence limits interpretation of results in this series, but smoking cessation was unaided and most patients exhibited decreases in smoking.

15.4 Aggressive and Self-Injurious Behavior

Neurosurgery has historically been employed to treat a range of disorders involving aggression and poor impulse control. Aggressive behavior is increasingly common in patients with a variety of brain insults in association with mental retardation and epilepsy.[38] Similarly, SIB is observed in similar patients, as well as those with severe autism. These behaviors are notoriously refractory to behavioral interventions and neuroleptic medications, at least at doses that are not excessively sedating.

The amygdala is a potential target for DBS in aggressive behavior. The amygdala and its projections have a role in anger processing, fear response, and relevance detection.[39] It also has a role in social processing, which is believed to be dysfunctional in autism. Historically, bilateral amygdala ablation was used in the treatment of epilepsy with comorbid aggression, but aberrant behavior eventually became the primary indication in the

Table 15.2 Selected studies of DBS for addiction and substance use disorders

Author	Patients	Study type	Abused substance	Target	Follow-up	Outcome
Zhou et al.[30]	1	Case report	Heroin	NAcc	6 years	The patient remained abstinent
Valencia-Alfonso et al.[31]	1	Case report	Heroin	NAcc	6 months	The patient remained abstinent
Voges et al.[35]	5[a]	Case series	Alcohol	NAcc	4 years	Two of five patients remained abstinent; all reported reduced craving and consumption
Müller et al.[34]	3	Cases series	Alcohol	NAcc	1 year	Two of three patients remained abstinent
Kuhn et al.[32]	1	Case report	Alcohol	NAcc	1 year	The patient decreased intake
Kuhn et al.[33]	1	Case report	Alcohol	NAcc	1 year	The patient remained abstinent
Mantione et al.[36]	1	Case report	Smoking	NAcc	2 years	Cessation in one patient
Kuhn et al.[37]	10	Case series	Smoking	NAcc	30 months	Cessation in three of ten patients (unaided)

Abbreviation: NAcc, nucleus accumbens.
[a]Includes three patients from Müller et al.[34]

Table 15.3 Selected studies of DBS for aggressive and self-injurious behavior

Author	Patients	Study type	Indication	Target	Follow-up	Outcome
Sturm et al.[40]	1	Case report	SIB with MR and autism	Amygdala	24 months	Improvement in SIB and autism symptoms
Franzini et al.[42]	7	Case series	Aggression and MR	PHR	1–9 years	Six of seven patients had reduced aggression and violent outbursts
Hernando et al.[43]	1	Case report	Aggression and MR	PHR	18 months	Significant improvement
Kuhn et al.[38]	1	Case report	SIB and TBI	PHR	4 months	Resolution of SIB
Giordano et al.[44]	1	Case report	Aggression and MR	VC/VS	22 months	Improvement in explosive outbursts
Taira et al.[45]	1	Case report	SIB and Lesch–Nyhan syndrome	GPi	24 months	Resolution of SIB

Abbreviations: GPi, globus pallidus internus; MR, mental retardation; PHR, posterior hypothalamic region; SIB, self-injurious behavior; TBI, traumatic brain injury.

1960s and 1970s.[2,39] These ablations were associated with reduced autonomic response to stressful stimuli and hypersexuality (i.e., Klüver–Bucy syndrome) and fell out favor with the growing use of pharmacologic restraint.[2] However, the growing applications of DBS and its reversible nature have renewed interest in the amygdala as a target. In one case report,[40] a 13-year-old boy with SIB, mental retardation, and autism, who had failed multiple trials of behavioral and pharmacotherapy, underwent bilateral DBS to the basolateral amygdala (BLA) (▶ Table 15.3). The patient experienced improvement in SIB as well as emotional, social, and cognitive symptoms of the autism spectrum over 24 months.

Another potential DBS target for aggression is the posterior hypothalamic region (PHR), an area with known connections to the amygdala and the medial limbic circuit. The PHR has also been a target for lesioning in patients with aggression, epilepsy, and mental retardation. DBS of the region was first reported by Franzini et al in the treatment of trigeminal autonomic cephalalgias to reduce pain and associated bouts of aggression.[41] The same group has since reported bilateral DBS in seven adult patients with aggression and severe mental retardation (IQ 20–40).[42] Six of seven patients had a reduction in aggression and violent outbursts. There are two other case reports of PHR DBS for aggression in the literature. Hernando et al[43] reported a 22-year-old patient with aggression and mental retardation who had significant improvement at 18 months with low-frequency (15 Hz) simulation. Kuhn et al[38] reported a 22-year-old woman with SIB and severe traumatic brain injury who had resolution of symptoms after 4 months of DBS.

Most recently, Giordano et al[44] performed bilateral VC/VS stimulation in a 21-year-old man with intermittent explosive disease and mild mental retardation secondary to hypoxia at birth. He had significant improvement at 22 months. Like the PHR, the VC/VS is a node in the mesolimbic pathway.

Finally, the SIB associated with Lesch–Nyhan syndrome may benefit from DBS targeting different pathways. Taira et al[45] reported a 19-year-old man with Lesch–Nyhan syndrome who underwent bilateral globus pallidus internus (GPi) DBS primarily for control of dystonic involuntary movements and had complete resolution of self-mutilating behavior at 24 months. The finding may be specific to patients with Lesch–Nyhan syndrome, suggesting that the self-mutilating behavior in this syndrome is mediated at least in part by basal ganglia pathways or is secondary to the dystonia.

15.5 Post-traumatic Stress Disorder

Post-traumatic stress disorder (PTSD) is characterized by a constellation of psychological and physical symptoms that occur after exposure to a traumatic event. Symptoms include intrusive thoughts or re-experiencing of the traumatic event, avoidance of associated stimuli, alterations in mood, and symptoms of hyperarousal.[46] It can cause significant distress, interfere with social and occupational functioning, and is associated with comorbid mood disorders, anxiety, and substance abuse. Lifetime prevalence in the United States is estimated between 5 and 8%[47] with significantly higher rates among soldiers who have experienced combat. Approximately 20 to 30% of patients are considered refractory to medication and psychotherapy.[48]

Numerous studies have found an association between PTSD and changes in the amygdala. The amygdala is believed to play a key role in fear conditioning and PTSD is a disorder of aberrant fear extinction. Functional imaging studies demonstrate increased amygdala activity in patients with PTSD that correlates with severity of symptoms and decreases with clinical improvement.[49] However, the amygdala has multiple subregions with other limbic and associative functions. The precise target and stimulation parameters will likely influence the effect of stimulation. Damage to the amygdala correlates with development of PTSD,[50] and stimulation of the amygdala can produce anger, fear, and anxiety in subjects without PTSD.[46] Preclinical animal models of conditioned fear and anxiety have suggested that stimulation of the BLA is anxiolytic and aids in fear extinction.[51,52,53]

A clinical of trial of DBS to the BLA is currently underway (NCT02091843).[54] In the only available case report, a combat veteran who underwent BLA DBS had a 37.8% reduction in the Clinician Administered PTSD Scale (CAPS) score at 8 months follow-up.[55] The frequency of nightmares decreased from daily to monthly, and average uninterrupted sleep increased from 2 to 5-hour intervals. Neuropsychological testing at 6 months was unaltered.

There are several other regions involved in fear conditioning and extinction that have been proposed as potential DBS targets. Some that have shown promise in animal models include the hippocampus,[56] VS,[57] and prefrontal cortex.[58]

15.6 Schizophrenia

Schizophrenia is a heterogeneous disorder characterized by varying degrees of psychotic positive symptoms, negative affective and social symptoms, and cognitive dysfunction.[59] The disease is a chronic, life-altering diagnosis. Many patients are unable to maintain a job or residence. Social isolation and medical comorbidities are common. The prevalence of schizophrenia in the United States is approximately 1.1%, and 10 to 30% of patients have little or no response to antipsychotic medication.[60] There are limited alternative treatments for these refractory patients.

Dopamine dysregulation plays a major role in schizophrenia. Positive delusions and hallucinations in schizophrenia are associated with excessive dopamine release from the VTA into the striatum. The dysregulation of tonic and phasic dopaminergic signals that normally have a role in prediction error and assignment of salience to stimuli may contribute to the downstream cortical development of hallucinations.[61] Incentive salience also involves a broader cortical network including the anterior cingulate cortex, insula, and inferior frontal gyrus.

Clinical trials of DBS for schizophrenia have thus far focused on the SCC and the NAcc in the VS. In an abstract presented at the American Association of Neurological Surgeons (AANS) Annual Scientific meeting, Roldán et al presented preliminary results from a trial of DBS to the SCC or NAcc for treatment-resistant schizophrenia (NCT02377505) in Barcelona, Spain.[62,63] Seven patients with treatment-resistant, chronic paranoid schizophrenia were randomized to DBS of either the SCC or the NAcc. Patients were followed under open conditions, and if they maintained clinical improvement at 6 months they entered a double-blind crossover phase in which stimulation was turned on or off every 3 months. All patients had progressive improvement in social isolation symptoms and auditory hallucinations at 12 months. Final results are pending with one additional patient planned.

An open-label trial of DBS to the NAcc/VS and VTA for treatment of negative symptoms from Toronto, Canada was withdrawn prior to enrollment (NCT01725334). The Johns Hopkins University is currently recruiting for a trial focused on treating positive symptoms with DBS of the substantia nigra pars reticulata (NCT02361554). No results have yet been reported from this trial.

Another proposed target for DBS in schizophrenia is the hippocampus.[61] Hippocampal activation in response to novel stimuli is associated with dopamine release from the VTA into the striatum. Hippocampal hyperactivity and long-term atrophy are seen in patients with schizophrenia and may be associated with aberrant dopamine release. No clinical trials have yet been reported. Further details regarding theories of circuit dysfunction in schizophrenia and the relative suitability of these targets for DBS is available in a recent review by Mikell, et al.[61]

15.7 Conclusion

Inspired by the success of DBS for movement disorders and advances in the understanding of neural circuit dysfunction underlying brain disease, the last decade has seen a tremendous renewal of interest in neurosurgical interventions for the treatment of psychiatric disorders. Interest has converged on several key brain structures and pathways involved in reward, prediction error, salience, and anxiety. This convergence likely reflects the high degree of comorbidity seen in many of the aforementioned psychiatric disorders, and future directions may focus on treating more specific symptom complexes and functional or structural imaging abnormalities, rather than broad disease categories defined by diagnostic criteria.[64] While the growing experience with DBS suggests that it can be performed in a wide variety of brain targets with minimal and largely reversible side effects, DBS remains an invasive procedure with associated surgical risks (i.e., hemorrhage, infection, hardware malfunction) as well as significant potential neurologic side effects, which are also target-dependent.

Demonstration of efficacy remains challenging if the threshold is an adequately powered sham-controlled, double-blind, randomized trial. The emerging indications for DBS described here are at very early proof-of-principle stages. A large trial would be very expensive and run a high risk of failing to demonstrate efficacy. An overly zealous rush to a large trial has been blamed for the two halted DBS for depression trials.[65] An important lesson learned from that experience is that a deeper understanding of the underlying circuitry is essential before embarking on a large, expensive trial. Developing this understanding is particularly challenging for these disorders, as they involve very human emotions and experiences and are therefore difficult to study in animal models. The starting step would be to design a smaller trial to test whether DBS has the intended physiological effect on the network. Such a trial would show that the desired target has been engaged and demonstrate the network's response properties to stimulation across a range of parameters. This information is critical to informing the design of a later pivotal trial. Large trials must also be efficient in the strategy they employ for programming adjustments. They are already expensive, and spending an inordinate amount of time exploring the parameter space would make them unfeasible, as well as increase the risk of biased dropout of non-responders before the cross-over phase and unblinding during it. A smaller trial would be "quick to fail" if the chosen target did not respond as predicted, allowing the field to nimbly move on to other ideas.

DBS for these emerging indications faces significant challenges. Patient recruitment, cost, identification and consistency of neurosurgical targeting, and the requirement of sufficient multidisciplinary expertise are just a few to name. Nevertheless, the extreme refractoriness and disability burden of these disorders, alongside the promise shown to date with DBS, continue to propel efforts worldwide. It is, therefore, highly likely that future efforts will continue to carve significant inroads in DBS as a treatment option for an increasing number of psychiatric indications.

References

[1] Youngerman BE, Chan AK, Mikell CB, McKhann GM, Sheth SA. A decade of emerging indications: deep brain stimulation in the United States. J Neurosurg. 2016; 125(2):461–471

[2] Cleary DR, Ozpinar A, Raslan AM, Ko AL. Deep brain stimulation for psychiatric disorders: where we are now. Neurosurg Focus. 2015; 38(6):E2–E24

[3] Hamani C, Pilitsis J, Rughani AI, et al. Deep brain stimulation for obsessive-compulsive disorder: systematic review and evidence-based guideline sponsored by the American Society for Stereotactic and Functional Neurosurgery and the Congress of Neurological Surgeons (CNS) and endorsed by the CNS and American Association of Neurological Surgeons. Neurosurgery. 2014; 75 (4):327–33–333

[4] Zipfel S, Giel KE, Bulik CM, Hay P, Schmidt U. Anorexia nervosa: aetiology, assessment, and treatment. Lancet Psychiatry. 2015; 2(12):1099–1111

[5] Hoek HW, van Hoeken D. Review of the prevalence and incidence of eating disorders. Int J Eat Disord. 2003; 34(4):383–396

[6] Zipfel S, Löwe B, Reas DL, Deter HC, Herzog W. Long-term prognosis in anorexia nervosa: lessons from a 21-year follow-up study. Lancet. 2000; 355 (9205):721–722

[7] Strober M, Freeman R, Morrell W. The long-term course of severe anorexia nervosa in adolescents: survival analysis of recovery, relapse, and outcome predictors over 10–15 years in a prospective study. Int J Eat Disord. 1997; 22 (4):339–360

[8] Wagner A, Ruf M, Braus DF, Schmidt MH. Neuronal activity changes and body image distortion in anorexia nervosa. Neuroreport. 2003; 14(17):2193–2197

[9] Fladung A-K, Grön G, Grammer K, et al. A neural signature of anorexia nervosa in the ventral striatal reward system. Am J Psychiatry. 2010; 167(2):206–212

[10] Friederich H-C, Wu M, Simon JJ, Herzog W. Neurocircuit function in eating disorders. Int J Eat Disord. 2013; 46(5):425–432

[11] Morgan JF, Crisp AH. Use of leucotomy for intractable anorexia nervosa: a long-term follow-up study. Int J Eat Disord. 2000; 27(3):249–258

[12] Zamboni R, Larach V, Poblete M, et al. Dorsomedial thalamotomy as a treatment for terminal anorexia: a report of two cases. Acta Neurochir Suppl (Wien). 1993; 58:34–35

[13] Lipsman N, Woodside DB, Giacobbe P, et al. Subcallosal cingulate deep brain stimulation for treatment-refractory anorexia nervosa: a phase 1 pilot trial. Lancet. 2013; 381(9875):1361–1370

[14] Lipsman N, Lam E, Volpini M, et al. Deep brain stimulation of the subcallosal cingulate for treatment-refractory anorexia nervosa: 1 year follow-up of an open-label trial. Lancet Psychiatry. 2017; 4(4):285–294

[15] Drevets WC, Savitz J, Trimble M. The subgenual anterior cingulate cortex in mood disorders. CNS Spectr. 2008; 13(8):663–681

[16] Delvenne V, Goldman S, De Maertelaer V, Lotstra F. Brain glucose metabolism in eating disorders assessed by positron emission tomography. Int J Eat Disord. 1999; 25(1):29–37

[17] Wang J, Chang C, Geng N, Wang X, Gao G. Treatment of intractable anorexia nervosa with inactivation of the nucleus accumbens using stereotactic surgery. Stereotact Funct Neurosurg. 2013; 91(6):364–372

[18] Wu H, Van Dyck-Lippens PJ, Santegoeds R, et al. Deep-brain stimulation for anorexia nervosa. World Neurosurg. 2013; 80(3–4):29.e1–29.e10

[19] Mc, Cl, aughlin NCR, Didie ER, Machado AG, Haber SN, Eskandar EN, Greenberg BD. Improvements in anorexia symptoms after deep brain stimulation for intractable obsessive-compulsive disorder. Biol Psychiatry. 2013; 73 (9):e29–e31

[20] Le Moal M, Koob GF. Drug addiction: pathways to the disease and pathophysiological perspectives. Eur Neuropsychopharmacol. 2007; 17(6–7):377–393

[21] United Nations Office on Drugs and Crime. World Drug Report 2016. Available at: https://www.unodc.org/wdr2016/. Accessed January 7, 2019.

[22] Koob GF, Simon EJ. The Neurobiology of Addiction: Where We Have Been and Where We Are Going. J Drug Issues. 2009; 39(1):115–132

[23] Stelten BML, Noblesse LHM, Ackermans L, Temel Y, Visser-Vandewalle V. The neurosurgical treatment of addiction. Neurosurg Focus. 2008; 25(1):E5

[24] Koob GF. The neurobiology of addiction: a neuroadaptational view relevant for diagnosis. Addiction. 2006; 101 Suppl 1:23–30

[25] Gao G, Wang X, He S, et al. Clinical study for alleviating opiate drug psychological dependence by a method of ablating the nucleus accumbens with stereotactic surgery. Stereotact Funct Neurosurg. 2003; 81(1–4):96–104

[26] Vassoler FM, Schmidt HD, Gerard ME, et al. Deep brain stimulation of the nucleus accumbens shell attenuates cocaine priming-induced reinstatement of drug seeking in rats. J Neurosci. 2008; 28(35):8735–8739

[27] Goto Y, Grace AA. Limbic and cortical information processing in the nucleus accumbens. Trends Neurosci. 2008; 31(11):552–558

[28] Knapp CM, Tozier L, Pak A, Ciraulo DA, Kornetsky C. Deep brain stimulation of the nucleus accumbens reduces ethanol consumption in rats. Pharmacol Biochem Behav. 2009; 92(3):474–479

[29] Holtzheimer PE, Mayberg HS. Deep brain stimulation for psychiatric disorders. Annu Rev Neurosci. 2011; 34(1):289–307

[30] Zhou H, Xu J, Jiang J. Deep brain stimulation of nucleus accumbens on heroin-seeking behaviors: a case report. Biol Psychiatry. 2011; 69(11):e41–e42

[31] Valencia-Alfonso C-E, Luigjes J, Smolders R, et al. Effective deep brain stimulation in heroin addiction: a case report with complementary intracranial electroencephalogram. Biol Psychiatry. 2012; 71(8):e35–e37

[32] Kuhn J, Lenartz D, Huff W, et al. Remission of alcohol dependency following deep brain stimulation of the nucleus accumbens: valuable therapeutic implications? J Neurol Neurosurg Psychiatry. 2007; 78(10):1152–1153

[33] Kuhn J, Gründler TOJ, Bauer R, et al. Successful deep brain stimulation of the nucleus accumbens in severe alcohol dependence is associated with changed performance monitoring. Addict Biol. 2011; 16(4):620–623

[34] Müller UJ, Sturm V, Voges J, et al. Successful treatment of chronic resistant alcoholism by deep brain stimulation of nucleus accumbens: first experience with three cases. Pharmacopsychiatry. 2009; 42(6):288–291

[35] Voges J, Müller U, Bogerts B, Münte T, Heinze H-J. Deep brain stimulation surgery for alcohol addiction. World Neurosurg. 2013; 80(3–4):28.e21–28.e31

[36] Mantione M, van de Brink W, Schuurman PR, Denys D. Smoking cessation and weight loss after chronic deep brain stimulation of the nucleus accumbens: therapeutic and research implications: case report. Neurosurgery. 2010; 66(1):E218–, discussion E218

[37] Kuhn J, Bauer R, Pohl S, et al. Observations on unaided smoking cessation after deep brain stimulation of the nucleus accumbens. Eur Addict Res. 2009; 15(4):196–201

[38] Kuhn J, Lenartz D, Mai JK, Huff W, Klosterkoetter J, Sturm V. Disappearance of self-aggressive behavior in a brain-injured patient after deep brain stimulation of the hypothalamus: technical case report. Neurosurgery. 2008; 62(5):E1182–, discussion E1182

[39] Mpakopoulou M, Gatos H, Brotis A, Paterakis KN, Fountas KN. Stereotactic amygdalotomy in the management of severe aggressive behavioral disorders. Neurosurg Focus. 2008; 25(1):E6

[40] Sturm V, Fricke O, Bührle CP, et al. DBS in the basolateral amygdala improves symptoms of autism and related self-injurious behavior: a case report and hypothesis on the pathogenesis of the disorder. Front Hum Neurosci. 2013; 6:341

[41] Franzini A, Ferroli P, Leone M, Broggi G. Stimulation of the posterior hypothalamus for treatment of chronic intractable cluster headaches: first reported series. Neurosurgery. 2003; 52(5):1095–1099, discussion 1099–1101

[42] Franzini A, Broggi G, Cordella R, Dones I, Messina G. Deep-brain stimulation for aggressive and disruptive behavior. World Neurosurg. 2013; 80(3–4):S29.e11–14

[43] Hernando V, Pastor J, Pedrosa M, Peña E, Sola RG. Low-frequency bilateral hypothalamic stimulation for treatment of drug-resistant aggressiveness in a young man with mental retardation. Stereotact Funct Neurosurg. 2008; 86 (4):219–223

[44] Giordano F, Cavallo M, Spacca B, et al. Deep brain stimulation of the anterior limb of the internal capsule may be efficacious for explosive aggressive behaviour. Stereotact Funct Neurosurg. 2016; 94(6):371–378

[45] Taira T, Kobayashi T, Hori T. Disappearance of self-mutilating behavior in a patient with Lesch–Nyhan syndrome after bilateral chronic stimulation of the globus pallidus internus. Case report. J Neurosurg. 2003; 98(2):414–416

[46] Reznikov R, Hamani C. Posttraumatic Stress Disorder: Perspectives for the Use of Deep Brain Stimulation. Neuromodulation. 2017; 20(1):7–14

[47] Kessler RC, Berglund P, Demler O, Jin R, Merikangas KR, Walters EE. Lifetime prevalence and age-of-onset distributions of DSM-IV disorders in the National Comorbidity Survey Replication. Arch Gen Psychiatry. 2005; 62(6):593–602

[48] Breslau N. Outcomes of posttraumatic stress disorder. J Clin Psychiatry. 2001; 62 Suppl 17:55–59

[49] Francati V, Vermetten E, Bremner JD. Functional neuroimaging studies in posttraumatic stress disorder: review of current methods and findings. Depress Anxiety. 2007; 24(3):202–218

[50] Koenigs M, Huey ED, Raymont V, et al. Focal brain damage protects against post-traumatic stress disorder in combat veterans. Nat Neurosci. 2008; 11(2):232–237

[51] Langevin J-P, De Salles AAF, Kosoyan HP, Krahl SE. Deep brain stimulation of the amygdala alleviates post-traumatic stress disorder symptoms in a rat model. J Psychiatr Res. 2010; 44(16):1241–1245

[52] Stidd DA, Vogelsang K, Krahl SE, Langevin J-P, Fellous J-M. Amygdala deep brain stimulation is superior to paroxetine treatment in a rat model of posttraumatic stress disorder. Brain Stimul. 2013; 6(6):837–844

[53] Saldívar-González JA, Posadas-Andrews A, Rodríguez R, et al. Effect of electrical stimulation of the baso-lateral amygdala nucleus on defensive burying shock probe test and elevated plus maze in rats. Life Sci. 2003; 72(7):819–829

[54] Koek RJ, Langevin J-P, Krahl SE, et al. Deep brain stimulation of the basolateral amygdala for treatment-refractory combat post-traumatic stress disorder (PTSD): study protocol for a pilot randomized controlled trial with blinded, staggered onset of stimulation. Trials. 2014; 15(1):356

[55] Langevin J-P, Koek RJ, Schwartz HN, et al. Deep brain stimulation of the basolateral amygdala for treatment-refractory posttraumatic stress disorder. Biol Psychiatry. 2016; 79(10):e82–e84

[56] Deschaux O, Thevenet A, Spennato G, Arnaud C, Moreau JL, Garcia R. Low-frequency stimulation of the hippocampus following fear extinction impairs both restoration of rapid eye movement sleep and retrieval of extinction memory. Neuroscience. 2010; 170(1):92–98

[57] Rodriguez-Romaguera J, Do Monte FHM, Quirk GJ. Deep brain stimulation of the ventral striatum enhances extinction of conditioned fear. Proc Natl Acad Sci U S A. 2012; 109(22):8764–8769

[58] Milad MR, Vidal-Gonzalez I, Quirk GJ. Electrical stimulation of medial prefrontal cortex reduces conditioned fear in a temporally specific manner. Behav Neurosci. 2004; 118(2):389–394

[59] Howes OD, Murray RM. Schizophrenia: an integrated sociodevelopmental-cognitive model. Lancet. 2014; 383(9929):1677–1687

[60] Lehman AF, Lieberman JA, Dixon LB, et al. American Psychiatric Association, Steering Committee on Practice Guidelines. Practice guideline for the treatment of patients with schizophrenia, second edition. Am J Psychiatry. 2004; 161(2) Suppl:1–56

[61] Mikell CB, Sinha S, Sheth SA. Neurosurgery for schizophrenia: an update on pathophysiology and a novel therapeutic target. J Neurosurg. 2016; 124(4):917–928

[62] Corripio I, Sarró S, McKenna PJ, et al. Clinical improvement in a treatment-resistant patient with schizophrenia treated with deep brain stimulation. Biol Psychiatry. 2016; 80(8):e69–e70

[63] Salgado L, Roldán A, Rodríguez R, et al. A Pilot Study of Deep Brain Stimulation in Treatment Resistant Schizophrenia. In: Los Angeles; 2017. https://aans.eventsential.org/Sessions/Details/265568

[64] Widge AS, Deckersbach T, Eskandar EN, Dougherty DD. Deep brain stimulation for treatment-resistant psychiatric illnesses: what has gone wrong and what should we do next? Biol Psychiatry. 2016; 79(4):e9–e10

[65] Bari AA, Mikell CB, Abosch A, et al. Charting the road forward in psychiatric neurosurgery: proceedings of the 2016 American Society for Stereotactic and Functional Neurosurgery workshop on neuromodulation for psychiatric disorders. J Neurol Neurosurg Psychiatr. 2018; 89:886–896

16 Intraoperative Research during Deep Brain Stimulation Surgery

Shane Lee, Meghal Shah, Peter M. Lauro, Wael F. Asaad

Abstract

In this chapter, we discuss the process of conducting intraoperative research during deep brain stimulation surgery. Microelectrode recordings, which are routinely used for intraoperative mapping, present a unique opportunity to listen to and record from neurons in the brain. These recordings, with or without a behavioral task, offer a window into human neuronal circuit function with a granularity that is not otherwise available. This chapter will go over the types of research questions that are amenable to intraoperative neurophysiology research, patient selection, and the additional equipment needed. Considerations such as task development, data analysis, and related neuroimaging are covered. Finally, limitations and ethical considerations are discussed.

Keywords: deep brain stimulation, neurophysiology, microelectrode recordings, intraoperative research, methods, behavioral task, spiking activity

16.1 Introduction

Deep brain stimulation (DBS) surgery presents neurosurgeons with a rare opportunity to observe neural activity in the brain. DBS electrode targeting typically relies upon a combination of imaging and neurophysiology. Though magnetic resonance imaging (MRI) and computed tomography (CT) techniques are becoming more powerful, many gross structures and especially subregions within a therapeutic target of interest still remain difficult to visualize.[1] In conjunction with preoperative—and increasingly intraoperative—imaging, microelectrode recordings (MERs) are often used for intraoperative mapping to delineate structural borders and identify subareas within a region of interest (ROI) that may lead overall to improved patient outcomes.[2,3,4,5,6]

In combination with carefully designed behavioral assays, recording and analysis of intraoperative neuronal data can provide insight into the functions of these structures and how their activity relates to other areas of the brain, behaviors, or disease processes. This approach has been employed in a growing number of studies, helping to improve understanding of basic and pathological neural activity in essential tremor,[7,8] Parkinson's disease,[8,9,10] Tourette syndrome,[11,12,13] obsessive-compulsive disorder,[14,15,16] and others. Other types of neural recordings are also being used increasingly in conjunction with MER, including electroencephalography (EEG) and electrocorticography (ECoG), adapting techniques largely pioneered within the context of epilepsy monitoring.[17,18,19]

For Parkinson's disease, the subthalamic nucleus (STN) and globus pallidus pars interna (GPi) are the most common therapeutic targets. Patients have performed tasks manipulating joysticks or haptic gloves while single neuron, multiunit, and local field potentials (LFPs) were recorded in STN or GPi.[5,20] Single neurons in these areas have demonstrated movement-related and direction-specific spike rate modulations, and STN neurons further showed oscillations at 3 to 5 Hz "tremor" frequencies or 15 to 30 Hz "beta" frequencies.[5,6,21] Other studies have engaged awake patients with tasks designed specifically to correlate neural activity with precise aspects of behavior. Both Zavala et al and Zaghloul et al demonstrated in distinct decision-making tasks that neuronal firing in the STN is correlated with conflict.[22,23] Using simultaneously recorded scalp EEG, Zavala et al showed that this STN activity was driven by activity in the frontal cortex.

In this chapter, practical considerations for conducting human intraoperative neurophysiology research are discussed.

16.2 Formulating Hypotheses

In developing a neurophysiology research study with human subjects, investigators must address the following questions while designing an experiment:

1. What cortical or subcortical structures are of interest?
2. What disease processes are of interest or would provide access to the structure in question?
3. Will this be an observational study or will there be behavioral task or measure?
4. What type(s) of neurophysiological recordings will be acquired?

The greatest potential limitation of intraoperative research is that by nature of the procedure, only patients with neurological disease will undergo DBS surgery. This may limit the interpretation of the data and may also limit the structures available for MER. Thus, the most common targets accessible in this fashion are the STN and GPi (patients with Parkinson's, the latter also for primary dystonia)[24] and the ventral intermediate nucleus (Vim) of the thalamus (patients with essential tremor).[8,25] MER can help localize specific substructures within these areas that are most desirable for electrode implantation.

In addition to these movement disorders that are now routinely treated with DBS, treatment of a number of psychiatric conditions has been explored with DBS therapy. For example, in extreme cases of obsessive-compulsive disorder and Tourette syndrome (a combination of both motor and psychiatric pathology) the ventral internal capsule/ventral striatum or cingulate cortex has been targeted for DBS with potentially impressive benefits in some patients.[14,15,16] For intractable obsessive-compulsive disorder, others have targeted the STN or the ventral anterior internal capsule/inferior thalamic peduncle.[26]

Recordings can be made through nontarget structures that are encountered along the trajectory to the target structure, such as frontal cortex and striatum, and in some cases just beyond the target structure, such as the substantia nigra, if such regions are routinely mapped to define a target's distal border.[27] In some cases, with the proper approvals, cortical recordings can be made with subdural electrodes, not typically required for DBS surgery, inserted through the standard burr holes.[10]

Often, a roadmap regarding what types of behaviors may be mediated by particular structures is available in the form of prior human or nonhuman primate functional MRI (fMRI) studies and in the wide body of literature describing electrophysiological correlates of behavior in animal studies. Adapting these behavioral paradigms to humans offers the opportunity to extend our knowledge of the neural correlates of behavior, especially those behaviors which may be elaborated in or are unique to humans.

16.3 Patient Selection and IRB Approval

Approval of the research protocol by an institutional review board (IRB) is mandatory even for observational studies. Patients who are considered for DBS are ideally first evaluated by a multidisciplinary team of clinicians. Appropriateness and fitness for surgery is determined by the surgeon, neurologist, anesthesiologist, and any other clinicians who are involved in the patient's care. Once patients are considered appropriate for surgery, they can be approached by a member of the clinical or research team per their specific IRB protocol to obtain voluntary consent after explaining the potential risks of the research-specific procedures (outlined in greater detail below). Because patients typically desire to please their physicians, especially in situations where they think this could improve the care or attention they receive, one should explain clearly that the quality of care provided will not depend on their participation. In addition, respecting a patient's decision-making autonomy extends throughout the process such that they should be allowed to withdraw from participation at any time, including during the procedure.[28]

Potential risks of intraoperative research include those related to additional time incurred during surgery to carry out the experimental procedures, such as behavioral tasks, the placement of additional electrodes (e.g., subdural electrodes) that are not typically required for the clinical procedure, and discomfort of the patient or anxiety related to task performance. Particular research protocols may incur other risks. In general, risks accrue as a result of any nonstandard surgical maneuvers or deviations from the clinical procedure. For example, the placement of subdural ECoG electrodes is not required for routine DBS procedure. While placement has been reported as generally safe, there is nonetheless a nonzero risk associated with any additional maneuver, and there may be risks not immediately considered (e.g., the additional time required to insert an ECoG electrode may result in increased pneumocephalus which could affect the accuracy of final DBS electrode placement).[29] While in some studies ECoG electrodes are used in hopes of improving the future efficacy of neuromodulation (such as a source of control signals for closed-loop DBS), in other cases the goal may be basic science. It may be easier, therefore, to justify the additional maneuver in the former case than in the latter, so careful deliberation over these issues is mandatory. Simply because an IRB may be convinced that a particular protocol is reasonable does not mean that the protocol is necessarily in a patient's best interest.

16.4 Equipment and Setup

In most of human acute recordings, the operating theater also serves as the laboratory. In this unique arrangement, some of the equipment serve a principally clinical purpose but may also serve research goals with no or minimal modification.

MER in DBS allows an assessment of somatotopic responses, in which high bandpass filtered neural recordings at multiple sites are monitored over audio speakers while a clinician elicits various neural responses by manipulating the face/jaw and limbs. Typically, 1 to 5 microelectrodes arranged in a Ben-Gun array are advanced toward a predefined target structure while somatotopic assessments performed at various locations along the trajectories.

In general, neural data recording requires electrodes, signal amplifiers, and an acquisition system. Depending on the research questions, additional systems may be necessary to measure movement or administer tasks to awake patients while recording. An example of multichannel neural and behavioral recording is shown in ▶ Fig. 16.1.

Typical sharp tungsten or platinum-iridium electrodes with impedances around 300 to 1000 kΩ are typically used to record single- and multiunit spiking activity. Online during a case, signals measured with these electrodes are typically bandpass filtered from approximately 300 Hz to around 10 kHz, appropriate for isolating action potentials from neurons surrounding the recording tip.

The Nyquist sampling theorem sets a lower bound on the appropriate sampling rate of the digital acquisition system. Nyquist states that the sampling rate must be two times greater than the maximum frequency of the activity of interest. For example, if one wants to sample single-unit activity at 10 kHz, then the minimum sampling rate according to the Nyquist theorem would be 20 kHz. In practice, due to the noisy nature of these data, it is generally advised to allocate spectral "overhead" to this calculation which helps to guarantee that the signal of interest will be recorded faithfully; though higher sampling rates require greater data storage and an analog-to-digital interface capable of handling these rates. Data storage is relatively inexpensive, and acquisition systems' capabilities are growing, so sampling rates of 30 to 50 kHz are commonly employed.

If one wishes to test hypotheses about single- or multiunit spiking activity, then the typical 300 Hz to 10 kHz band will be appropriate. If one is testing hypotheses involving lower frequency LFPs (approximately 0.5–600 Hz), the neural recordings must be filtered appropriately with a very low high pass band stop (~ 0.1 Hz) and a low pass band stop of at least 1200 Hz to capture the highest frequency signal (2 × 600 Hz). Alternatively, if filtered data is not needed "online" as it is being acquired, data can be saved in its "raw" form, with the bandpass filter characteristics set to be the most permissive, for offline filtering as needed.

There are sometimes options available for online spike detection. Though they may be useful for rapid online analysis, in principle there are no benefits to online-only spike detection if not immediately required for closed-loop control or feedback. Saving raw data and performing offline spike sorting is preferable, because spike sorting can be performed in a more systematic manner without the limitations of the often-busy surgical environment.

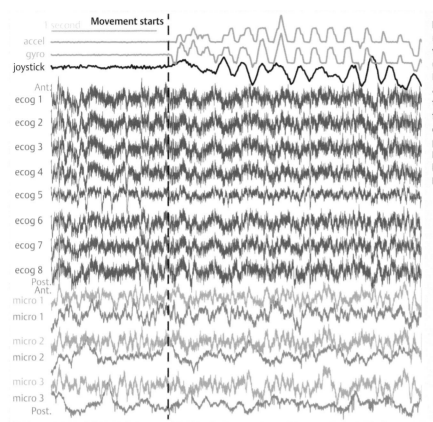

Fig. 16.1 Synchronization of behavioral and neural data. Intraoperative data recorded from ventral intermediate nucleus of the thalamus (LFPs) and somatomotor cortices (ECoG). Examples of 3.5 seconds of composite three-axis accelerometer and three-axis gyroscope (*green*), task joystick (*black*), 8 channels of ECoG (*blue*, from anterior to posterior), and 3 channels of depth electrodes (*orange/red*, from anterior to posterior). Macro tip is 3 mm above the micro. Electrodes are 2 mm from each other. LFP on both, also single unit responses on micro. Movement starts at the black line.

Signal amplifiers and acquisition systems should be selected to suit current and anticipated future requirements. The role of the signal amplifier is to faithfully capture very small, noisy neural signals with high fidelity, while the acquisition system must be able to write multiple channels of data rapidly with no loss. The number of channels also depends on the specific clinical and research aims. For a minimal system, the number of channels might equal the number of microelectrodes implanted for recording, but it is more likely that a research system requires additional analog and digital inputs. Having a primary, clinical system that can serve as a data hub for other recording streams is convenient, as this will implicitly synchronize any data streams for which it is responsible (see later). These additional channels often come in a wide range of connector types and can be sampled at widely varying sampling rates, often with both an upper limit on the maximal signal amplitude or a bound on the amplitude resolution.

As an example, accelerometers can be placed on patient limbs to assess movements, and these signals can be sent to the amplifier and acquisition systems. But because relevant limb movements are biomechanically limited in speed and frequency, 10 kHz or greater sampling is potentially superfluous. Therefore, these inputs should be software-limited to an appropriate sampling rate that accounts for the trade-offs with storage mentioned previously. At our site, we routinely record accelerometer activity at 1000 to 3000 Hz, which results in manageably small data sizes but faithfully captures the fine details of movement.[30]

Routinely, the data recorded for three full-bandwidth channels of microelectrode data, three lower rate field recordings, and eight analog channels at lower sampling rates results in approximately 10 GB of data for 2 to 3 hours of recording. Including additional high-bandwidth channels, such as ECoG, can triple these data sizes for each case. Neurophysiology systems capable of recording high-bandwidth data should be capable of rapid transfer of these data to an external device for offline analysis.

Another important consideration in selecting a neurophysiology monitoring system is the software. Though hardware specifications may seem to be appropriate, it is the software that provides the interface that will be critical for both providing quality patient care as well as efficiency in processing the recorded data. Equipment and interfaces approved by a country's health and safety regulatory commissions may impose restrictions on how frequently software is updated, despite a company's best intentions, so the shipping product must be free of major issues. Good commercial vendors who appreciate the importance of intraoperative research and are committed to supporting it will work to mitigate issues with their hardware and software as they are identified. Wherever possible, open-source and cross-platform data formats and software tools are preferable to closed formats, as this will ensure longevity in data archival and future access.

16.5 Behavioral Task Control

In most cases, research involving human intracranial recordings requires quantitatively rigorous behavioral and precisely time-stamped metrics for correlation with neural signals. A simple accelerometer attached to a patient's wrist may be sufficient for some questions about the relationship of movement to neural activity, but for other behavioral activity, more interesting questions addressing complex motor behaviors and cognition will likely require a dedicated behavioral task control system. For example, our system uses a portable case with rack mounted hardware to house a standard desktop computer, a digital acquisition system used for behavior that is different from the neurophysiological system, and a multi-monitor mount. This system includes a monitor that can be positioned in front of the patient, as well as a joystick that controls the tasks. We present visual tasks to the patients while they manipulate a joystick or button box to provide behavioral responses. For other types of tasks, haptic gloves or other unique manipulanda might be employed for patient interaction. Irrespective of the input device selected for the tracking of behavioral data, patient comfort and reproducible placement are crucial to capturing performance accurately and reliably.

In our laboratory, tasks are programmed in MonkeyLogic, a free, MATLAB-based software toolbox[31,32,33] that enables millisecond precision in our psychophysical experiments (MonkeyLogic is currently supported and maintained at the NIH: https://www.nimh.nih.gov/labs-at-nimh/research-areas/clinics-and-labs/ln/shn/monkeylogic). Importantly, this software also sends precisely timed digital event codes to the neurophysiology acquisition system, enabling synchronization between the two systems. The goal of behavioral–neural synchronization in neurophysiology is to be accurate to ~1 millisecond timescale; in contrast, synchronization between behavior and slower modalities, such as fMRI, is often performed manually (the experimenter simultaneously initiates both systems by striking a key on each system, one with a finger of each hand).

16.6 Data Analysis

Creating a robust data processing and analysis pipeline is critical for an efficient and reliable research workflow. Even though most analyses can be performed post hoc and not online in the operating room, the acquisition system's hardware and data format serve as the starting point. When dealing with separate systems that are synchronized, custom software is often necessary to align the data according to the synchronizing signal.

Modern neuroscientific data analysis generally falls into two categories: continuous and point process. Continuous data consists of any time series, such as neurophysiological field potentials or accelerometer output. Point process data consists of discrete events, such as spiking activity or activity counts (e.g., number of choices A versus B). Specific methods exist for each class of data, though it is often necessary or desirable to convert between the two data types. Several neural data-specific guides are available that are balanced in presenting both theory and practical implementation.[34,35]

One of the most common and critical preprocessing steps in neurophysiology is spike sorting, which takes a continuous time series recording as input and converts it to a set of events that are labeled into one or many single "units." In general, spike sorting is a procedure to isolate an individual neuron's spikes from other neurons' spikes in an MER. Typically, MERs sampled at a high rate[3] (30 kHz) are bandpassed (approximately 0.3–10 kHz), resulting in a zero-mean noise baseline. A threshold is calculated based on the noise distribution and spike waveforms are isolated as threshold crossings. These waveforms are then analyzed using automated or semiautomated methods, such as principle components analysis and clustering algorithms (e.g., k-means algorithm). Manual methods that categorize waveforms on the basis of waveform features, fully automated methods, or a hybrid of approaches are commonly used, but knowing the ground truth is difficult, so accurate spike sorting remains an active area of research.[36] Both open-source and commercial solutions exist to perform spike sorting.

Even within a data type, different techniques that are commonly employed can lead to different qualitative and quantitative interpretations of neural activity. In ▶ Fig. 16.2, 2 seconds of ECoG data recorded from human somatomotor cortex of a patient with essential tremor are shown with different spectral techniques demonstrating different results. The choice of analysis can make a substantial difference in the interpretation of the results. ▶ Fig. 16.2a shows the time series, referenced and z-scored. There was clear oscillatory activity that occurred at different times in the epoch, but the precise frequency characteristics need to be quantified. ▶ Fig. 16.2b shows a discrete Fourier transformed (DFT) power spectrum in which two distinct peaks were seen at 1.5 and 22 Hz. The DFT analysis assumed that the data were constant within the analysis window—a property called stationarity—which may be a poor assumption here, considering that different oscillatory activity was variable within this epoch.

Multiple methods are available for investigating time-varying spectral features. The most common is the short-time Fourier transform (STFT), which is also commonly referred to as a spectrogram (▶ Fig. 16.2c). In the STFT, small segments of time (in this case 0.5 s) were analyzed, and the window was slid across at short intervals (0.025 s) to provide a time-varying estimate of the activity. As the frequency interval is inversely proportional to the amount of time in the analyzed window, shorter time windows result in a larger frequency interval or poorer frequency resolution. The trade-off of frequency resolution, amount of data, and stationarity of data should be considered when using the STFT. Here, both low- and higher-frequency activities were seen, but the activity around 25 Hz was mostly limited near 1.2 s. Furthermore, the first estimate of data is centered around 0.25 s, and the last sample was centered around 0.75 s, and no estimates were available outside of those, meaning the data of interest needed to be within the boundaries set by the temporal window parameters. The timing information seen in the STFT was lost with a power spectrum (▶ Fig. 16.2b).

Wavelet-based time-varying spectral analyses are also commonly employed. These can provide estimates for an entire short window but also have their own shortcomings. In ▶ Fig. 16.2d, the power was calculated from a family of Morlet wavelets convolved with the time series. This method showed a consistent result with the STFT for the higher-frequency activity and its timing, but the lower- frequency activity was not clearly captured.

Finally, in ▶ Fig. 16.2e, a Hilbert transform spectral method was applied in a similar manner to the Morlet wavelets. This method captured the activity around 22 Hz well along with the lower-frequency activity which appeared to be primarily isolated to the first 0.5 s of the data. The power spectrum (▶ Fig. 16.2b) picked up this activity but not the timing, while

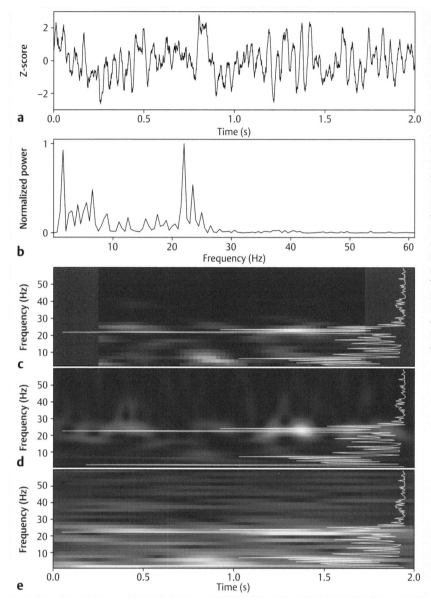

Fig. 16.2 Choice of analysis affects interpretation. **(a)** Two seconds of human somatomotor ECoG data recorded from essential tremor patient. Recorded at 11 kHz. Downsampled to 1 kHz. Referenced, normalized. **(b)** Discrete Fourier Transform shows stationary peaks of similar height at 1.5 and 22 Hz. The stationarity assumption misses time-varying spectral changes. **(c)** Short-time Fourier Transform (STFT). 0.5 s windows, 0.025 s overlap for temporal estimates. Low-frequency peak and high-frequency peaks are observed with temporal information. No estimates for beginning and end of a short time series. Frequency resolution is limited by length of window. At 0.75 s, 5–10 Hz activity appears briefly. 1.5 Hz activity is not visible here. Mostly consistent with the Hilbert (E). **(d)** Morlet wavelet spectrogram. σ = 7. Due to scaling, only activity at ~ 25 Hz is visible, within a narrow temporal window. No low-frequency activity is resolved here. **(e)** Hilbert transformed power spectrum. Low-frequency and high-frequency activity is captured; suffers from potentially poor temporal resolution but estimates for entire sample of data. Mostly consistent with the STFT.

the STFT (▸ Fig. 16.2c) picked up this activity in its first estimate, though it was difficult to see represented in the figure, and the Morlet (▸ Fig. 16.2d) had these spectral features washed out by the much higher powered activity around 25 Hz. In general, the choice of spectral technique comes down to empirical questions about one's hypothesis and represents a trade-off between temporal precision and frequency precision. This example illustrates the necessity for these analyses to be selected on the basis of the hypothesis prior to analysis of one's data.

A substantial amount of data analysis can be done now on widely available computer hardware on all major computing platforms. In addition, depending on the type of analysis necessary, multiple commercial software solutions may exist, though these are often operating system (OS)-limited. Many free and non-free high-level programming languages (e.g., Python: https://www.python.org/) have fewer OS limitations and also have a large number of extensions or modules that are specifically tailored for scientific computing. Commercial programs (e.g., MATLAB, from

Mathworks, Inc.) often have the benefit of customer support, while open-source solutions have third party paid support vendors who may be able to provide assistance. Both free and commercial software have large communities of users from which one might be able to get help.

16.7 Image-Based Reconstruction of Recording Sites

Offline analysis of MER data often requires the reconstruction of recording and/or stimulation sites in order to verify appropriate electrode placement and to understand the potential anatomical distribution of neural and/or behavioral data. Imaging data (cortical thickness, diffusion-tensor imaging) may also provide additional insight into the neural or behavioral features observed in intraoperative experiments. Clinical imaging used for surgical targeting and placement confirmation can be used, but multiple processing steps are needed for reproducible calculation of stereotactic coordinates.

16.7.1 Image Acquisition Considerations

Preoperative MRI is typically used to plan DBS implantation surgical trajectories and targets. Potential research-relevant sequences include:

- High-resolution T1-weighted images (e.g., MPRAGE) prior to gadolinium contrast to visualize anatomical structures.
- T2- or T2*-weighted images, ideally with fat suppression, for structural template for diffusion weighted images (DWI).
- DWI sequence for calculating tractography either for preoperative planning or postoperative analysis.
  - T1- and T2-weighted images are typically acquired as part of standard clinical imaging workflows. These images should be of high resolution (voxels should be 1.0 mm isotropic). DW images have several additional, important acquisition parameters. In general, DW images are formed by applying paired magnetic gradient pulses to the tissue, allowing the diffusion-related properties of tissue to emerge. Typically, the isotropy of spatial diffusion of protons in water (or lack thereof) is examined to differentiate white and gray matter, as it is assumed that proton diffusion is more constrained in fatty myelin sheaths. Tractography uses this anisotropic diffusion, assigning the diffusion orientation with the highest anisotropy in each voxel (i.e., the direction in which diffusion was the most constrained—this is thought to occur when this diffusion orientation is parallel with axons). These voxel-based orientations are then combined to form long-reaching estimations of white matter "tracts." This technique can help to identify target structures by their connections to other structures or provide additional anatomical context to neurophysiological or clinical data (e.g., stimulation to specific white matter tracts associated with more paresthesias). To estimate accurately the orientation of white matter tracts, multiple diffusion gradient directions are used during the acquisition sequence. For research purposes, a minimum of 64 gradient directions are recommended.[37] DWI sequences typically have one or more so-called B-values (expressed in seconds/mm^2), which describe the degree of diffusion weighting applied to tissue. Specifically, the B-value is the product of diffusion gradient amplitude, the duration of applied diffusion gradient pulses, and the duration between the first and second paired pulses. Different B-values allow different comparisons of diffusion-based tissue contrast.
  - For example, a DWI sequence with a single shell (b = 1000) is used for standard tensor-model diffusion tensor imaging (DTI). Multishell acquisition sequences (b = 1000, 2850) can be used for more advanced diffusion imaging techniques (e.g., neurite orientation dispersion and density imaging [NODDI] or diffusion spectrum imaging [DSI]). These latter techniques are typically used for disentangling neurite density, orientation dispersion index, and axonal coherence.

The surgical frame used for the DBS implantation surgery can also influence preoperative image sequences. Patient-specific frames, such as FHC's STarFix platform, typically require a preoperative CT scan, which is registered to preoperative MR images prior to planning. Patients with an Integra CRW or Leksell frame can also be imaged with preoperative CT. If patients are using an MR-compatible frame, magnetic field distortion of the frame and tissue should be considered and accounted for. In addition, affixed stereotactic frames may impact the duration of time patients will tolerate an MRI scan, which may limit the ultimate resolution of scans. A good review of frames, image registration, and other sources of error in stereotactic surgical planning is available.[38]

Intraoperative imaging provides valuable data for deep or surface electrode location and/or pneumocephalus. Intraoperative fluoroscopy and CT are fairly simple modalities for DBS surgery of awake patients. Intraoperative MRI (typically used for DBS procedures under general anesthesia) can provide more anatomical detail but is typically incompatible with MER.

Postoperative imaging (CT or MRI) can help to confirm the final location of electrodes. For direct visualization of DBS electrodes, postoperative CT can be acquired and registered back to preoperative MR images. Pneumocephalus-related brain shift (if a concern) is better identified with postoperative MRI. If postoperative MRI is used, it must be performed in a 1.5 T magnet, and performed sequences must have a specific absorption rate less than 0.4 W/kg in the head. Postoperative fMRI sequences are typically approved on a case-by-case basis and may require IRB approval.

16.7.2 Reconstructing the Recording Locations

Image processing steps are unique to the software package one decides to use. Software packages include the Analysis of Functional Neuroimages (AFNI; https://afni.nimh.nih.gov)[39,40] the FMRIB Software Library (FSL; https://fsl.fmrib.ox.ac.uk/fsl/fslwiki),[41,42,43] the MATLAB-based Lead-DBS (http://www.lead-dbs.org),[44] and Statistical Parametric Mapping (SPM; http://www.fil.ion.ucl.ac.uk/spm) software packages. Many of the steps described below use AFNI, as it provides command-line flexibility for manipulating datasets, is compatible with other modality-specific software toolkits (TORTOISE, Freesurfer), and is free and open source.

Reconstructing DBS contact or MER coordinates can be useful for overlaying/understanding clinical, behavioral, or neural data in anatomical space. Generally speaking, the "bottom" or "final" location coordinate of a DBS electrode is typically considered the bottom of DBS contact 0 of a Medtronic 3387 or 3389 electrode or similar device. Semiautomated methods using AFNI for reconstructing postoperative DBS contacts[45] or MER locations from patient-specific platforms exist.[1]

To perform reconstructions, all images should be brought to a standard stereotactic coordinate space. Intra- or postoperative images can be registered to a preoperative plan in order to understand the location of recording or stimulating electrodes relative to planned implantation coordinates. However, this depends on the choice of stereotactic frame or platform. For example, Leksell frames are typically integrated with the Medtronic StealthStation or Brainlab systems, while FHC STarFix platforms require Waypoint software. At the time of writing, the former software does not export the registration matrices between images or any other information, while Waypoint can export registration matrices between images and coordinates of anterior commissure (AC), posterior commissure (PC), and targets as a plain text file that can be processed in external software packages.

To create a stereotactic coordinate space outside a surgical plan, AC and PC coordinates can also be manually determined in preoperative images. The preoperative volume should then be affinely transformed so that the midsagittal plane is aligned to the AC-PC axis. AC/PC determination can be performed using software such as AFNI, Medical Image Processing, Analysis, and Visualization (MIPAV; https://mipav.cit.nih.gov), or 3D Slicer (https://www.slicer.org). Consistent criteria are required for AC/PC delineation; for this, the neurosurgeon's determination can be used. From there, electrode coordinates can be manually delineated by navigating through planning software and locating the bottom of electrodes present within the images. Alternatively, coordinates can be reconstructed from Leksell frame arc and ring angles with the depth of the recording probe.

When reporting coordinates, it is important to differentiate between patient-specific and atlas coordinates. Patient-specific coordinates allow for the faithful reporting of targets relative to a patient's individualized surgical plan, while using a standardized atlas allows for reporting of group-level coordinates to account for anatomical or surgical variability. To normalize patient anatomy to an atlas, perform a nonlinear registration (e.g., AFNI's 3dQwarp) between the patient's high-resolution preoperative images (typically T1-weighted) and the atlas template volume. Montreal Neurological Institute (MNI) atlases are typically used, such as the 2009 152-subject average brain (http://www.bic.mni.mcgill.ca/ServicesAtlases/ICBM152NLin2009).[46,47,48] Disease-specific and more subcortically oriented atlases also exist, including the multi-contrast PD25 atlas, which is based on the Schaltenbrand atlas (http://nist.mni.mcgill.ca/?p=1209).[49,50,51] The Lead-DBS project maintains comprehensive listings of subcortical (http://www.lead-dbs.org/?page_id=45) and cortical (http://www.lead-dbs.org/?page_id=1004) atlases. Each atlas has its own limitations, so validation of group-level results may require two or more atlases (▶ Fig. 16.3).

Reconstruction of ECoG electrode locations is typically done with intra- or postoperative CT images. As ECoG electrodes conform to the cortical surface, they are more susceptible to brain shift and deformation due to pneumocephalus or the electrodes themselves. While electrode position can be approximated with sensory- or motor-evoked cortical potentials, there remains a research need to accurately determine electrode position.

Some groups have used fluoroscopy to localize ECoG electrodes,[52] and others have used image-based methods to reconstruct cortical surfaces and spring energy functions to characterize the deformation of tissue and electrodes.[17]

16.7.3 Additional Image-Based Analyses

Investigating the topographic properties of a specific target nuclei (e.g., the difference between dorsal and ventral STN) can be performed with patient-specific anatomical segmentation or with atlas-based ROIs. Patient-specific cortical and subcortical segmentation can be performed using Freesurfer's "recon-all" command (https://surfer.nmr.mgh.harvard.edu).[53] For ease of use, the input T1-weighted volume should be already registered to the preferred coordinate space. If Freesurfer does not adequately delineate the ROIs/structures of interest, atlas-based ROIs in patient or atlas space can be used. Regardless of method, one can delineate topographic distribution of recording or stimulation coordinates by comparing them to the ROI's center-of-mass coordinates.

16.7.4 Diffusion-Weighted Imaging Analysis

For DTI analysis, one should affinely register T2- and DW images to the surgical plan coordinate space. Preprocessing of DWI data can be performed by TORTOISE's "DIFFPREP" function (https://science.nichd.nih.gov/confluence/display/nihpd/TORTOISE).[54] As DW images are prone to various forms of distortion (see review[37]), it is important to correct these sources of error. Preprocessing steps include (but are not limited to) eddy

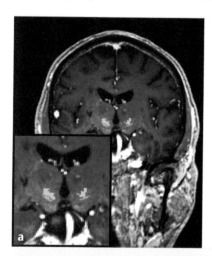
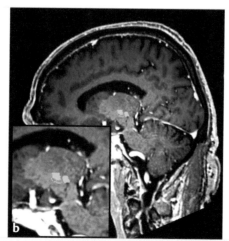
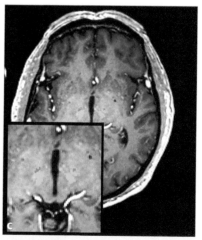

Fig. 16.3 Subthalamic nucleus (STN) volumes from two separate atlases (TT_N27, MNI PD25) overlaid in patient's T1-weighted volume native space in **(a)** coronal, **(b)** sagittal, and **(c)** axial views. Insets in lower-left corners represent the center of each panel. *Orange voxels* represent STN volume from MNI PD25 atlas, *green voxels* represent STN volume from TT_N27 atlas, and *red voxels* indicate overlap between the two.

current correction, motion correction, and noise reduction. Regardless of the selected DTI software, these preprocessing steps should be performed with analogous functions.

With tractography estimation in AFNI, a network of ROIs must be specified to characterize what each tract "connects" to. Again, a patient-specific segmentation from Freesurfer can be used or atlas-based ROIs. In addition, ROIs can be generated around a coordinate of interest (e.g., a 2 mm radius sphere centered on a particular recording coordinate) or from voxels where a specific neural/behavioral feature was observed (e.g., high beta oscillatory activity). For research purposes, probabilistic tractography should be performed, as deterministic tractography can be susceptible to bias within the source DWIs and mask multiple fiber crossings.

16.8 Limitations

Though DBS surgery presents a fairly unique opportunity to observe neurons directly from the human brain, there are notable limitations. Perhaps the greatest limitation is the ability to record only from patients with neurological illness. Thus, activity related to apparently "normal" functions may be distorted by the pathological context, even if behavioral metrics appear grossly normal. In some cases, it may be possible to record data from the same structure in the setting of different diseases (such as the GPi in patients with Parkinson's disease or dystonia); this may add some measure of generalizability to the interpretation of the data, but even in such cases, the diseases may share common pathological mechanisms (such as the frequently observed presence of dystonic movements in patients with Parkinson's disease) that limit our ability to generalize results beyond these patient populations.

The data collected from single-neuron MERs provide relatively limited spatial sampling, so it may not be representative of the circuit as a whole. This is not unique to human electrophysiology but is rather a long-appreciated trade-off between the high spatial and temporal resolution of this method and broader sampling of neural activity at coarse resolution by other methods, such as noninvasive imaging. Indeed, the combination of these modalities may be especially interesting.[55]

Furthermore, the nature of the intraoperative environment may pose challenges. For example, patient positioning can make it difficult to comfortably allow the patient to move freely in order to complete the task and may contribute to accelerated fatigue during task performance. In addition, awkward patient positioning may distort motor symptoms. As patients are not free to stand and walk, testing of major subgroups of symptoms, such as those affecting gait, is not possible. Similarly, intraoperative eye-tracking is challenging due to the positioning and lighting constraints, as well as electrical and mechanical noise within the intraoperative environment. Modifying the behavioral tasks, when appropriate, may be a necessary compromise for the operating room.

The duration of a behavioral experiment is limited during surgery compared to the typical length of similar experiments in a nonsurgical environment. As neuronal responses (especially those of single units) are variable (or "noisy"), many repetitions of a behavioral condition are typically desirable in such experiments. Therefore, ideal tasks for intraoperative experiments may have relatively few conditions and may be simpler in overall structure. This may limit the ability to study more complex cognitive functions or nonstationary cognitive phenomena such as learning.

In addition, rapidly identifying and holding reliable neurons is challenging because signals can drift due to physical changes in the positioning of the tissue relative to the electrode (physical drift) or as a result of slow changes in excitability or neuronal integrity (physiological drift). In nonhuman electrophysiological experiments, isolated neurons may be allowed to stabilize for hours in the case of acute recordings or for many days or weeks in the case of chronic recordings. Semichronic, extraoperative recordings in patients undergoing invasive electrophysiological monitoring for epilepsy also allows for longer stabilization of neural signals. In contrast, intraoperative human neurophysiology often allows only a few minutes for recording stabilization.

Patients may experience subtle, prolonged changes in alertness, cognition, or affect due to transiently administered anxiolytic medications at the beginning of a case or may develop such changes during the surgical procedure, perhaps due to anxiety, somnolence, or physical discomfort (such as due to the pressure of a standard stereotactic frame). In case of Parkinson's disease, patients are typically off their anti-Parkinsonian medications for several hours and often experience increasing discomfort as the time since the last dose increases, due to the primary symptoms of the disease (such as painful dystonias). These factors can result in unreliable behavioral data or abandonment of the task. The reliability of even simple motor task behavior is contingent upon the patient's state that can be influenced by seemingly mundane variables such as the patient's position on the bed. Every aspect of intraoperative research must, therefore, be designed to optimize these often-challenging conditions so as to record meaningful data.

16.9 Conclusion

Although there are many potential limitations and pitfalls that complicate the undertaking of intraoperative neurophysiological experiments, the rare opportunity to observe the human brain in action on the level of individual neuronal spikes is, nonetheless, enormously attractive and important. Well-designed and executed experiments can shed light on patho-neurophysiological mechanisms directly, without the need for an intermediate animal model. Likewise, well-designed tasks that investigate abstract concepts may elucidate cognitive functions that are unique to or elaborated in humans at the neuronal level.

References

[1] Lauro PM, Lee S, Ahn M, Barborica A, Asaad WF. DBStar: An open-source toolkit for imaging analysis with patient-customized deep brain stimulation platforms. Stereotact Funct Neurosurg. 2018; 96(1):13–21

[2] Seifried C, Weise L, Hartmann R, et al. Intraoperative microelectrode recording for the delineation of subthalamic nucleus topography in Parkinson's disease. Brain Stimul. 2012; 5(3):378–387

[3] Reck C, Maarouf M, Wojtecki L, et al. Clinical outcome of subthalamic stimulation in Parkinson's disease is improved by intraoperative multiple trajectories microelectrode recording. J Neurol Surg A Cent Eur Neurosurg. 2012; 73: 377–386

[4] Gross RE, Krack P, Rodriguez-Oroz MC, Rezai AR, Benabid AL. Electrophysiological mapping for the implantation of deep brain stimulators for Parkinson's disease and tremor. Mov Disord. 2006; 21 Suppl 14:S259–S283

[5] Williams ZM, Neimat JS, Cosgrove GR, Eskandar EN. Timing and direction selectivity of subthalamic and pallidal neurons in patients with Parkinson disease. Exp Brain Res. 2005; 162(4):407–416

[6] Moran A, Bergman H, Israel Z, Bar-Gad I. Subthalamic nucleus functional organization revealed by parkinsonian neuronal oscillations and synchrony. Brain. 2008; 131(Pt 12):3395–3409

[7] Holdefer RN, Cohen BA, Greene KA. Intraoperative local field recording for deep brain stimulation in Parkinson's disease and essential tremor. Mov Disord. 2010; 25(13):2067–2075

[8] Hubble JP, Busenbark KL, Wilkinson S, Penn RD, Lyons K, Koller WC. Deep brain stimulation for essential tremor. Neurology. 1996; 46(4):1150–1153

[9] Weinberger M, Mahant N, Hutchison WD, et al. Beta oscillatory activity in the subthalamic nucleus and its relation to dopaminergic response in Parkinson's disease. J Neurophysiol. 2006; 96(6):3248–3256

[10] Miocinovic S, de Hemptinne C, Qasim S, Ostrem JL, Starr PA. Patterns of cortical synchronization in isolated dystonia compared with Parkinson disease. JAMA Neurol. 2015; 72(11):1244–1251

[11] Israelashvili M, Loewenstern Y, Bar-Gad I. Abnormal neuronal activity in Tourette syndrome and its modulation using deep brain stimulation. J Neurophysiol. 2015; 114(1):6–20

[12] Priori A, Giannicola G, Rosa M, et al. Deep brain electrophysiological recordings provide clues to the pathophysiology of Tourette syndrome. Neurosci Biobehav Rev. 2013; 37(6):1063–1068

[13] Hampson M, Tokoglu F, King RA, Constable RT, Leckman JF. Brain areas coactivating with motor cortex during chronic motor tics and intentional movements. Biol Psychiatry. 2009; 65(7):594–599

[14] Mian MK, Campos M, Sheth SA, Eskandar EN. Deep brain stimulation for obsessive-compulsive disorder: past, present, and future. Neurosurg Focus. 2010; 29(2):E10

[15] Visser-Vandewalle V, Kuhn J. Deep brain stimulation for Tourette syndrome. Handb Clin Neurol. 2013; 116:251–258

[16] Kim W, Pouratian N. Deep brain stimulation for Tourette syndrome. Neurosurg Clin N Am. 2014; 25(1):117–135

[17] Trotta M, Cocjin J, Whitehead E, et al. Surface based electrode localization and standardized regions of interest for intracranial EEG. Hum Brain Mapp. 2018; 39:709–721

[18] Yang T, Hakimian S, Schwartz TH. Intraoperative ElectroCorticoGraphy (ECog): indications, techniques, and utility in epilepsy surgery. Epileptic Disord. 2014; 16(3):271–279

[19] Greiner HM, Horn PS, Tenney JR, et al. Preresection intraoperative electrocorticography (ECoG) abnormalities predict seizure-onset zone and outcome in pediatric epilepsy surgery. Epilepsia. 2016; 57(4):582–589

[20] Hanson TL, Fuller AM, Lebedev MA, Turner DA, Nicolelis MA. Subcortical neuronal ensembles: an analysis of motor task association, tremor, oscillations, and synchrony in human patients. J Neurosci. 2012; 32(25):8620–8632

[21] Levy R, Hutchison WD, Lozano AM, Dostrovsky JO. High-frequency synchronization of neuronal activity in the subthalamic nucleus of parkinsonian patients with limb tremor. J Neurosci. 2000; 20(20):7766–7775

[22] Zavala BA, Tan H, Little S, et al. Midline frontal cortex low-frequency activity drives subthalamic nucleus oscillations during conflict. J Neurosci. 2014; 34(21):7322–7333

[23] Zaghloul KA, Weidemann CT, Lega BC, Jaggi JL, Baltuch GH, Kahana MJ. Neuronal activity in the human subthalamic nucleus encodes decision conflict during action selection. J Neurosci. 2012; 32(7):2453–2460

[24] Vidailhet M, Vercueil L, Houeto JL, et al. French Stimulation du Pallidum Interne dans la Dystonie (SPIDY) Study Group. Bilateral deep-brain stimulation of the globus pallidus in primary generalized dystonia. N Engl J Med. 2005; 352(5):459–467

[25] Kumar R, Lozano AM, Kim YJ, et al. Double-blind evaluation of subthalamic nucleus deep brain stimulation in advanced Parkinson's disease. Neurology. 1998; 51(3):850–855

[26] Tierney TS, Abd-El-Barr MM, Stanford AD, Foote KD, Okun MS. Deep brain stimulation and ablation for obsessive compulsive disorder: evolution of contemporary indications, targets and techniques. Int J Neurosci. 2014; 124(6):394–402

[27] Ramayya AG, Zaghloul KA, Weidemann CT, Baltuch GH, Kahana MJ. Electrophysiological evidence for functionally distinct neuronal populations in the human substantia nigra. Front Hum Neurosci. 2014; 8:655

[28] Patel SR, Sheth SA, Martinez-Rubio C, et al. Studying task-related activity of individual neurons in the human brain. Nat Protoc. 2013; 8(5):949–957

[29] Panov F, Levin E, de Hemptinne C, et al. Intraoperative electrocorticography for physiological research in movement disorders: principles and experience in 200 cases. J Neurosurg. 2017; 126(1):122–131

[30] Schaeffer EL, Liu DY, Guerin J, Ahn M, Lee S, Asaad WF. A low-cost solution for quantification of movement during DBS surgery. J Neurosci Methods. 2018; 303:136–145

[31] Asaad WF, Eskandar EN. A flexible software tool for temporally-precise behavioral control in Matlab. J Neurosci Methods. 2008; 174(2):245–258

[32] Asaad WF, Eskandar EN. Achieving behavioral control with millisecond resolution in a high-level programming environment. J Neurosci Methods. 2008; 173(2):235–240

[33] Asaad WF, Santhanam N, McClellan S, Freedman DJ. High-performance execution of psychophysical tasks with complex visual stimuli in MATLAB. J Neurophysiol. 2013; 109(1):249–260

[34] Cohen M. Analyzing Neural Time Series Data: Theory and Practice. MIT Press; 2014

[35] Kass R, Eden U, Brown E. Analysis of Neural Data. In: New York, NY: Springer; 2014

[36] Wood F, Black MJ, Vargas-Irwin C, Fellows M, Donoghue JP. On the variability of manual spike sorting. IEEE Trans Biomed Eng. 2004; 51(6):912–918

[37] Jones DK, Knösche TR, Turner R. White matter integrity, fiber count, and other fallacies: the do's and don'ts of diffusion MRI. Neuroimage. 2013; 73:239–254

[38] Zrinzo L. Pitfalls in precision stereotactic surgery. Surg Neurol Int. 2012; 3 Suppl 1:S53–S61

[39] Cox RW. AFNI: software for analysis and visualization of functional magnetic resonance neuroimages. Comput Biomed Res. 1996; 29(3):162–173

[40] Saad ZS, Reynolds RC. SUMA. Neuroimage. 2012; 62(2):768–773

[41] Smith SM, Jenkinson M, Woolrich MW, et al. Advances in functional and structural MR image analysis and implementation as FSL. Neuroimage. 2004; 23 Suppl 1:S208–S219

[42] Woolrich MW, Jbabdi S, Patenaude B, et al. Bayesian analysis of neuroimaging data in FSL. Neuroimage. 2009; 45(1) Suppl:S173–S186

[43] Jenkinson M, Beckmann CF, Behrens TE, Woolrich MW, Smith SM. FSL. Neuroimage. 2012; 62(2):782–790

[44] Horn A, Kühn AA. Lead-DBS: a toolbox for deep brain stimulation electrode localizations and visualizations. Neuroimage. 2015; 107:127–135

[45] Lauro PM, Vanegas-Arroyave N, Huang L, et al. DBSproc: An open source process for DBS electrode localization and tractographic analysis. Hum Brain Mapp. 2016; 37(1):422–433

[46] Collins D, Zijdenbos A, Baaré W, Evans A. ANIMAL+INSECT: Improved Cortical Structure Segmentation. In: Information Processing in Medical Imaging. Berlin, Heidelberg: Springer; 1999

[47] Fonov V, Evans A, McKinstry R, Almli C, Collins D. Unbiased nonlinear average age-appropriate brain templates from birth to adulthood. Neuroimage. 2009; 47(Suppl)(1):S102

[48] Fonov V, Evans AC, Botteron K, Almli CR, McKinstry RC, Collins DL, Brain Development Cooperative Group. Unbiased average age-appropriate atlases for pediatric studies. Neuroimage. 2011; 54(1):313–327

[49] Xiao Y, Bériault S, Pike GB, Collins DL. Multicontrast multiecho FLASH MRI for targeting the subthalamic nucleus. Magn Reson Imaging. 2012; 30(5):627–640

[50] Xiao Y, Fonov V, Bériault S, et al. Multi-contrast unbiased MRI atlas of a Parkinson's disease population. Int J CARS. 2015; 10(3):329–341

[51] Xiao Y, Fonov V, Chakravarty MM, et al. A dataset of multi-contrast population-averaged brain MRI atlases of a Parkinson's disease cohort. Data Brief. 2017; 12:370–379

[52] Randazzo MJ, Kondylis ED, Alhourani A, et al. Three-dimensional localization of cortical electrodes in deep brain stimulation surgery from intraoperative fluoroscopy. Neuroimage. 2016; 125:515–521

[53] Fischl B. FreeSurfer. Neuroimage. 2012; 62(2):774–781

[54] Pierpaoli C, Walker L, Irfanoglu M, et al. TORTOISE: An Integrated Software Package for Processing of Diffusion MRI Data. Stockholm, Sweden; 2010

[55] Sheth SA, Mian MK, Patel SR, et al. Human dorsal anterior cingulate cortex neurons mediate ongoing behavioural adaptation. Nature. 2012; 488(7410):218–221

17 Deep Brain Stimulation: Techniques and Practice for Pediatrics Indications

Travis S. Tierney, William S. Anderson, H. Isaac Chen, Shenandoah Robinson

Abstract

Motor dysfunction in childhood usually manifests as spasticity or dystonia. By far the most common cause of motor problems in children is cerebral palsy, and varying degrees of both spasticity and dystonia are usually present. We examine the surgical options for treating either condition. Pallidal deep brain stimulation (DBS) is highly effective for most forms of primary dystonia including DYT1 +, DYT6 +, and DYT11 + genetic subtypes. Pallidal DBS or intrathecal baclofen is moderately effective for secondary dystonia associated with the heredodegenerative dystonias or dystonic cerebral palsy. Spasticity is common and its treatment is individually tailored according to age, severity, and limb distribution. Under the age of 6 years, children with cerebral palsy are best treated with botulinum toxin because spasticity often abates with age. On the other hand, most forms of childhood dystonia usually progress and early surgical intervention may be desirable. Optimal age and selection of the most effective surgical modality has not been well studied for any etiology, but the decision to proceed with most surgery is usually elective. However, two life-threatening conditions associated with movement disorders require urgent medical and often emergent surgical intervention: baclofen withdrawal and status dystonicus. Surgeons need to be aware of early and subtle signs of either condition as these are occasionally overlooked. Finally, selected pediatric neuropsychiatric conditions such as Tourette syndrome and obsessive-compulsive disorder are now being investigated in children, a natural evolution of the field.

Keywords: ablation, baclofen, deep brain stimulation, dystonia, neuromodulation, pediatric, spasticity, surgery

17.1 Introduction

Movement disorders that occur during childhood are mainly hyperkinetic.[1] Many of these are transient (e.g., stereotypies, tics, myoclonus), but the few that progress or persist sometimes come to neurosurgical attention (e.g., the dystonias, choreoathetosis). Although spasticity is characterized by motor dysfunction, it is not considered a "movement disorder" by convention[2] Nonetheless, spasticity associated with cerebral palsy is by far the most common condition referred to the pediatric movement disorders clinic. Nearly all of these referrals are nonurgent and often involve extensive discussion with an experienced multidisciplinary movement disorders team. On the other hand, two life-threating conditions require rapid recognition and surgical attention: *intrathecal baclofen (ITB) withdrawal* and *status dystonicus*. Baclofen overdose, while an emergency when not anticipated, is rarely fatal but often requires ventilator support for a few days and possibly cerebrospinal fluid (CSF) barbotage. This chapter will discuss these emergencies, interventions for primary and secondary dystonia, and briefly touch on Tourette syndrome (TS), a quintessential pediatric neuropsychiatric condition. Surgical management of related conditions such as obsessive-compulsive disorder (OCD) and various other psychiatric disorders that can occur in childhood but have not been well studied in the pediatric population and so remain for future investigation. This chapter emphasizes deep brain stimulation (DBS) therapy for a number of pediatric indications and the differences compared to adult patients.

17.2 Pediatric Movement Disorders: Neurosurgical Emergencies

Some movement disorders in children can present dramatically, and occasionally urgent surgical referrals are made to the clinic or come from the emergency department with concerns about a serious underlying condition. Examples include benign paroxysmal torticollis mimicking rotary subluxation, or Sandifer's syndrome mimicking seizure or dystonic storm. Often the history and physical exam, together with basic imaging and electrodiagnostic studies are reassuring, and further urgent neurosurgical management can be deferred.

Baclofen overdose is typically iatrogenic and occurs at refilling/reprogramming intervals or after surgical repair of an ITB system without adequate dose adjustment. Overdose can lead rapidly to hypoventilation, flaccid paralysis, and coma. However, baclofen even at high doses is not neurotoxic and complete recovery within a few days with supportive care should be expected. Ventilatory support with intensive care unit (ICU) monitoring is often required. There is no specific pharmacological antidote for baclofen overdose, although some have recommended the acetylcholinesterase inhibitor physostigmine or the benzodiazepine receptor antagonist flumazenil for symptomatic relief.[3,4] Neither of these agents have been found to be effective,[5,6,7] and a recent consensus statement suggests they should not be used for ITB overdose.[8] The most effective therapy seems to be stopping the pump and aspirating 20 to 30 ml of CSF from the access port.

On the other hand, delayed diagnoses of status dystonicus[9,10] or baclofen withdrawal[8,11] may be lethal. Suspicion of these two life-threating conditions should prompt an urgent surgical visit and rapid mobilization of combined medical and surgical care. General initial management of either condition usually involves a low threshold for intubation or insertion of an oral airway followed by admission to the pediatric ICU, aggressive hydration to prevent renal compromise from myoglobinuria, rapid correction of electrolytes, and administration of intravenous benzodiazepine. ► Table 17.1 presents a simple algorithm to guide initial diagnosis and management of these two closely related conditions.

To avoid progression of baclofen withdrawal, prompt intervention to re-establish ITB therapy is necessary. Even high-dose oral/enteral baclofen cannot be reliably used to temporize

Table 17.1 1 Initial management steps for treating status dystonicus and ITB withdrawal

	Status dystonicus	ITB withdrawal
1. Note mental status	Usually unchanged	Early agitation, delirium, seizures
2. Recognize key clinical features	Rapidly evolving painful spasms, often retrocollis opisthotonos Hyperthermia without prominent autonomic symptoms Early bulbar spasm leading to respiratory failure	Pruritis, piloerection (goose bumps), severe rebound spasticity Hyperthermia with autonomic instability (tachycardia, tachypnea, labile BP) Early DIC leading to rapid multiple organ failure
3. Initiate acute management (maintenance of airway, respiration, and circulation)	Low threshold for intubation 1.5 X maintenance fluids A-line, pulse oximetry, cardiac monitor	IV diazepam (or midazolam) May require intubation Aggressive IV hydration (keeping urine output > 0.5 ml/kg/hour) A-line, pulse oximetry, cardiac monitor (with initial 12 lead EKG) Enteral baclofen and cyproheptadine
4. Order preliminary studies	ABG, CXR, CBC, CMP, serum CK, urine myoglobin, blood and urine gram stain and culture	ABG, CXR and Abd X-ray, CBC, CMP, serum CK, urine myoglobin, blood and urine gram stain and culture, LFTs, coagulation profile including fibrinogen and d-dimers
5. Give initial medications	IV diazepam or midazolam, titrated to muscle relaxation (may require ventilator support) Clonidine infusion (0.25–2.0 mcg/kg/hour) if not intubated Antipyretics Dantrolene and urine alkalization if rhabdomyolysis develops Broad-spectrum antibiotics if infection suspected	IV diazepam or midazolam, titrated to muscle relaxation (may require ventilator support) IT bolus via lumbar puncture, or infusion via lumbar catheter at pre-withdrawal rate, if severe Antipyretics Dantrolene and urine alkalization if rhabdomyolysis develops Broad-spectrum antibiotics if infection suspected
6. Search for correctable triggers	Gastroenteritis Diarrhea Occult infection Recent medication adjustment	Catheter discontinuity (40%) Pump malfunction (check logs) Reservoir empty (check last refill and replace drug to exclude pocket fill) Infection, meningitis
7. Determine disposition	ICU admission	ICU or OR for pump revision
8. Immediate therapeutic goal	Avoid rhabdomyolysis	Re-establish ITB as soon as possible

Abbreviations: ABG, arterial blood gas; BP, blood pressure; CBC, complete blood count; CK, creatine kinase; CMP, complete metabolic panel; CSF, cerebrospinal fluid; CXR, chest X-ray; DIC, disseminated intravascular coagulopathy (aka, death is coming); ICU, intensive care unit; ITB, intrathecal baclofen; LFT, liver function tests; MOR, multi-organ failure; OR, operating room.

definitive care because oral routes do not achieve high enough CSF levels.[12,13] Only 1 to 2% of enteral baclofen crosses the blood–brain barrier, and it cannot prevent central nervous system (CNS) signs of withdrawal such as seizures. Enteral baclofen and cyproheptadine can be used to reduce non-CNS symptoms such as pruritis. $GABA_B$ receptor modulation with intravenous benzodiazepine (see ▶ Table 17.1 for doses) or propofol[14] has been shown to be highly effective against symptomatic progression, and both agents protect against withdrawal seizure. Sustained use of propofol has a risk of propofol infusion syndrome in children so it is not recommended. Like baclofen overdose, withdrawal also tends to occur around refill times. Often, pump interrogation for confirmation of correct drug concentrations and rates together with bolus dosing may be all that is required to resolve the under dose. Pump logs should be checked to exclude pump stall, which is rare, but does occur and can be quickly excluded. There is no test for a pocket refill; to exclude an empty pump, prompt refill of the pump with fresh drug can be performed. A bolus can be programmed to provide faster relief. After human factors, catheter problems are the most common cause of withdrawal. Disconnection and kinking can often be detected on plain films. Occlusion cannot

always be detected by a bolus test or aspiration. If a catheter problem is suspected, operative exploration is often the most expeditious route to return of drug delivery. While dye studies were performed in the past, they were often nondiagnostic and simply delayed operative exploration. In unfortunate cases of meningitis or implant infection, device explantation probably will be necessary together with broad-spectrum antibiotics. For complex patients on high ITB doses with pump infection, rapid taper of ITB over a few days, while on broad-spectrum antibiotics, can reduce the overlap of severe infection and withdrawal and improve the overall safety. Here, case reports have suggested that re-establishment of external ITB therapy via lumbar infusion is feasible.[15,16] Inflammatory granuloma formation has been observed in patients receiving intrathecal opiate therapy, but has not been reported with ITB infusion.

Similar to baclofen withdrawal, status dystonicus (also called dystonic storm or crisis) can rapidly escalate into a life-threating condition in children and may require urgent surgical intervention if it is refractory to medically induced coma.[17] The goal of rapid therapeutic escalation is to avoid the development of rhabdomyolysis and respiratory collapse. In most cases, the diagnosis of dystonia is previously known, but in the rare syndrome of glutaric aciduria type I, status dystonicus may be the presenting condition and can be mistaken for status epilepticus.[18] The acquired (so-called secondary) dystonias are most likely to develop into dystonic storm,[19,20] although any form of dystonia has the potential to escalate. Factors triggering a crisis include infection, fever, dehydration, and DBS or ITB failure.[21,22] In these latter triggers, therapeutic failures often occur after depletion of the implanted pulse generator (IPG) or baclofen reservoir. System interrogation and re-establishment of therapy is again urgently indicated. Surgical intervention to place bilateral pallidal leads should be considered when specific medical therapy and paralytic coma fail to control status dystonicus.[21,23,24,25,26,27] The youngest patient in the literature so far to have DBS for storm was 4 years of age.[28] Attempts to control refractory status dystonicus with ITB have also been made.[22,29,30,31] Some centers have reported significantly less success with ITB than DBS,[32,33] especially in cases originating from secondary dystonia. However, ITB therapy has been successful in the authors' experience. Unilateral pallidotomy[10,34] or even bilateral staged procedures[35,36] are effective, though historical,[37,38] treatments for status dystonicus that might still be considered in cases where ongoing infection or other technical complications preclude hardware implantation.[39,40]

17.3 Dystonia

The dystonias are a heterogeneous group of conditions that share a common formal definition[1]: "a movement disorder in which involuntary sustained or intermittent muscle contractions cause twisting and repetitive movements, abnormal postures, or both." Clinically, dystonia manifests as involuntary cocontraction of opposing muscle groups that often causes a smooth lead pipe type rigidity which differs substantially in quality from the so-called knife-clasp rigidity of spasticity (see later). Age-related progression of disability, progressive pain, and social isolation that often accompany the disease in children represent important indications for early surgical intervention. Unlike adult-onset dystonia that tends to remain relatively focal,[41] dystonia in childhood usually generalizes shortly after it is diagnosed, especially in cases of primary dystonia.[42] The classic but now antiquated term *dystonia musculorum deformans* is synonymous with the currently used term *primary dystonia* where genetic analyses have yielded a number of abnormalities leading to various subtypes of primary dystonia.[43,44] In general these are rare disorders with prevalence rates ranging from 1 in 10,000 to 1 in 30,000 children. This prevalence is many times higher in the Ashkenazi Jews.

The *secondary dystonias* are differentiated from the primary dystonia when a structural lesion within the brain (usually involving the internal segment of the pallidum) is evident on magnetic resonance imaging (MRI)[20] (▶ Fig. 17.1). They also have a broad spectrum of causes including both genetic and acquired etiologies, but by far the most common is cerebral palsy-associated dystonia with a prevalence of 2 to 3 per 1,000 or about 15 to 25% of all children with cerebral palsy.[45] In general, the secondary dystonias are thought to be less responsive to DBS compared with the primary dystonia, however open-label studies and case reports indicate that tardive dystonia,[46,47,48] well-selected cases of dystonic cerebral palsy[49,50] and certain heredodegenerative disease including pantothenate kinase-associated neurodegeneration (PKAN)[51,52] may respond to bilateral pallidal stimulation. ITB can improve the comfort and function of many, but not all, patients with secondary dystonia.

The initial clinical presentation of dystonia in children is usually subtle, but in rare instances noted above, dystonic storm is the first indication of disease where rapid surgical intervention may be required. Often the forme fruste of the condition is intermittently present and usually involves torsion of a limb. Here, home videos are helpful. An experienced childhood movement disorders specialist is even more helpful. From guiding the initial genetic diagnoses of the primary and heredodegenerative dystonias to coordinating ongoing medical management, multidisciplinary teams are essential. To follow these patients over the long-term and to ensure a smooth transition to adult providers, a dedicated multidisciplinary pediatric team that includes neurology, physiatry, and/or developmental pediatrics is essential for successful care of these complex patients.

Although full consideration of the diagnosis of dystonia lies outside the scope of this chapter, the neurosurgeon should be aware of a few pitfalls in the diagnosis of dystonia, recognize

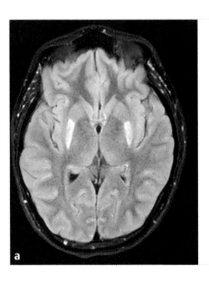
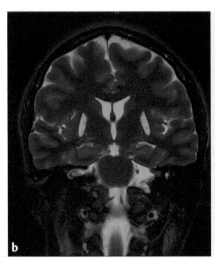

Fig. 17.1 (a, b) Axial fluid-attenuated inversion recovery and coronal T2-weighted images of a 19-year-old female with cerebral palsy secondary to an anoxic brain injury showing hyperintense signal in the putamen and pallidum characteristic of patients presenting with generalized secondary dystonia.

those genetic subtypes that seem to respond best to DBS, or ITB therapy, and be familiar with the basic rating scales. Rating scales for primary dystonia (Burke–Fahn–Marsden Dystonia Rating Scale, BFMDRS) and secondary dystonia (Barry–Albright Dystonic Scale, BAD) have been validated in children.[53,54,55,56] These scales can serve as a benchmarks to gauge treatment effects and compare outcomes between centers.

Segawa syndrome,[57] also called *dopa-responsive dystonia* (DYT5 +), has features of spasticity and parkinsonism with childhood onset and is occasionally misdiagnosed as dystonic cerebral palsy.[58,59] Most experts recommend a trial of levodopa in all children who develop dystonic posturing since Segawa syndrome, as well as a number of other dystonias, responds dramatically to a low dose of levodopa.[43] In cases where the diagnosis of dystonic cerebral palsy is not unequivocally supported by historical and radiographic data, delaying surgical interventions for a trial of levodopa over several weeks is warranted to avoid an error in diagnosis and unnecessary surgery.

In general, the primary dystonias are thought to be more responsive to DBS than the secondary dystonias.[47] There are now a number of genetically identified etiologies of the primary dystonias, making the once synonymous term *idiopathic generalized dystonia* now somewhat of a misnomer. Genetic screening for the 20 or so various subtypes of torsion dystonia (DTY) is available, as is genetic testing for the heredodegenerative secondary dystonias.[60] Once the diagnosis of dystonia is suspected and high-resolution images have excluded various forms of secondary dystonia (e.g., dystonic cerebral palsy, Rett syndrome, Leigh's disease, metal accumulation diseases, trauma, tumors, and stroke), this testing is usually undertaken in conjunction with a medical geneticist. Fortunately, the most common form of early-onset primary dystonia is also among the most responsive dystonias to bilateral pallidal stimulation. Dystonia with DYT1 gene mutation, caused by *TOR1A* gene CAG deletion on chromosome 9q, accounts for 40 to 60% of childhood-onset primary dystonia.[61] Autosomal dominant dystonia with cranio-cervical predilection (DYT6 +) and myoclonic dystonia (DYT11 +) have also been noted in open-label studies to be similarly responsive to DBS.[62,63] Several studies have also shown that genetically undetermined causes of primary dystonia, so called non-DYT cases, may also respond well to pallidal stimulation.[64]

Consideration of nonpallidal targets, for example, the ventrolateral thalamus and the subthalamic nucleus, has been suggested in childhood dystonia,[65] but these nuclei are generally reserved for cases where optimally placed pallidal electrodes are ineffective or cause hypokinetic side effects.[66] Although the United States Food and Drug Administration (FDA) Humanitarian Device Exemption does allow for placement of electrodes at the subthalamic nucleus (STN), the posteroventral pallidum remains, by far, the most commonly selected target for both pediatric primary[67] and secondary dystonia.[68] Note that secondary dystonia is an off- label use and it does not require applications to the FDA or approval by an institutional review board if conducted on a case-by-case basis. No comparative studies in children exist to guide selection of an optimal target in childhood dystonia, but it seems intuitive that the STN might be a favorable site in children with damaged pallidum that commonly accompanies the secondary dystonias.[20] However, for primary dystonias, the posteroventral pallidum should remain the favored site. Secondary dystonias are often responsive to ITB treatment.[69] In some patients, ITB therapy can significantly improve function and comfort. Those with severe dystonia may benefit from ITB therapy supplemented by DBS.

17.4 Spasticity

Compared with dystonia, spasticity is much more common, affecting about 300,000 people under 18 years of age in the United States alone. Paradoxically perhaps, advances in perinatal care seem to be increasing the incidence of cerebral spasticity as the survival of at-risk low birth weight infants, who go on to develop cerebral palsy, increases.[70,71] Defined as velocity-dependent increase in muscle resistance to passive stretch, limb spasticity can be clinically classified into four useful groups based on location: quadriparesis (also called tetraplegia), paraparesis (also called diplegia), hemiparesis, and monoparesis. The extent of limb function disruption largely guides the selection of therapy. For example, monoparesis may respond well to botulinum toxin injections, whereas quadriparesis might be best treated with ITB therapy. In well-selected cases of spastic diplegia, selective dorsal rhizotomy is often ideal. It is important to note that spasticity is not always harmful. Many patients use their spasticity to maintain trunk support and supplement weak leg muscles. While the initial insult that precipitates spasticity was likely a static injury, the impact of spasticity on function and comfort can change with time.[72] On one hand, "worsening spasticity" may be a red flag for a missed diagnosis of hypertonicity associated with dystonia or hereditary spastic paraparesis (also called familial spastic paraplegia or Strumpell–Lorrain disease).[73] The pattern of severity of cerebral palsy is changing in the United States over time,[74] which likely reflects the improvements in obstetrical and neonatal care. With these improvements in care, some infants are left with fewer deficits, while others who previously may not have survived now experience significant deficits.

Spasticity can be graded clinically and treatment effects may be followed using one of two rating scales: the simpler and validated Modified Ashworth Scale[75,76] or the more comprehensive but less studied Tardieu Scale[77] (▶ Table 17.2). Both provide a method for assessing the degree of spasticity across limb joints and are an important criterion in patient selection.

The child is usually tested lying down and each joint is evaluated methodically with particular attention being paid to flexors and internal rotators of the lower extremities. It is also important to test muscle strength in the legs and trunk as some children may supplement weakened muscles with involuntary spastic contractions to improve their gait and pivot transfers. In these cases, interventions to improve spasticity may actually reduce overall functional mobility. When a joint has been subjected to severe spasticity for many months, the muscle and tendon tend to progressively shorten into a fixed contracture that does not improve with treatment of the spasticity. Commonly, this occurs at the plantar flexors, knee flexors, and hip adductors, the latter of which often leads to progressive hip subluxation and acetabular deformity. The goal of treating spastic diplegia, in particular, is to avoid the development of this painful condition. Orthopedic treatment of fixed contractures is not discussed in detail in this chapter but consists of various

Table 17.2 Two common rating scales for pediatric dystonia: Burke–Fahn–Marsden Dystonia Rating Scale motor subscale (BFMDRS-M) for primary dystonia and the Barry-Albright Dystonia (BAD) scale for secondary dystonia

Region and description	BFMDRS-M (score range 0–120[a])	BADS (score range 0–32[b])
Eyes—signs of dystonia of the eyes include: prolonged eyelid spasms and/or forced eye deviations	0 No dystonia present 1 Slight: occasional blinking 2 Mild: frequent blinking without prolonged spasms of eye closure 3 Moderate: prolonged spasms of eyelid closure, but eyes open most of the time 4 Severe: prolonged spasms of eyelid closure, with eyes closed at least 30% of the time	0 Absent 1 Slight: dystonia less than 10% of the time and does not interfere with tracking 2 Mild: frequent blinking without prolonged spasms of eyelid closure, and/or eye movements less than 50% of the time 3 Moderate: prolonged spasms of eyelid closure, but eyes open most of the time, and/or eye movements more than 50% of the time that interfere with tracking, but able to resume tracking 4 Severe: prolonged spasms of eyelid closure, with eyelids closed at least 30% of the time, and/or eye movements more than 50% of the time that prevent tracking
Mouth—signs of dystonia of the mouth include grimacing, clenched or deviated jaw, forced open mouth, and/or forceful tongue thrusting	0 No dystonia present 1 Slight: occasional grimacing or other mouth movements (e.g., jaw open or clenched, tongue movement) 2 Mild: movement present less than 50% of the time 3 Moderate: dystonic moderate movements or contractions present most of the time 4 Severe: severe dystonic movements or contractions present most of the time	0 Absent 1 Slight: dystonia less than 10% of the time and does not interfere with speech and/or feeding 2 Mild: dystonia less than 50% of the time and does not interfere with speech and/or feeding 3 Moderate: dystonia more than 50% of the time and/or dystonia that interferes with speech and/or feeding 4 Severe: dystonia more than 50% of the time and/or dystonia that prevents speech and/or feeding
Speech and swallowing	0 Normal 1 Slightly involved; speech easily understood or occasional choking 2 Some difficulty in understanding speech or frequent choking 3 Marked difficulty in understanding speech or inability to swallow firm foods 4 Complete or almost complete anarthria, or marked difficulty swallowing soft foods or liquids	
Neck—signs of dystonia of the neck include pulling of the neck into any plane of motion: extension, flexion, lateral flexion or rotation	0 No dystonia present 1 Slight: occasional pulling 2 Obvious torticollis, but mild 3 Moderate pulling 4 Extreme pulling	0 Absent 1 Slight: pulling less than 10% of the time and does not interfere with lying, sitting, standing and/or walking 2 Mild: pulling less than 50% of the time and does not interfere with lying, sitting, standing and/or walking 3 Moderate: pulling more than 50% of the time and/or dystonia that interferes with lying, sitting, standing and/or walking 4 Severe: pulling more than 50% of the time and dystonia that prevents sitting in a standard wheelchair (e.g., requires special head rest), standing and/or walking
Arm—signs of dystonia of the upper extremities include sustained muscle contractions causing abnormal postures, score each limb separately	0 No dystonia present 1 Slight: clinically insignificant 2 Mild: obvious dystonia but not disabling 3 Moderate: able to grasp, with some manual function 4 Severe: no useful grasp	0 Absent 1 Slight: dystonia less than 10% of the time and does not interfere with normal positioning and/or functional activities 2 Mild: dystonia less than 50% of the time and does not interfere with normal positioning and/or functional activities 3 Moderate: dystonia more than 50% of the time and/or dystonia that interferes with normal positioning and/or upper extremity function 4 Severe: dystonia more than 50% of the time and/or dystonia that prevents normal positioning and/or upper extremity function (e.g., arms restrained to prevent injury)

Table 17.2 (*Continued*) Two common rating scales for pediatric dystonia: Burke–Fahn–Marsden Dystonia Rating Scale motor subscale (BFMDRS-M) for primary dystonia and the Barry-Albright Dystonia (BAD) scale for secondary dystonia

Region and description	BFMDRS-M (score range 0–120[a])	BADS (score range 0–32[b])
Trunk—signs of dystonia of the trunk include pulling of the trunk into any plane of motion: extension, flexion, lateral flexion or rotation	0 No dystonia present 1 Slight bending; clinically insignificant 2 Definite bending but not interfering with standing or walking 3 Moderate bending; interfering with standing or walking 4 Extreme bending of trunk preventing standing or walking	0 Absent 1 Slight: pulling less than 10% of the time and does not interfere with lying, sitting, standing and/or walking 2 Mild: pulling less than 50% of the time and does not interfere with lying, sitting, standing and/or walking 3 Moderate: pulling more than 50% of the time and/or dystonia that interferes with lying, sitting, standing and/or walking 4 Severe: pulling more than 50% of the time and dystonia that prevents sitting in a standard wheelchair (e.g., requires adapted seating system), standing and/or walking
Leg—signs of dystonia of the lower extremities include sustained muscle contractions causing abnormal postures, Score each limb separately	0 No dystonia present 1 Slight: dystonia but not causing impairment; clinically insignificant 2 Mild: walks briskly and unaided 3 Moderate: severely impairs walking or requires assistance. 4 Severe: unable to stand or walk on involved leg	0 Absent 1 Slight: dystonia less than 10% of the time and does not interfere with normal positioning and/or functional activities 2 Mild: dystonia less than 50% of the time and does not interfere with normal positioning and/or functional activities 3 Moderate: dystonia more than 50% of the time and/or dystonia that interferes with normal positioning and/or lower extremity weight bearing and/or function 4 Severe: dystonia more than 50% of the time and/or dystonia that prevents normal positioning and/or lower extremity weight bearing and/or function

[a] The above severity score in each region of the BFMDRS is multiplied by a provoking factor score as follows: **0**: No dystonia at rest or with action, **1**: dystonia on a particular action, **2**: dystonia on many actions, **3**: dystonia on action of distant part of body, or intermittently at rest **4**: dystonia at rest. For speech and swallowing the provoking factor score is **0**: none, **1** occasional speech and/or swallow difficulty, **2**: frequent speech or swallow difficulty, **3**: frequent speech or swallow difficulty, and occasional speech or/and swallow difficulty, **4**: frequent speech and swallowing difficulty. Additionally, a weight of ½ is given for severity and provoking products of eye, mouth and neck. The total summed adjusted maximum score is 120.

[b] The BADS score is simply the sum of severity scores in each of the 8 body regions for a maximum of 32.

surgeries for musculoskeletal release followed by extensive rehabilitative therapy to maintain enhanced mobility.[78,79]

Before any surgical therapy, a candid discussion with the child, parents, and associated care givers should clearly establish postoperative expectations and set a few common goals. In general, the therapeutic goal should include: (1) reduction of pain, (2) facilitation of routine care such as bathing and feeding, (3) prevention of contractures, and (4) some degree of functional improvement. Often high expectations on the part of the patient with regard to functional improvement must be tempered in order to offer realistic hope. In general, this last goal encompasses greater ease in activities of daily living such as dressing, transfers, and ambulation. No studies have yielded more specific predictors of improvements in fine motor or midline control required for improved handwriting or augmented speech intelligibility or swallowing capability. No screening trial has been developed to accurately predict functional improvement after selective dorsal rhizotomy or ITB therapy. Current clinical selection criteria for surgical intervention depend heavily on severity and distribution of spasticity as well as the child's age (▶ Table 17.3).

17.5 Tourette Syndrome

TS is a quintessential pediatric neuropsychiatric condition in the sense that tics and urges phenomenologically bridge neurology and childhood psychiatry. Characterized by prepubertal onset of motor and vocal tics, TS is often associated with attention deficit hyperactivity disorder and OCD, but its relationship to these comorbid conditions remains controversial.[24,80,81] Like spasticity, tic severity tends to decrease during adolescence, and by early adulthood as many as one-third of children with TS become tic free.[82,83] Despite this regressive natural history, a number of centers have now treated pediatric patients with severely disabling motor/vocal tics with surgery.[84,85,86,87] The most common procedures involve bilateral placement of thalamic (centromedian-parafascicular and ventralis oralis complex) or pallidal (pars internus) DBS leads. In general, the results of DBS for the treatment of TS in children from these studies seem to be on par with those outcomes from the adult cohort. Some have offered important ethical as well as biological reasons to remain cautious in treating pediatric neuropsychiatric disease surgically.[88] On the other hand, children with medically

Table 17.3 Comparison of two common scales for evaluating spasticity in children

Modified Ashworth Scale Grade	Description	Tardieu Scale Grade[a]	Description
0	No increased muscle tone	0	No resistance to passive movement
1	Slight increase in muscle tone	1	Slight resistance to passive movement, but no "catch"
1+	Slight increase in muscle tone with a "catch" followed by minimal resistance	2	Clear "catch" at a precise angle followed by release
2	Marked increase in muscle tone, but joint moves easily	3	Fatigable clonus less than 10 seconds
3	Considerable muscle tone with difficult passive joint motion	4	Unfatigable clonus
4	Joint ridge (fixed) in flexion or extension	5	Joint immobile

[a] The Tardieu scales assess spasticity at three velocities (V1: as slow as possible, V2: velocity under gravity drop, V3: as fast as possible) and notes the angle at which joint catches appear. The "catch" is sudden increase in muscle resistance felt when moving the limb through passive range of motion.

intractable TS may be considered an extremely vulnerable group, in which surgical interventions shown to be safe and effective in adults should be studied in small-scale trials at dedicated pediatric research centers. A cautious but timely approach to childhood psychiatric conditions naturally follows from the many historical successes of DBS in treatment of pediatric movement disorders.[89,90] Still, no governmental regulatory agency has approved DBS for the treatment of tics associated with TS in children or adults. Some possible explanations include the paucity of cases referred for DBS even at larger academic medical centers, the lack of a major multisite randomized trial, and the diversity of surgical targets and outcomes observed in various studies (see Chapter 14, DBS in Tourette Syndrome). To this end, an international registry under the aegis of the Tourette Association of America has recently been established in the hope of systematically capturing all adverse events and efficacy data from a large number of cases worldwide.[91] Similar data was used to achieve a Humanitarian Device Exemption from the US FDA in 2009 for the treatment of OCD in adults, another developmental psychiatric condition with pediatric origins.[80]

17.6 Surgical Considerations

Although children have benefitted enormously from the technical advances in functional neurosurgery that are proposed, tested, and refined in adults, children require additional considerations.[92,93,94,95,96,97] Due to their complex medical conditions, many children who may benefit from surgical intervention are also at higher risk for complications, poor wound healing from inadequate nutrition, and infection.[98] Young children also have not reached skeletal maturity, which may impact surgical options.

To minimize the risk of poor wound healing, many multidisciplinary pediatric movement disorders programs include specialists in pediatric gastroenterology and nutrition. A few months of concerted efforts can raise the body mass index and reduce the risk of complications. Transient or permanent use of supplemental nutrition is often necessary to optimize wound healing. The concept of adequate nutrition to support brain growth as well as to ensure surgical healing should be emphasized from a young age as soon as the diagnosis of dystonia and spasticity is made and the likely need for surgery appears on the distant horizon. This will help to avoid delay of surgical interventions in a timely manner while nutrition is addressed urgently in preparation for surgery.

Infection reduction protocols are now in widespread use at most pediatric neurosurgical centers. While small variances in protocol details exist between institutions, recent use of such protocols has shown that device-related infections can be drastically reduced in children, with many centers achieving 1-year infection rates below 3%. Reducing the infection rate can markedly shift the risk–benefit ratio for those children in whom the benefit is not well known prior to implantation.

Since the purpose of surgical intervention is to improve comfort, function, and independence, intervention in young children may be particularly beneficial. For DBS to support the stereotactic frame, the skull needs to be fused and of adequate thickness. Due to the impact of neurogenetic disorders on skeletal growth, no specific weight or age can be considered adequate, and children need to be assessed on an individualized basis. Similarly, for insertion of an ITB pump, the specific body habitus and nutritional status of each child should be considered. In general, a stable weight above 15 kg is a useful, but not fixed threshold. For selective dorsal rhizotomy, because of the importance of motivation and cooperation for the intense postoperative rehabilitation protocol, each child is ideally mature enough to be self-motivated to improve his or her gait.

At the time of surgery, potential growth and weight gain over years should be considered at the time of hardware placement. Despite being an expected concern, growth rarely becomes an issue.

17.7 Illustrative Case of DBS Insertion

The patient is discussed at the multidisciplinary movement disorders conference. After the team and the patient and family agree to proceed, the patient is prepared for surgery in the intraoperative MRI suite. Under general anesthesia, the head is placed in a head holder with four pin contacts. After hair-clipping, prepping and draping, MR fiducial grids are placed on the scalp overlying the proposed bilateral frontal bur holes (▶ Fig. 17.2). The patient is placed in the MR scanner and 3D

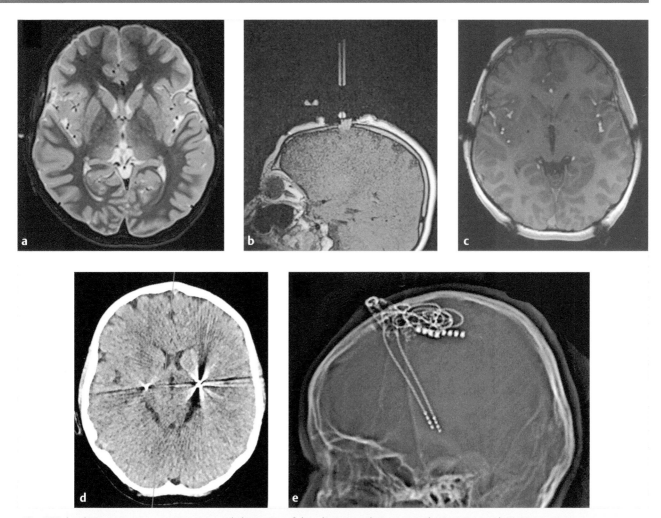

Fig. 17.2 (a–e) Magnetic resonance imaging-guided insertion of deep brain stimulation in a pediatric patient with DYT6 mutation.

volumetric T1 scan is obtained (▶ Fig. 17.2a). Using the stereotactic guidance system, the trajectory on each side is verified, and then made with the ceramic stylet (▶ Fig. 17.2b). Another MRI scan is obtained to confirm the localization of the ceramic stylets (▶ Fig. 17.2c), and then the leads are passed into the brain and then secured to the skull. A final scan is obtained for the leads at the conclusion of the surgery. A postoperative CT scan is obtained the evening of surgery to evaluate for potential complications. The leads are gently coiled in the subgaleal space and the wound is closed (▶ Fig. 17.2e). The patient returns at another surgery to have the leads connected to the generator.

17.8 Further Directions

In general, from a technical standpoint it seems that functional neurosurgical interventions in children have almost exclusively been driven by clinical experience gained from treating similar conditions in adults. It is likely that this natural progression of surgical innovation in our field will continue. From technical refinements such as image-guided lead placement without microelectrodes to new indications in the field of childhood psychiatric disease, innovation in pediatric functional neurosurgery

has largely been drive by challenges and interests of functional neurosurgeons at adult centers. More recently, a greater appreciation for the advantages of bringing the focused expertise from dedicated pediatric neurosurgical centers has become evident. Technical refinements continue to occur in the main treatment modalities (selective dorsal rhizotomy, DBS, and ITB therapy) making surgical interventions for movement disorders in children safer.

Genetic, imaging, and technical advances will expand the types of diseases and disorders that can be treated in children with functional neurosurgery. Certain conditions such as the autism spectrum disorders are beginning to be being suggested as surgical candidates.[99,100,101] These kinds of provocative directions in conditions that are so obviously development disorders are probably best explored first in dedicated children's hospitals where substantial subspecialized expertise exists. The field of functional pediatric neurosurgery is now emerging with a number of subspecialists dually trained in both pediatric and functional neurosurgery. The recent establishment the Pediatric International DBS (PEDiDBS) Registry Project[102] is strong evidence of nascent collaborative efforts being organized within the field of pediatric functional neurosurgery.

17.9 Some Pearls in Pediatric Functional Neurosurgery

- Pallidal DBS is highly effective for most forms of medically intractable primary dystonias including DYT1 +, DYT6 +, and DYT11 + genetic subtypes.
- Trials of levodopa are warranted in nonlesional imaging cases of childhood-onset dystonia to exclude dopa-responsive dystonias.
- Pallidal DBS or ITB therapy is moderately to very effective for secondary dystonia associated with the heredodegenerative dystonias and dystonic cerebral palsy.
- Spasticity is common in children and its treatment should be individually tailored according to age, severity, and limb distribution.
- ITB therapy efficiently treats upper and lower extremity spasticity.
- Selective dorsal rhizotomies for spastic diplegia can permanently improve gait in well-selected children with spastic diplegia and avoids implantation of hardware.

References

[1] Sanger TD, Delgado MR, Gaebler-Spira D, Hallett M, Mink JW, Task Force on Childhood Motor Disorders. Classification and definition of disorders causing hypertonia in childhood. Pediatrics. 2003; 111(1):e89–e97
[2] Singer. Movement Disorders in Childhood. 2010
[3] Greenberg MS. Handbook of neurosurgery. New York: Thieme; 2016
[4] Müller-Schwefe G, Penn RD. Physostigmine in the treatment of intrathecal baclofen overdose. Report of three cases. J Neurosurg. 1989; 71(2):273–275
[5] Byrnes SM, Watson GW, Hardy PA. Flumazenil: an unreliable antagonist in baclofen overdose. Anaesthesia. 1996; 51(5):481–482
[6] Delhaas EM, Brouwers JR. Intrathecal baclofen overdose: report of 7 events in 5 patients and review of the literature. Int J Clin Pharmacol Ther Toxicol. 1991; 29(7):274–280
[7] Rushman S, McLaren I. Management of intra-thecal baclofen overdose. Intensive Care Med. 1999; 25(2):239
[8] Saulino M, Anderson DJ, Doble J, et al. Best practices for intrathecal baclofen therapy: troubleshooting. Neuromodulation. 2016; 19(6):632–641
[9] Allen NM, Lin JP, Lynch T, King MD. Status dystonicus: a practice guide. Dev Med Child Neurol. 2014; 56(2):105–112
[10] Manji H, Howard RS, Miller DH, et al. Status dystonicus: the syndrome and its management. Brain. 1998; 121(Pt 2):243–252
[11] Watve SV, Sivan M, Raza WA, Jamil FF. Management of acute overdose or withdrawal state in intrathecal baclofen therapy. Spinal Cord. 2012; 50(2):107–111
[12] Fernandes P, Dolan L, Weinstein SL. Intrathecal baclofen withdrawal syndrome following posterior spinal fusion for neuromuscular scoliosis: a case report. Iowa Orthop J. 2008; 28:77–80
[13] Ross JC, Cook AM, Stewart GL, Fahy BG. Acute intrathecal baclofen withdrawal: a brief review of treatment options. Neurocrit Care. 2011; 14(1):103–108
[14] Ackland GL, Fox R. Low-dose propofol infusion for controlling acute hyperspasticity after withdrawal of intrathecal baclofen therapy. Anesthesiology. 2005; 103(3):663–665
[15] Bellinger A, Siriwetchadarak R, Rosenquist R, Greenlee JD. Prevention of intrathecal baclofen withdrawal syndrome: successful use of a temporary intrathecal catheter. Reg Anesth Pain Med. 2009; 34(6):600–602
[16] Duhon BS, MacDonald JD. Infusion of intrathecal baclofen for acute withdrawal. Technical note. J Neurosurg. 2007; 107(4):878–880
[17] Lumsden DE, King MD, Allen NM. Status dystonicus in childhood. Curr Opin Pediatr. 2017; 29(6):674–682
[18] Boy N, Mühlhausen C, Maier EM, et al. additional individual contributors. Proposed recommendations for diagnosing and managing individuals with glutaric aciduria type I: second revision. J Inherit Metab Dis. 2017; 40(1):75–101
[19] Fasano A, Ricciardi L, Bentivoglio AR, et al. Status dystonicus: predictors of outcome and progression patterns of underlying disease. Mov Disord. 2012; 27(6):783–788
[20] Tierney TS, Lozano AM. Surgical treatment for secondary dystonia. Mov Disord. 2012; 27(13):1598–1605
[21] Apetauerova D, Schirmer CM, Shils JL, Zani J, Arle JE. Successful bilateral deep brain stimulation of the globus pallidus internus for persistent status dystonicus and generalized chorea. J Neurosurg. 2010; 113(3):634–638
[22] Muirhead W, Jalloh I, Vloeberghs M. Status dystonicus resembling the intrathecal baclofen withdrawal syndrome: a case report and review of the literature. J Med Case Reports. 2010; 4:294
[23] Coubes P, Echenne B, Roubertie A, et al. Treatment of early-onset generalized dystonia by chronic bilateral stimulation of the internal globus pallidus. Apropos of a case. Neurochirurgie. 1999; 45(2):139–144
[24] Jankovic J, Kurlan R. Tourette syndrome: evolving concepts. Mov Disord. 2011; 26(6):1149–1156
[25] Jech R, Bares M, Urgosík D, et al. Deep brain stimulation in acute management of status dystonicus. Mov Disord. 2009; 24(15):2291–2292
[26] Walcott BP, Nahed BV, Kahle KT, Duhaime AC, Sharma N, Eskandar EN. Deep brain stimulation for medically refractory life-threatening status dystonicus in children. J Neurosurg Pediatr. 2012; 9(1):99–102
[27] Zorzi G, Marras C, Nardocci N, et al. Stimulation of the globus pallidus internus for childhood-onset dystonia. Mov Disord. 2005; 20(9):1194–1200
[28] Chakraborti S, Hasegawa H, Lumsden DE, et al. Bilateral subthalamic nucleus deep brain stimulation for refractory total body dystonia secondary to metabolic autopallidotomy in a 4-year-old boy with infantile methylmalonic acidemia: case report. J Neurosurg Pediatr. 2013; 12(4):374–379
[29] Grosso S, Verrotti A, Messina M, Sacchini M, Balestri P. Management of status dystonicus in children. Cases report and review. Eur J Paediatr Neurol. 2012; 16(4):390–395
[30] Mariotti P, Fasano A, Contarino MF, et al. Management of status dystonicus: our experience and review of the literature. Mov Disord. 2007; 22(7):963–968
[31] Narayan RK, Loubser PG, Jankovic J, Donovan WH, Bontke CF. Intrathecal baclofen for intractable axial dystonia. Neurology. 1991; 41(7):1141–1142
[32] Dalvi A, Fahn S, Ford B. Intrathecal baclofen in the treatment of dystonic storm. Mov Disord. 1998; 13(3):611–612
[33] Elkay M, Silver K, Penn RD, Dalvi A. Dystonic storm due to Batten's disease treated with pallidotomy and deep brain stimulation. Mov Disord. 2009; 24(7):1048–1053
[34] Justesen CR, Penn RD, Kroin JS, Egel RT. Stereotactic pallidotomy in a child with Hallervorden-Spatz disease. Case report. J Neurosurg. 1999; 90(3):551–554
[35] Balas I, Kovacs N, Hollody K. Staged bilateral stereotactic pallidothalamotomy for life-threatening dystonia in a child with Hallervorden-Spatz disease. Mov Disord. 2006; 21(1):82–85
[36] Kyriagis M, Grattan-Smith P, Scheinberg A, Teo C, Nakaji N, Waugh M. Status dystonicus and Hallervorden-Spatz disease: treatment with intrathecal baclofen and pallidotomy. J Paediatr Child Health. 2004; 40(5–6):322–325
[37] Cif L, Hariz M. Seventy years of pallidotomy for movement disorders. Mov Disord. 2017; 32(7):972–982
[38] Gross RE. What happened to posteroventral pallidotomy for Parkinson's disease and dystonia? Neurotherapeutics. 2008; 5(2):281–293
[39] Blomstedt P, Taira T, Hariz M. Rescue pallidotomy for dystonia through implanted deep brain stimulation electrode. Surg Neurol Int. 2016; 7 Suppl 35: S815–S817
[40] Marras CE, Rizzi M, Cantonetti L, et al. Pallidotomy for medically refractory status dystonicus in childhood. Dev Med Child Neurol. 2014; 56(7):649–656
[41] Weiss EM, Hershey T, Karimi M, et al. Relative risk of spread of symptoms among the focal onset primary dystonias. Mov Disord. 2006; 21(8):1175–1181
[42] Tabbal SD. Childhood dystonias. Curr Treat Options Neurol. 2015; 17(3):339
[43] Albanese A, Bhatia K, Bressman SB, et al. Phenomenology and classification of dystonia: a consensus update. Mov Disord. 2013; 28(7):863–873
[44] Fahn S. Concept and classification of dystonia. Adv Neurol. 1988; 50:1–8
[45] Winter S, Autry A, Boyle C, Yeargin-Allsopp M. Trends in the prevalence of cerebral palsy in a population-based study. Pediatrics. 2002; 110(6):1220–1225
[46] Damier P, Thobois S, Witjas T, et al. French Stimulation for Tardive Dyskinesia (STARDYS) Study Group. Bilateral deep brain stimulation of the globus pallidus to treat tardive dyskinesia. Arch Gen Psychiatry. 2007; 64(2):170–176
[47] Eltahawy HA, Saint-Cyr J, Giladi N, Lang AE, Lozano AM. Primary dystonia is more responsive than secondary dystonia to pallidal interventions: outcome after pallidotomy or pallidal deep brain stimulation. Neurosurgery. 2004; 54(3):613–619, discussion 619–621

[48] Macerollo A, Deuschl G. Deep brain stimulation for tardive syndromes: systematic review and meta-analysis. J Neurol Sci. 2018; 389:55–60

[49] Koy A, Timmermann L. Deep brain stimulation in cerebral palsy: challenges and opportunities. Eur J Paediatr Neurol. 2017; 21(1):118–121

[50] Vidailhet M, Yelnik J, Lagrange C, et al. French SPIDY-2 Study Group. Bilateral pallidal deep brain stimulation for the treatment of patients with dystonia-choreoathetosis cerebral palsy: a prospective pilot study. Lancet Neurol. 2009; 8(8):709–717

[51] Castelnau P, Cif L, Valente EM, et al. Pallidal stimulation improves pantothenate kinase-associated neurodegeneration. Ann Neurol. 2005; 57(5):738–741

[52] Timmermann L, Pauls KA, Wieland K, et al. Dystonia in neurodegeneration with brain iron accumulation: outcome of bilateral pallidal stimulation. Brain. 2010; 133(Pt 3):701–712

[53] Barry MJ, VanSwearingen JM, Albright AL. Reliability and responsiveness of the Barry-Albright Dystonia Scale. Dev Med Child Neurol. 1999; 41(6):404–411

[54] Burke RE, Fahn S, Marsden CD, Bressman SB, Moskowitz C, Friedman J. Validity and reliability of a rating scale for the primary torsion dystonias. Neurology. 1985; 35(1):73–77

[55] Johanna KM, Loïs V, et al. The Burke-Fahn-Marsden Dystonia Rating Scale is age-dependent in healthy children. Mov Disord Clin Pract (Hoboken). 2016; 3(6):580–586

[56] Mink JW. Special concerns in defining, studying, and treating dystonia in children. Mov Disord. 2013; 28(7):921–925

[57] Segawa M. Dopa-responsive dystonia. Handb Clin Neurol. 2011; 100:539–557

[58] Boyd K, Patterson V. Dopa responsive dystonia: a treatable condition misdiagnosed as cerebral palsy. BMJ. 1989; 298(6679):1019–1020

[59] Fletcher NA, Thompson PD, Scadding JW, Marsden CD. Successful treatment of childhood onset symptomatic dystonia with levodopa. J Neurol Neurosurg Psychiatry. 1993; 56(8):865–867

[60] Jinnah HA, Alterman R, Klein C, et al. Deep brain stimulation for dystonia: a novel perspective on the value of genetic testing. J Neural Transm (Vienna). 2017; 124(4):417–430

[61] Uc EY, Rodnitzky RL. Childhood dystonia. Semin Pediatr Neurol. 2003; 10(1):52–61

[62] Brüggemann N, Kühn A, Schneider SA, et al. Short- and long-term outcome of chronic pallidal neurostimulation in monogenic isolated dystonia. Neurology. 2015; 84(9):895–903

[63] Rughani AI, Lozano AM. Surgical treatment of myoclonus dystonia syndrome. Mov Disord. 2013; 28(3):282–287

[64] Zorzi G, Carecchio M, Zibordi F, Garavaglia B, Nardocci N. Diagnosis and treatment of pediatric onset isolated dystonia. Eur J Paediatr Neurol. 2018; 22(2):238–244

[65] Lumsden DE, Kaminska M, Ashkan K, Selway R, Lin JP. Deep brain stimulation for childhood dystonia: is 'where' as important as in 'whom'? Eur J Paediatr Neurol. 2017; 21(1):176–184

[66] Berman BD, Starr PA, Marks WJ, Jr, Ostrem JL. Induction of bradykinesia with pallidal deep brain stimulation in patients with cranial-cervical dystonia. Stereotact Funct Neurosurg. 2009; 87(1):37–44

[67] DiFrancesco MF, Halpern CH, Hurtig HH, Baltuch GH, Heuer GG. Pediatric indications for deep brain stimulation. Childs Nerv Syst. 2012; 28(10):1701–1714

[68] Koy A, Hellmich M, Pauls KA, et al. Effects of deep brain stimulation in dyskinetic cerebral palsy: a meta-analysis. Mov Disord. 2013; 28(5):647–654

[69] Albright AL, Ferson SS. Intraventricular baclofen for dystonia: techniques and outcomes. Clinical article. J Neurosurg Pediatr. 2009; 3(1):11–14

[70] Odding E, Roebroeck ME, Stam HJ. The epidemiology of cerebral palsy: incidence, impairments and risk factors. Disabil Rehabil. 2006; 28(4):183–191

[71] Reid SM, Meehan E, McIntyre S, Goldsmith S, Badawi N, Reddihough DS, Australian Cerebral Palsy Register Group. Temporal trends in cerebral palsy by impairment severity and birth gestation. Dev Med Child Neurol. 2016; 58 Suppl 2:25–35

[72] Nelson KB, Ellenberg JH. Children who 'outgrew' cerebral palsy. Pediatrics. 1982; 69(5):529–536

[73] Fink JK. Hereditary spastic paraplegia. Curr Neurol Neurosci Rep. 2006; 6(1):65–76

[74] Durkin MS, Benedict RE, Christensen D, et al. Prevalence of cerebral palsy among 8-year-old children in 2010 and preliminary evidence of trends in its relationship to low birthweight. Paediatr Perinat Epidemiol. 2016; 30(5):496–510

[75] Delgado MR, Albright AL. Movement disorders in children: definitions, classifications, and grading systems. J Child Neurol. 2003; 18 Suppl 1:S1–S8

[76] Platz T, Eickhof C, Nuyens G, Vuadens P. Clinical scales for the assessment of spasticity, associated phenomena, and function: a systematic review of the literature. Disabil Rehabil. 2005; 27(1–2):7–18

[77] Haugh AB, Pandyan AD, Johnson GR. A systematic review of the Tardieu Scale for the measurement of spasticity. Disabil Rehabil. 2006; 28(15):899–907

[78] Karol LA. Surgical management of the lower extremity in ambulatory children with cerebral palsy. J Am Acad Orthop Surg. 2004; 12(3):196–203

[79] Spiegel DA, Flynn JM. Evaluation and treatment of hip dysplasia in cerebral palsy. Orthop Clin North Am. 2006; 37(2):185–196, vi

[80] Tierney TS, Abd-El-Barr MM, Stanford AD, Foote KD, Okun MS. Deep brain stimulation and ablation for obsessive compulsive disorder: evolution of contemporary indications, targets and techniques. Int J Neurosci. 2014; 124(6):394–402

[81] Worbe Y, Mallet L, Golmard JL, et al. Repetitive behaviours in patients with Gilles de la Tourette syndrome: tics, compulsions, or both? PLoS One. 2010; 5(9):e12959

[82] Bloch MH, Leckman JF. Clinical course of Tourette syndrome. J Psychosom Res. 2009; 67(6):497–501

[83] Freeman RD, Fast DK, Burd L, Kerbeshian J, Robertson MM, Sandor P. An international perspective on Tourette syndrome: selected findings from 3,500 individuals in 22 countries. Dev Med Child Neurol. 2000; 42(7):436–447

[84] Motlagh MG, Smith ME, Landeros-Weisenberger A, et al. Lessons learned from open-label deep brain stimulation for Tourette syndrome: eight cases over 7 years. Tremor Other Hyperkinet Mov (N Y). 2013; 3:3

[85] Porta M, Brambilla A, Cavanna AE, et al. Thalamic deep brain stimulation for treatment-refractory Tourette syndrome: two-year outcome. Neurology. 2009; 73(17):1375–1380

[86] Servello D, Porta M, Sassi M, Brambilla A, Robertson MM. Deep brain stimulation in 18 patients with severe Gilles de la Tourette syndrome refractory to treatment: the surgery and stimulation. J Neurol Neurosurg Psychiatry. 2008; 79(2):136–142

[87] Zhang JG, Ge Y, Stead M, et al. Long-term outcome of globus pallidus internus deep brain stimulation in patients with Tourette syndrome. Mayo Clin Proc. 2014; 89(11):1506–1514

[88] Focquaert F. Pediatric deep brain stimulation: a cautionary approach. Front Integr Nuerosci. 2011; 5:9

[89] Cif L, Coubes P. Historical developments in children's deep brain stimulation. Eur J Paediatr Neurol. 2017; 21(1):109–117

[90] Leckman JF. Deep brain stimulation for Tourette syndrome: lessons learned and future directions. Biol Psychiatry. 2016; 79(5):343–344

[91] Deeb W, Rossi PJ, Porta M, et al. The International Deep Brain Stimulation Registry and Database for Gilles de la Tourette Syndrome: how does it work? Front Neurosci. 2016; 10:170

[92] Air EL, Ostrem JL, Sanger TD, Starr PA. Deep brain stimulation in children: experience and technical pearls. J Neurosurg Pediatr. 2011; 8(6):566–574

[93] Ghosh PS, Machado AG, Deogaonkar M, Ghosh D. Deep brain stimulation in children with dystonia: experience from a tertiary care center. Pediatr Neurosurg. 2012; 48(3):146–151

[94] Haridas A, Tagliati M, Osborn I, et al. Pallidal deep brain stimulation for primary dystonia in children. Neurosurgery. 2011; 68(3):738–743, discussion 743

[95] Keen JR, Przekop A, Olaya JE, Zouros A, Hsu FP. Deep brain stimulation for the treatment of childhood dystonic cerebral palsy. J Neurosurg Pediatr. 2014; 14(6):585–593

[96] Koy A, Lin JP, Sanger TD, Marks WA, Mink JW, Timmermann L. Advances in management of movement disorders in children. Lancet Neurol. 2016; 15(7):719–735

[97] Marks WA, Honeycutt J, Acosta F, Reed M. Deep brain stimulation for pediatric movement disorders. Semin Pediatr Neurol. 2009; 16(2):90–98

[98] Johans SJ, Swong KN, Hofler RC, Anderson DE. A stepwise approach: decreasing infection in deep brain stimulation for childhood dystonic cerebral palsy. J Child Neurol. 2017; 32(10):871–875

[99] Park HR, Kim IH, Kang H, et al. Nucleus accumbens deep brain stimulation for a patient with self-injurious behavior and autism spectrum disorder: functional and structural changes of the brain: report of a case and review of literature. Acta Neurochir (Wien). 2017; 159(1):137–143

[100] Sinha S, McGovern RA, Sheth SA. Deep brain stimulation for severe autism: from pathophysiology to procedure. Neurosurg Focus. 2015; 38(6):E3

[101] Sturm V, Fricke O, Bührle CP, et al. DBS in the basolateral amygdala improves symptoms of autism and related self-injurious behavior: a case report and hypothesis on the pathogenesis of the disorder. Front Hum Neurosci. 2013; 6:341

[102] Marks W, Bailey L, Sanger TD. PEDiDBS: The pediatric international deep brain stimulation registry project. Eur J Paediatr Neurol. 2017; 21(1):218–222

18 Establishing a Deep Brain Stimulation Practice

Charles B. Mikell, Joseph Adachi, Jennifer Cheng, Joseph S. Neimat

Abstract

This chapter is intended for newly trained functional neurosurgeons and describes key elements and considerations within the first years after training to establish a successful functional neurosurgery practice. This chapter lays out what a newly minted neurosurgeon can expect from the field of functional neurosurgery and helps to define the scope of personal and professional goals which will be achievable within the various practice settings. The pros and cons of private practice, hospital, and academic practices will be discussed. Further, the chapter dispenses advice relevant to the finer details of negotiating a contract, building a research lab, clinical team, referral network, and professional reputation. Although the chapter is focused on the early stage of a neurosurgical career, elements will certainly be applicable to those further along in their practice or those wishing to begin a new facet of their career.

Keywords: practice-building, functional neurosurgery, DBS, practice-management, professional development, 2018, referral networks, neurosurgery residency, neurosurgery

18.1 Introduction

Among the first things a newly hired functional neurosurgeon has to do is build a practice. This is invariably a more complex process than in some more traditional practices, because it necessarily involves the organizing and motivating a large and multidisciplinary group. Notwithstanding these increased challenges, we believe that the creation of such an effort can be one of the most rewarding aspects of a functional neurosurgery career.

Despite the ultimate importance of this activity, new graduates have often received little training or guidance in how practices are built. Although each environment has unique challenges and opportunities, we feel there are some common themes that merit discussion and incorporation early in the process of building individual practice. This chapter is an attempt to summarize those common strategies and think constructively about the goals that such practice elements serve.

We suggest three main elements to successful practice building. First, it is important to know *what you want*. Ask yourself what your "dream job" actually looks like. The second element of a successful practice is the *right environment*: the right department, right partners, right neurologists, and right chairperson. The final element is the *right approach* to your patients, your collaborators, your institution, and your practice environment.

18.2 What Do I Actually Want?

γνῶθι σεαυτόν - "Know thyself"

-A Delphic maxim, inscribed on the wall of the Temple of Apollo.

Neurosurgeons, no exception to the population at large, are quite capable of resisting self-examination. The beginning of one's career is an especially important time to pause and reflect on the specific aspects of a surgical career that will be most important to you. A failure to be introspective and deliberate about how a career is built invites the inevitable chaos of a surgical practice to make its own determinations.

Most people who are interested in functional neurosurgery are fascinated by the science of the nervous system and by the opportunity to manipulate and investigate its functions. Nonetheless, the cases themselves can be tiresome, and are not as well-compensated as other procedures in neurosurgery. It is, therefore, important to know *what cases* you want to do, and *how often*. If you do not have clear goals, you will inevitably have difficulty arranging your priorities and may eventually find your schedule strangled by obligations not of your choosing.

The next question to ask yourself is *how much money will be enough for you*. In functional neurosurgery, "[they're] electrodes, not screws. Nobody's getting rich," as one colleague recently reflected. Therefore, almost all functional neurosurgeons incorporate other elements of neurosurgical practice into their career. Establishment of these ancillary elements are outside the scope of this book, but should not be overlooked in helping an individual achieve both financial and intellectual balance. Ultimately, functional neurosurgery is not so poorly compensated as it is widely believed to be—although spine surgery certainly pays more. A recent survey of functional neurosurgeons found that their salaries tend to be commensurate with the 50th percentile of academic neurosurgeons. The Goldilocks zone that balances the: case mix, research time, and compensation that is "just right" for you, is the key to long-term happiness. And it will be important that you have a frank and honest discussion with your chair about these goals before you sign your contract. When you believe you have answered these questions, you are ready to start making more specific decisions to build your future practice.

18.2.1 What Do I Want: Joining a Program, or Starting a Program?

Job opportunities can be divided into two categories: either a department is looking for a junior partner to add to an existing functional neurosurgery practice or a department is planning to build its own functional neurosurgery program from the ground up. There are pros and cons to each (► Table 18.1). In the first scenario, joining the practice of an experienced senior functional neurosurgeon has a number of advantages. An established program will allow a new partner to get started quickly and without many of the initial challenges of practice building. Your senior partners have done the spadework of establishing referral networks, clinical multidisciplinary teams have already been built, and the hospital has all of the relevant equipment and needed support staff. On the other hand, if you are building a new program, you alone will be responsible for establishing relationships along with referring neurologists, buying equipment, and training support staff such as electroencephalography (EEG) technicians. Nonetheless, you can build the program the way you want it, meaning you can buy whatever toys you

Table 18.1 Pros and cons of starting a new practice

	The upside	The downside
Joining an established practice	1. Allows a new partner to get started quickly 2. Avoids the initial challenges of practice building 3. Senior partners have already established referral networks 4. Hospital already has all necessary equipment and support staff	1. Reduced control of practice decisions 2. An established and immutable organizational culture 3. Entrenched and inefficient practices which may be resistant to change
Starting a new practice	1. Ability to construct the practice as you see fit 2. Control over purchase decisions: equipment, staff, schedule, etc.	1. Required to establish referral network and relationships with referring neurologists 2. An initial lack of equipment and facilities 3. Responsible for hiring, administrating and training support staff

want, define the workplace culture you want, and make key personnel decisions at your own discretion. If you are starting a new program, it is important that your chair and hospital be committed to the enterprise. The startup costs for a functional neurosurgery program are significant (including microelectrode recording equipment, head frame, laser, etc.), and the chair will have to be willing to make these initial investments in order for the program to be successful.

18.2.2 What Do I Want: Teaching, Research, Surgery?

For many of us in academic medicine, success is predicated not only on excellence in the clinic and operating room (OR), but in the conquest of the domains of research and teaching as well. This classic three-legged stool—a rare feat, has long served as the precarious metaphor for achievement in academic medicine. Inevitably, as career progresses, administrative roles become an important fourth leg of one's endeavors. In the private practice setting, formal roles in education and research are less common but can nevertheless be pursued and successfully integrated into one's practice.

If such endeavors are important to your job satisfaction, recognize that they will take considerable time and commitment. Teaching can be a satisfying activity; watching your trainee perform a simple or complex procedure for the first time, independently, can give a tremendous sense of accomplishment. Most new graduates have had some experience teaching junior residents and will have a sense of whether they are drawn to education. In academic medicine, most departments will have some expectation that you lecture a few times each year, but if you want to do more, this will almost certainly be accommodated. Early in your career, it can be challenging to share responsibility with residents, as you yourself are consolidating operative confidence. Striking this balance is ultimately rewarding and becomes easier with a few years of experience. Most surgeons become better teachers over time, if they are willing to listen and attend to the feedback they receive from their trainees early on. There are some drawbacks of a major teaching role. These include the time required to prepare educational materials, as well as the constant and taxing requirements to provide documentation of how your trainees are progressing. In 2013, as a response to criticism from previous years that educational requirements in neurosurgery were "fuzzy," the American College of Graduate Medical Education (ACGME) in consultation with the Society of Neurological Surgeons (SNS) developed a curriculum of milestones required for each

resident to achieve. These milestones have indeed improved the standardization of training but are quite paperwork-intensive. In short, there is no doubt that a committed role in education will require the dedication of significant time. Moreover, for those who wish to be a teacher or mentor, few time investments are personally fulfilling.

Likewise, a serious research career can be both satisfying and frustrating simultaneously. You should decide early on if you are going to initiate your own research or collaborate with other scientists. If you want to be a principal investigator yourself, you will need to have an explicit conversation with your chair about the time and resources that will be available. Competition for your time will be great and you will need to protect your dedicated research time vigilantly. The most critical support will come in the form of personnel. One full-time employee is probably a bare minimum requirement. You will also need lab space and money for resources (animals, computers, or whatever else). While starting out, most chairs are able to furnish you with some resources... *with the expectation that you soon establish your own grant funding.* Resources in academic centers are increasingly scarce; there will be a defined period for which a "startup" package will be available and after that point you will need to secure your own money to keep things going. In addition to working toward publications, your early time should be spent obtaining pilot data for grants. Until you have your own grants, you should expect to spend an equal amount of time writing pilot grants, just so you can stay in the game. You should also expect significant paperwork associated with Institutional Review Board submissions, animal care, and other related activities. As funding is established, either from the National Institutes of Health (NIH) or private foundations, pressure on you will start to ease; however, the challenge of funding will last as long as the lifetime of the lab.

An alternative to running a lab independently is to seek out collaborators who will share the lead on your projects and grants. Although you may have to share in your dictatorial power, you may gain the novel expertise of capable researchers with experience that compliments your own. The ability to share lab management responsibilities will reduce the time commitment on your part and may be more commensurate with keeping a busy surgical practice. Valued collaborators need not necessarily be at your institution. Modern data sharing has made collaboration between centers far more achievable than before. If these collaborations are successful, and you are getting grants and publishing papers, you may be able to make a case to your chair to recruit these collaborators to your department. Having collaborators close at hand can compound the value of an already productive relationship. Delegating authority to these collaborators will additionally free up more of your time for surgery and patient care.

Despite the time commitment and challenges associated with doing research, the opportunity a functional neurosurgeon has to learn about the nervous system is unique. Your position will grant you daily, direct access to human neural activity which, until the recent birth of our discipline, no human in history has ever had. You will also have the unique ability to integrate the latest advances in electronics and neuroscience to manipulate brain pathology with electrical stimulation. It is an auspicious time for clinical researchers in this small field that shows great promise in revolutionizing the landscape of neurological and psychiatric illness.

18.2.3 What Do I Want: My Schedule?

Once you have decided how much teaching and research you want to do, you should briefly think about how your week will be arranged. Most neurosurgeons start out with 1 to 2 clinic days, 1 to 2 OR days, leaving an unscheduled day or two for academic activities. Maybe you want to have two research days, but are willing to make less money. Or maybe you want to be the guy who does 300 cases a year. You should think through all of these possibilities carefully, and discuss this with your chair. In private practice, less flexibility is available because your job is chiefly to do cases. But even in the private setting, your schedule should reflect your priorities.

18.3 Practice Types

18.3.1 Practice Types: Private Practice

The majority of neurosurgeons in the United States are in private practice. However, only larger, subspecialized private groups of 10 or more surgeons are able to support a dedicated functional neurosurgeon. It is fairly unusual for small private groups to employ a full-time functional neurosurgeon, but it is not uncommon for one surgeon in a smaller practice to have an interest and offer deep brain stimulation (DBS) and epilepsy surgeries as a subset of his otherwise general practice.

In either environment, the incorporation of functional neurosurgery will allow a practice to market themselves to payors and hospitals as "comprehensive" providers of neurosurgical care, and it may translate to better leverage when negotiating reimbursement. If the group is large enough, you will have peers with whom to discuss complex cases. These large groups may also employ dedicated administrative staff to assist with practice building. As we will see, many of these advantages are shared with hospital-employed positions.

18.3.2 Practice Types: Hospital-Employed

Over the past decade, large academic groups that have staffed large hospitals have faced pressure from the hospital to join their employed staff. Likewise, hospitals have also sought to hire their own neurosurgical staff to secure financial advantages over private groups. There is probably no reversing this trend; each year a larger and larger proportion of neurosurgeons in the United States are working for hospitals. The hospital-employed model does have some benefits but has a few drawbacks also. As with a large private group, it handles a lot of the administrative work for you; but this, of course, is a double-edged sword. A professional administrator may take on these responsibilities for you, but this change may be felt acutely as a loss of autonomy. You may have little control over who is helping you in the OR or whether you have physician extenders for the floor. Finally, hospitals are generally able to offer higher initial salaries than their academic counterparts due to their size and resources; however, they will typically make significant demands on clinical productivity, and if high targets are not met, they can play "hardball" in contract renegotiations. Ultimately the success of a position, be it private, hospital-employed, or academic, will depend on shared goals between you and your employer. If aspects such as teaching or research are important to you, be certain that the hospital administration understands the value you bring to their program and is committed to supporting your extra-clinical goals. It is critical that your employer's expectations are compatible with your identified goals.

18.3.3 Practice Types: Academic

Academic departments typically employ one or more functional neurosurgeons, as functional cases are now a part of the ACGME requirement for residency training programs. Academic departments are the traditional centers for teaching and research, and you may find there is increased prestige with being linked to an academic center. The cases that come to academic institutions are typically more complex and may include those that are passed over by community physicians. Other advantages over community practice include better ancillary services at large academic facilities, and more direct access to collaborators in neurology and other specialties. Partnership with neurology collaborators, in particular, is critical for building effective teams in a functional neurosurgery practice.

Although academic salaries are somewhat less than the private salaries, these positions typically emphasize research and education as an important part of your activities. Although most academic departments still incentivize clinical productivity, the best positions strike a balance between clinical duties and academic opportunities to achieve a salary that is fair. Again, it is critical to establish what benchmarks your chair will use to evaluate your productivity when the time for contract negotiations and/or promotion comes.

18.4 How to Get Started?

18.4.1 How to Get Started: Building Your Team?

Once you have started your job, the work of building a practice really begins. If there is an existing functional neurosurgeon, and your job is to be a release valve for the backlog of his or her patients, a lot of the team building has already been done for you. In this case, it will be critical to have a good communication with your partner or partners. Make sure you understand how cases and responsibilities will be shared and all the partners are comfortable with this arrangement.

If you are starting a new program, you will face the challenge of building from the ground up. The foundation of a good functional program begins with establishing collaboration between neurology and neurosurgery. In the beginning, you should have conversations with your referring neurologists. Programs are built most easily if there is a specialized subgroup of neurologists in your institution's Department of Neurology. Most neurology departments will have divisions of "Movement Disorders" and "Epilepsy." In an ideal situation, these divisions already exist and may have a significant backlog of potential surgical patients. You should approach these people first and begin working with them to structure your programs. In most cases, these physicians will be excited to have a surgeon offering services that augment their own programs. You should speak at their division meetings and make an effort to establish a standing date for a *surgical conference* (i.e., the first Tuesday of the month) to discuss treatment options for patients in each department. In this way, you get their buy-in and define your relationship as partners with a shared commitment to the effort. These approaches can be specially tailored to movement disorders, pain, or epilepsy practices.

Movement disorder neurologists have traditionally been the most eager neurologists to embrace surgical treatment for their patients. DBS can have such a dramatic effect for Parkinson's disease and tremor patients that they are usually enthusiastic about a new surgical program. However, program building will require a significant time commitment with your neurology partners and it is important to recognize this. If your neurology colleagues have an academic interest in DBS surgery, this relationship can be tremendously synergistic. As a bonus, their clinical time expenditure is usually offset, to some degree by the ability to bill for high-complexity visits when they program, in addition to billing the programming codes. Ultimately, collaboration with movement disorders neurologists is natural and the rewards are mutual and substantial.

Pain physicians have related but distinct considerations to those of movement disorder neurologists, but they should be equally enthusiastic about your presence. Pain physicians typically perform initial percutaneous spinal cord stimulation (SCS) trials, and subsequently refer patients for permanent implantation. If they have been sending patients outside for treatment, they are typically happy to have someone at their home institution. An important distinction from movement disorder neurologists is that percutaneous spinal cord stimulators simply lack the efficacy of DBS and the patient population has lower satisfaction levels in general. SCSs also have significant rates of migration requiring revision, so it is important that the pain physicians understand that not every patient will be a "home run." Good pain partners understand this and make allowances for suboptimal outcomes in preoperative counseling. In general, pain physicians are acutely aware of the lack of safe therapeutic options for intractable pain, and are pleased to have your services available within the team.

Epilepsy has traditionally been the most challenging area to make inroads. Resective epilepsy surgery lacks the immediate gratification of DBS implantation and is perceived to carry significantly more risk. For this reason, some epileptologists have been hesitant to recommend surgery for their patients. Recently however, attractive surgical options have become available that are substantially less invasive at the time when it is increasingly accepted that serial medication trials are unlikely to provide meaningful improvement. For this reason, we expect to see substantial growth in epilepsy surgical practice in future years. In a growing program, referrals will typically increase as your neurologists gain familiarity with the new options available for treatment (for MRI-negative epilepsy in particular), such as laser ablation and responsive neurostimulation (RNS). You should meet with the division chief of epilepsy surgery early on, and come prepared with evidence from recent trials demonstrating the benefit of surgery over continued medical management. You should try to agree on which patients should receive surgery, and to establish a recurring conference date to discuss new cases. As you successfully treat more and more patients with surgical therapy, your referrals will likely grow.

18.4.2 How to Get Started: Other Team Members?

To successfully screen surgical patients, you will need additional team members other than your neurology colleagues. For DBS programs, the multidisciplinary team typically includes one or more neuropsychologists. These staff are often divided conceptually into preoperative and postoperative roles. Preoperatively, these individuals interpret functional tests and provide guidance to patients regarding specific risks of surgical intervention such as functional deficits and disability. Preoperative evaluation is often part of the workup for seizure focus localization and may reveal additional cognitive deficits and latent mood disorders prior to surgery. These insights can be critical for judicious patient selection and successful management. Postoperatively, neurophysiologists monitor clinical outcomes, arrange follow-ups, and assist with the smooth transition of care to specialists in rehabilitation.

A surgical patient coordinator, dedicated epilepsy monitoring unit, and team of experienced EEG technicians are also crucial. Because of the complexities of managing DBS patients, many groups have incorporated advanced practice nurses trained specifically to assess and program DBS patients, as well as patient navigators who coordinate patient access to the many specialists within the DBS team. It is commonplace for programs to utilize a psychiatrist, either as a standing member of the committee or as a frequent consult who is called in on an ad hoc basis. Their insights are invaluable when, as is often the case, psychiatric comorbidities are present. In addition, neuroimaging capabilities such as those provided by experienced neuroradiologists are key in the identification of subtle abnormalities, such as mesial temporal sclerosis, cortical dysplasias, migration abnormalities, and encephaloceles. Finally, a dedicated neurophysiologist or scientific partner may assist in the OR if you prefer to not always perform the neurophysiology yourself.

18.4.3 How to Get Started: Hospital Partnership?

The support of your hospital will be critical to the success of your functional program. From the very beginning, the hospital will need to support your program by purchasing specialized surgical equipment,such as a stereotactic frame, a neurophysiology system, specialized imaging systems etc. They will also need to work with you to schedule multistage surgeries and provide resources commensurate with the complexities of awake surgeries and complex intraoperative mapping. It is important to understand and attend to the hospital's side of this equation. While the calculation of the contribution margin for any case will vary across institutions (based on the way the surgery is done, payer mix, accounting methods, etc.), DBS cases typically produce a positive contribution margin overall. It may be less remunerative than other neurosurgery types (e.g., spine surgery) but the performance of such specialized surgery may benefit the hospital in contracting, or it may provide a halo effect to the institute as a whole. As with all things, communication on these points with the hospital administration will be important at the outset.

18.4.4 How to Get Started: The Role of Industry?

DBS surgery, in addition to vagus nerve stimulation, RNS and SCS, features an implanted device, hence the companies producing these devices have an important synergistic interest in promoting your surgeries. Whether you choose to engage them or not, there are representatives from almost every company in your market working to promote the surgeries that you perform. Among physicians, there has been a general mistrust directed towards these corporate interests and sales people. Fundamentally, however, it is our belief that their conflict of interest is no greater than our own conflict as physicians who are ultimately paid to perform surgery. We, therefore, feel that working with these agents is mutually productive, provided we encourage them to apply the same integrity that we hold ourselves to in selecting appropriate patients and withholding surgery for those we feel will not be helped.

With this in mind, corporate partners can be invaluable allies in patient education and practice growth. They can assist you with introductions to potential referring physicians (they typically have access to data on high-volume referrers); access to patient groups; and an ability to get your name out to these groups. Since there is now competition among several device manufacturers (as there has been in the SCS space for some time), it is important to be forthright in your interactions with each representative. In our practices, we have worked to select devices based on their clinical merits and allow our patients to independently decide which implant they will have, after the advantages of each are dispassionately presented.

18.4.5 How to Get Started: Community Outreach?

As a more centralized model of healthcare delivery has developed in the past 20 years, centers have grappled with how best to move patients between centers and yet ultimately return them to care in their community setting. DBS surgery has been a prime example of this type of tertiary care model. There was a time, 20 years ago, when it was assumed that every community hospital would perform a limited number of DBS surgeries, prompting the development of systems for portable intraoperative neurophysiology and remote monitoring (Medtronic Inc., unpublished communications). Although there are presently many outstanding community hospitals performing DBS, the general consensus has, for

a variety of reasons including a study at the University of Florida Movement Disorders Center,[1] migrated to the opposite pole, stating that larger centers are able to deliver the nuanced and specialized surgical technique required for DBS more efficiently. Some centers have even made a point of addressing and marketing their skill at addressing DBS failures. This has led to the adoption of a "spoke and hub" model by many centers in which community hospitals refer DBS cases to a designated regional center of excellence for surgery.

DBS surgery is not alone, nor was it first in offering this specialized care model. The spoke and hub model is commonly credited to the development of specialized hepatitis C treatment delivery pioneered by "Project Echo"[2] at the University of New Mexico that subsequently spread across the country and internationally. This spoke and hub model has been proven as substantially beneficial to centralized DBS practice. The model helps invested practitioners in the community offer their patients specialized DBS therapy (or pain, epilepsy, etc.) by partnering with a larger academic center for the most specialized part of that delivery. They then refer patients in for surgery but assume subsequent care of monitoring and programming the patient. This approach combines the unique and complementary strengths of community physicians and their superspecialized academic counterparts. The community neurologist becomes an integral part of a larger conceptual network of providers and can (formally or informally) claim a link to a higher profile academic center. At one of our own centers, we grew such a program to include more than 10 dedicated spoke centers associated with our program. This resulted in one of the busiest DBS centers in the country. The model utilized for patient referral, review, and surgical treatment is featured in ▶ Fig. 18.1.

18.4.6 How to Get Started: Building Your Reputation?

Everyone has heard the three A's: affability, availability, and ability (in that order). However, you should think carefully about what these words actually mean for you. Everybody wants to refer to a nice person. Affability means being nice to other providers, and maintaining a polite and professional attitude at all times. When you start out, you should make every effort to reach out to referring providers when they send you an operative case. If you provide a positive experience for operative referrals, more referrals will come to you. If you are easy-going and polite to everyone, they will remember that and seek out your help next time. Whereas, if you get a reputation as a person who is difficult to talk to on the phone, people won't want to refer to you. Of course, this is easier said than done, especially when the ER attending calls you at 3 AM to admit a nonoperative patient to your service. But you should try anyway. This also speaks to availability.

Availability is a more slippery concept. You want to be available, but not so much that you compromise your personal livelihood. Early on, you should talk to whoever manages your outpatient schedule with the goal of prioritizing operative referrals. In our group, brain tumors get seen as soon as possible, for instance. You should make similar allowances for epilepsy and DBS patients. You should also make an effort to prioritize personal referrals over referrals to the "first available" neurosurgeon. Again, when someone sends you an operative case, call him or

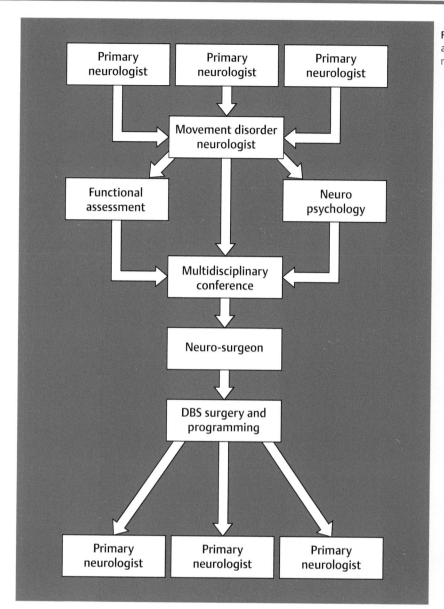

Fig. 18.1 A referral flow diagram illustrating appropriate transfer of care from a community neurologist to functional neurosurgeon and back.

her. If someone calls you to see a patient, see the patient as soon as possible. You can even offer to visit the patient at the referring physician's office if circumstances allow. Some practices have shared clinics where movement disorder patients see their neurologist and neurosurgeon in the same day, greatly facilitating patient flow. Patients who experience a smoothly run preoperative and postoperative course are typically happier and may convey this to their primary physician or other potential patients.

As your practice grows and you continue to provide successful outcomes, it is important to "close the loop" with referring doctors. Let them know after surgery that everything went well and the patient is happy. If the patient is happy, he or she will also go back to the referring physician and reinforce your message. Patients are generally your best form of advertising. DBS patients will tell other Parkinson's patients how much the therapy has changed their life, resulting in more referrals. In this way, good outcomes lead to more referrals which in turn lead to more good outcomes, continuing as a "virtuous cycle."

18.5 Summary and Conclusion

Knowing what you want from your job is the beginning of a successful practice. Codifying these goals and making them consonant with your chair's expectations is the second step. As you embark on your practice, being nice to referring doctors and patients will lead to more referrals, and maintaining excellent outcomes will cause those referrals to multiply along with your reputation. After a while, you will find that practice building is just a natural consequence of doing your job, and it is a rewarding and effortless part of your practice.

References

[1] Arora S, Thornton K, Murata G, et al. Outcomes of treatment for hepatitis C virus infection by primary care providers. N Engl J Med. 2011; 364(23): 2199–2207

[2] Okun MS, Tagliati M, Pourfar M, et al. Management of referred deep brain stimulation failures: a retrospective analysis from 2 movement disorders centers. Arch Neurol. 2005; 62(8):1250–1255

Index